Decision Making in Perioperative Medicine

Clinical Pearls

SECOND EDITION

T0357594

Decision Making in Perioperative Medicine
Clinical Pearls

SECOND EDITION

EDITOR

Steven L. Cohn, MD, MACP, SFHM, FRCP
Professor Emeritus
Department of Medicine
University of Miami Miller School of Medicine
Miami, Florida
Clinical Professor of Medicine Emeritus
SUNY Downstate Health Sciences University
Brooklyn, New York

Decision Making in Perioperative Medicine: Clinical Pearls, Second Edition

1 2 3 4 5 LBC 29 28 27 26 25

ISBN 978-1-266-07296-3
MHID 1-266-07296-9

This book was set in Minion Pro by MPS Limited.
The editors were Kay Conerly and Sylvia Choi.
The production supervisor was Catherine Saggese.
Project management was provided by Poonam Bisht, MPS Limited.

Library of Congress Control Number: 2024951650

McGraw Hill books are available at special quantity discounts to use as premiums and sales promotions, or for use in corporate training programs. To contact a representative please visit the Contact Us pages at www.mhprofessional.com.

To my family, I would like to thank my wife, Debbie, and children, Alison and Jeff, for their love and encouragement. And to my parents, I dedicate this book to you in recognition of the unfaltering support you provided throughout my educational and professional career; I share this latest accomplishment in your memory.

Contents

Contributors

Moises Auron, MD, FAAP, FACP, SFHM, FRCP (Lon), FRCPCH

Professor of Medicine and Pediatrics
Cleveland Clinic Lerner College of Medicine of Case Western Reserve University
Staff Physician Departments of Hospital Medicine and Pediatric Hospital Medicine
Cleveland Clinic
Cleveland, Ohio
Chapter 22

Christine E. Boxhorn, MD, DABA

Assistant Professor of Anesthesiology
Medical College of Wisconsin
Milwaukee, Wisconsin
Chapters 30, 45

Frances Chung MD, MBBS, SAMBAf, FRCPC

Professor
Department of Anesthesiology and Pain Medicine
University of Toronto
ResMed Chair in Anesthesiology, Sleep, and Perioperative Medicine Research
University Health Network
Faculty
Institute of Medical Science, Temerity Faculty of Medicine
University of Toronto
Toronto, Ontario, Canada
Chapter 17

Steven L. Cohn, MD, MACP, SFHM, FRCP

Professor Emeritus
Department of Medicine
Former Medical Director—UHealth Preoperative Assessment Center (UPAC)
Former Director—Medical Consultation Service—Jackson Memorial Hospital
University of Miami Miller School of Medicine
Miami, Florida
Clinical Professor of Medicine Emeritus
SUNY Downstate Health Sciences University
Brooklyn, New York
Chapters 1, 2, 4, 8, 9, 11, 37

James D. Douketis, MD, FRCPC

Professor and David Braley Nancy Gordon Chair in Thromboembolic Disease
McMaster University
Hamilton, Ontario, Canada
Chapters 5, 40

Emmanuelle Duceppe, MD, PhD

Associate Clinical Professor of Medicine
Faculty of Medicine
University of Montreal
Montreal, Quebec, Canada
Chapter 10

Leonard S. Feldman, MD, FACP, FAAP, MHM

Associate Professor of Internal Medicine and Pediatrics
Johns Hopkins School of Medicine
Baltimore, Maryland
Chapter 19

Tong J. Gan, MD, MBA, MHS, FASA, FRCA

*Professor and Mildred M. Oppenheimer Distinguished
Endowed Chair and Head
Division of Anesthesiology, Critical Care and Pain
Medicine
University of Texas MD Anderson Cancer Center
Houston, Texas
Chapter 43*

Paul J. Grant, MD, SFHM, FACP

*Professor of Medicine
Director, Medicine Preoperative Clinic
Division of Hospital Medicine, Department of Internal
Medicine
University of Michigan Medical School
Ann Arbor, Michigan
Chapters 4, 42*

**Michael P.W. Grocott, BSc, MSc, MBBS, MD,
FRCA, FRCP, FFICM, GChPOM**

*Professor of Anaesthesia and Critical Care Medicine
Director, NIHR Southampton Biomedical Research
Centre
University Hospital Southampton/University of
Southampton
Southampton, United Kingdom
Chapters 15, 36*

**Alexander I.R. Jackson, BMedSci(Hons),
MBChB, MSc**

*NIHR Doctoral Fellow
NIHR Southampton Biomedical Research Centre,
University Hospital Southampton
University of Southampton
Southampton, United Kingdom
Chapters 15, 36*

Kay M. Johnson, MD, MPH

*Hospital and Specialty Medicine, VA Puget Sound
Health Care System
Professor, Division of General Internal Medicine
University of Washington School of Medicine
Seattle, Washington
Chapter 26*

Scott Kaatz, DO, MSc, FACP, SFHM

*Clinical Professor of Medicine, Michigan State
University—College of Human Medicine and Wayne
State University—School of Medicine
Division of Hospital Medicine
Co-director, Anticoagulation Clinics
Henry Ford Hospital
Detroit, Michigan
Chapters 5, 40*

Smita K. Kalra, MD, FACP, SFHM

*Director, Preoperative Hospitalist Clinic
Associate Professor of Medicine
University of California Irvine Medical School
Irvine, California
Chapter 6*

Gregary D. Marhefka, MD, FACP, FACC

*The Howard H. Weitz, MD, Professor of Cardiology
Director, Medical Cardiovascular Intensive Care Unit
Sidney Kimmel Medical College at Thomas Jefferson
University Hospital
Jefferson Heart Institute
Philadelphia, Pennsylvania
Chapters 12, 13*

Karen F. Mauck, MD, MSc, FACP

*Associate Professor of Medicine
Mayo Clinic
Rochester, Minnesota
Chapter 4*

Daniel I. McIsaac, MD, MPH, FRCPC

*Professor of Anesthesiology & Pain Medicine,
Epidemiology & Public Health
University of Ottawa
Ottawa, Ontario, Canada
Chapters 31, 44*

Heather E. Nye, MD, PhD, SFHM, FACP

*Professor of Medicine
University of California
San Francisco, California
Chapters 31, 44*

Avital Y. O'Glasser, MD, FACP, SFHM, DFPM

Professor of Medicine
Oregon Health & Science University
Portland, Oregon
Chapters 24, 26, 30

Kurt Pfeifer, MD, FACP, SFHM, DFPM

Chief and Professor of Medicine, Section of
Perioperative & Consultative Medicine
Medical College of Wisconsin
Milwaukee, Wisconsin
Chapters 16, 17, 18, 23

Deborah C. Richman, MBChB, FFA(SA)

Clinical Associate Professor of Anesthesiology
Stony Brook Medicine
Stony Brook, New York
Chapter 43

Nidhi Rohatgi, MD, MS, SFHM

Clinical Professor of Medicine
Clinical Professor of Neurosurgery (by courtesy)
Clinical Professor of Anesthesiology, Perioperative and
Pain Medicine (by courtesy)
Faculty Affiliate
Center for Artificial Intelligence in Medicine and
Imaging and Center for Digital Health
Stanford University School of Medicine
Palo Alto, California
Chapters 14, 24, 27, 28, 38

Linda A. Russell, MD

Anne and Joel Ehrenkranz Chair in Perioperative
Medicine
Vice Chair of Clinical Affairs, Department of Medicine
Director of Perioperative Medicine
Hospital for Special Surgery
Associate Professor of Clinical Medicine
Weill Cornell Medical College
New York, New York
Chapter 29

Sunil K. Sahai, MD, FAAP, FACP, SFHM

Professor & Division Chief, General Internal Medicine
The John Sealy School of Medicine
The University of Texas Medical Branch
Galveston, Texas
Chapters 21, 32, 33, 34

Angela Roberts Selzer, MD, FASA, DFPM

Associate Professor of Anesthesiology
University of Colorado
Aurora, Colorado
Chapter 18

Jeffrey W. Simmons, MD, MSHQS, FASA

Professor of Anesthesiology and Perioperative Medicine
UAB Medicine
Birmingham, Alabama
Chapters 3, 32

Barbara Slawski, MD, MS, SFHM

Professor of Medicine and Orthopaedic Surgery
Chief, Section of Hospital Medicine
Interim Chief, Division of General Internal Medicine
Medical College of Wisconsin
Chief of Staff
Froedtert Memorial Lutheran Hospital
Milwaukee, Wisconsin
Chapters 22, 25, 41

Gerald W. Smetana, MD, MACP

Professor of Medicine
Harvard Medical School
Division of General Medicine
Beth Israel Deaconess Medical Center
Boston, Massachusetts
Chapters 2, 16

Guillermo E. Umpierrez, MD, CDCES, FACE, MACP

Professor of Medicine
Department of Medicine
Emory University School of Medicine
Atlanta, Georgia
Chapter 19

J. Njeri Wainaina, MD, FACP, FHM, FIDSA

Associate Professor of Medicine and Surgery
Vice Chair for Quality
Department of Medicine
Medical College of Wisconsin
Milwaukee, Wisconsin
Enterprise Medical Director for Antimicrobial
Stewardship
Froedtert Health and Thedacare Health South Region
Chapters 7, 24, 35, 39

Paul J. Wang, MD, FAHA, FACC, FHRS, FESC

Director
Cardiac Arrhythmia Service
Professor of Medicine and Bioengineering (by Courtesy)
The John R. and Ai Giak L. Singleton Co-Director of
the Stanford Center for Arrhythmia Research
Department of Medicine
Stanford University School of Medicine
Stanford, California
Chapters 14, 38

Howard H. Weitz, MD, MACP, FRCP, FACC

Bernard Segal Professor of Medicine (Cardiology)
Senior Associate Dean
Sidney Kimmel Medical College at Thomas Jefferson
University
Philadelphia, Pennsylvania
Chapters 12, 13

Christopher M. Whinney, MD, FACP, SFHM

Chairman
Division of Hospital Medicine
Cleveland Clinic
Clinical Assistant Professor of Medicine
Cleveland Clinic Lerner College of Medicine
Cleveland, Ohio
Chapters 20, 21, 33

Preface

Worldwide, over 300 million people undergo surgery every year. It is estimated that 1–4% of these patients will die, up to 15% will have serious postoperative morbidity, and 5–15% will be readmitted within 30 days.[1] Although patients are unlikely to die from anesthesia, the burden of perioperative complications falls more on exacerbations of underlying medical conditions, in part because we are operating on older and sicker patients. While it is unrealistic to believe that perioperative deaths and complications can be eliminated, our goal is to minimize this risk as much as possible.

With the explosion of medical knowledge, treatment innovation, and increasing specialization, it is difficult for any physician to keep current with the constant influx of information. While surgeons, anesthesiologists, and some hospitalists may spend a major portion of their clinical time caring for patients in the perioperative period, many other hospitalists, primary care physicians, and their teams of nurse practitioners and physician assistants may need guidance to address specific issues for their patients before and/or after surgery. The goal of this book is to provide a simple, direct guide to the medical, as opposed to surgical and anesthetic, aspects of perioperative care. It is not intended to be a comprehensive textbook, and references have deliberately been limited to keep the focus on the practical aspects of patient care. This book is intended for use by all members of the perioperative team—hospitalists, general internists and specialists, family medicine physicians, anesthesiologists, surgeons, advanced practice providers, and residents in-training who are caring for patients before and after surgery.

The genesis of this book comes from a lecture I gave at the annual meeting of the American College of Physicians. Attendees at the session asked many questions—which risk calculator should I use, who needs a stress test, how long should surgery be delayed after percutaneous coronary intervention (PCI), should aspirin be continued, how long before surgery should I stop a direct-acting oral anticoagulant (DOAC), who needs bridging, should surgery be delayed for a sleep study, and many more. They also repeatedly requested lists of risk factors, tables for medication management, and algorithms for the approach to evaluation and management of various comorbid conditions. This book is a response to these requests. I invited leading experts to distill their vast knowledge and experience into focused, need-to-know information that will be useful to clinicians at the point-of-care. For this second edition, I added eight anesthesiologists as coauthors to provide their perspectives, as well as five other experts in internal medicine. In contrast to many other books, over 85% of contributors to this book are senior faculty members with professor or associate professor appointments and extensive clinical experience, serving as section chiefs and perioperative clinic or consult service directors. All chapters were revised, and in particular, new recommendations from the 2022 ESC and 2024 ACC/AHA guidelines have been incorporated in the cardiac chapters. Several new chapters were added including cardiac biomarkers, postoperative nausea and vomiting, and postoperative urinary retention. The result is this practical decision-making reference which consolidates updated information from multiple guidelines, clinical trials, and expert opinion. It uses

---

[1] World Health Organization (WHO) Fact Sheets—Patient Safety. September 11, 2023. Available at https://www.who.int/news-room/fact-sheets/detail/patient-safety#:~:text=Over%20300%20million%20surgical%20procedures,each%20year%20worldwide%20(6). Accessed January 30, 2025.

algorithms, tables, and clinical pearls to summarize the key concepts and takeaways.

Our collective goal is to navigate clinicians to the best evidence-based and most cost-effective decisions that will in turn ensure quality, patient-safety, and optimal perioperative outcomes. To this end, the content has been organized into four sections:

1. Key takeaways on perioperative evaluation, testing, anesthesia, and medication management
2. Prophylaxis to prevent venous thromboembolism, surgical site infection, and endocarditis
3. Guidance on specific risk factors by organ system to help clinicians evaluate the effect of various comorbidities on surgical outcome and provide perioperative management to minimize risk
4. A brief review of common postoperative medical complications and their treatment

The field of perioperative medicine continues to evolve, and new information may make previous guidelines and recommendations obsolete. Errors, inaccuracies, and omissions are an inevitable part of any human endeavor, and the reader is urged to use this book in the context of clinical judgment and confirm information, particularly as it relates to medications and dosing. The first edition of this book was written during a difficult time—the COVID-19 pandemic.

The coronavirus affects multiple organ systems, and we do not fully know the extent of its aftereffects. Scheduling, preoperative testing, and operating room procedures have changed and continue to evolve, guided by recommendations from various societies. Because there were no specific guidelines for changes to perioperative evaluation and testing of patients who have had COVID-19, and the rapidly evolving nature of the problem, I chose not to include a chapter on this topic in the first edition. Although there are still many unknowns, we now have more information, and I decided to include COVID-19 as part of the infectious disease chapter in the second edition.

With over 30 years of experience in perioperative medicine, having evaluated over 30,000 patients preoperatively and having served as the director of preoperative clinics and medical consultation services at two major academic medical centers (SUNY Downstate Medical Center/Kings County Hospital and University of Miami Miller School of Medicine/Jackson Memorial Hospital), I have dedicated my medical career to the field of perioperative medicine. I hope that this book will provide key information to increase knowledge and instill confidence in clinicians providing perioperative care, and as a result help ensure optimal patient outcomes.

–Steven L. Cohn, MD, MACP, SFHM, FRCP

Acknowledgments

I would like to acknowledge James Shanahan from McGraw Hill and Diane Scott-Lichter from ACP for inviting me to edit this book, and Kay Conerly and Jennifer Bernstein for their advice and support in keeping this project on track. Special thanks to Dr. Robert Lavender, Professor of Medicine at the University of Arkansas for his review of and critical feedback on the entire manuscript. I am also grateful to Sylvia Choi and Poonam Bisht for their meticulous work and management to give the book chapters their appealing design. I would also like to thank all the contributors for their commitment and thoroughness in writing, revising, and updating their chapters.

About the Editor

Dr. Cohn is Professor Emeritus in the Department of Medicine at the University of Miami Miller School of Medicine. He is the former Director of the Medical Consultation Service at Jackson Memorial Hospital and Medical Director of the UHealth Preoperative Assessment Center (UPAC) and Medical Consultation Service at the University of Miami Hospital, having relocated to Miami after 30 years at the State University of New York—Downstate Medical Center in Brooklyn where he is also Clinical Professor of Medicine Emeritus. He served as the Chief of the Division of General Internal Medicine and Associate Medical Director for Performance Improvement at Downstate, and the Director of the Preoperative Medical Consultation Clinic and Medical Consultation Service at Kings County Hospital Center. He was responsible for education and supervision of over 1,100 senior medical residents in both inpatient and ambulatory care settings, and he has evaluated over 30,000 patients preoperatively. After receiving his medical degree from the University of Monterrey, Dr. Cohn completed his residency in internal medicine at SUNY—Downstate Medical Center. He is a Master of the American College of Physicians (ACP), a senior fellow of the Society for Hospital Medicine (SHM), a fellow of the Royal College of Physicians (RCP), and a board member of the Society for Perioperative Assessment and Quality Improvement (SPAQI). He has given over 400 CME lectures, authored/edited four books and over 100 book chapters and peer-reviewed manuscripts, and in 2017, he received the Society for Hospital Medicine award for Excellence in Teaching.

INTRODUCTION TO PERIOPERATIVE PATIENT CARE

Role of the Perioperative Medical Consultant

Steven L. Cohn, MD, MACP, SFHM, FRCP

COMMON CLINICAL QUESTIONS

1. What are the goals of the perioperative medical consultant?
2. What information should be included in the consultation report?
3. How can the consultant improve compliance with the recommendations?

INTRODUCTION

Preoperative medical consultation and perioperative management of the surgical patient are important roles in the clinical practice of internists, hospitalists, and subspecialists. The role of the hospitalist has expanded to include comanagement for orthopedic, neurosurgical, vascular, and other surgical patients, and even the role of the anesthesiologist has evolved, focusing on perioperative medicine outside the operating room setting as well. This chapter discusses the principles of medical consultation and the role of the perioperative medical consultant. Specifics regarding risk assessment and management are discussed in subsequent chapters.

ROLE OF THE PERIOPERATIVE MEDICAL CONSULTANT

The role of the perioperative medical consultant can be described as having three main goals:

1. *Preoperative risk stratification*—to define and evaluate the patient's current medical conditions, uncover previously unrecognized problems, and estimate the patient's surgical risk
2. *Medical optimization*—to recommend risk reduction strategies, perioperative medication management, and any additional testing if indicated
3. *Postoperative follow-up*—to re-evaluate medical problems, ensure compliance with recommendations and medical therapy, provide advice, and anticipate, recognize, and treat any postoperative medical complications

GENERAL PRINCIPLES OF MEDICAL CONSULTATION

In 1983, Goldman and colleagues[1] published their "Ten Commandments" for effective consultation which were modified in 2007 by Salerno and colleagues[2] (Table 1-1). These basic principles included: (1) Determine the question. (2) Establish urgency. (3) Look for yourself. (4) Be as brief as appropriate. (5) Be specific and concise. (6) Provide contingency plans. (7) Honor thy turf. (8) Teach with tact. (9) Talk is cheap and effective. (10) Follow-up. The basic meaning of these concepts is noted in Table 1-1, and they will be highlighted throughout this discussion.

Types of Consultation

It is important to recognize different types of consultation requests. The *traditional or standard* medical

	1983 COMMANDMENTS[1]	2007 MODIFICATIONS[2]	MEANING AND MODIFICATION
	TABLE 1-1. Original and Modified Ten Commandments for Effective Consultations		
1	Determine the question.	Determine *your customer.*	If the specific question is not obvious, call the requesting physician—*and ask if they want comanagement.*
2	Establish urgency.	Establish urgency.	Determine whether the consultation is emergent, urgent, or elective.
3	Look for yourself.	Look for yourself.	Gather data independently to be most effective.
4	Be brief as appropriate.	Be brief as appropriate.	No need to repeat in full detail the data that were already documented.
5	Be specific.	Be specific, *be thorough, and descend from thy ivory tower to help when requested.*	Limit recommendations to improve likelihood of compliance vs. *leave as many specific recommendations as needed but offer assistance in order writing if needed.*
6	Provide contingency plans.	Provide contingency plans *and discuss their execution.*	Anticipate potential problems, document therapeutic options *and contingency plans, and provide 24-hour contact information for help if needed.*
7	Thou shalt not covet thy neighbor's turf.	Thou *may negotiate joint title* to thy neighbor's turf.	In most cases, consultants should play a subsidiary role; *however, consultants can and should comanage any facet of patient care the requesting physician desires (but clarify who is responsible for what).*
8	Teach with tact.	Teach with tact *and pragmatism.*	Sharing your expertise is appreciated—*although decisions on leaving references should be tailored to the requesting physician's specialty, level of training, and urgency of the consult.*
9	Talk is cheap and effective.	Talk is *essential.*	There is no substitute for direct personal contact with the primary physician.
10	Provide appropriate follow-up.	Follow-up *daily.*	Recognize when to fade into a background role, but that time is almost never on the same day as the consult. *Daily written follow-up notes are desirable, but when problems are no longer active, sign-off after discussing with the requesting physician.*

Data from Salerno et al. *Arch Intern Med.* 2007;167:271-275 and Goldman et al. *Arch Intern Med.* 1983;143(9):1753-1755.

consult is a formal request from the patient's attending physician/surgeon to evaluate the patient and answer a specific question. In this role, the consultant is expected to address the question and provide advice and recommendations, but not to write orders, request additional consultants, or assume primary care of the patient. The consultant focuses on the specific problem rather than other medical issues, follows up briefly in the postoperative period, and then signs off. More recently, many surgeons are requesting the medical consultant to assume more of a *comanagement role* taking a more global approach, addressing all necessary medical issues, writing orders, and providing daily follow-up. The responsibilities of the consultant and the surgical team need to be clearly defined in advance. Another type of consultation is the so-called *"curbside" or informal consult* in which the consultant is asked to provide an opinion or advice without personally seeing the patient. These should be discouraged from a medicolegal standpoint as there is no formal doctor–patient relationship although at times this has been challenged in court. Instead, the consultant should offer to perform a formal consultation, but if any advice is given, it should be generic and simple. The "consultant" should also inform the requesting physician not to refer to him in the medical record.

Determining the Question

Although incumbent on the requesting physician to clearly define the reason for the consultation and provide relevant information, this is often not the case. Many consult requests only state "medical clearance" or "preoperative evaluation" without mentioning the medical problems or even the type of surgery planned. Therefore, it is imperative for the consultant to determine what is being requested to be able to respond appropriately. The best way to clarify the question is by direct verbal communication with the requesting physician.

Answering the Question

In order to decide whether the patient is medically optimized for surgery, the consultant must identify and address any specific medical problem mentioned as well as any others that may impact surgical risk. As noted above, there has been a shift from the traditional consult to more of a comanagement request,

and the consultant now tends to address more than just the specific disease that was initially mentioned. The basic approach on how to answer the question is listed in Table 1-2. The consultant should also avoid use of the phrase "cleared for surgery," even if that was the request, as it implies that the procedure carries no risk for the particular patient when all patients are potentially at some risk when they undergo anesthesia and surgery. The consultant cannot and should not guarantee a complication-free outcome.

The Consultation Report

Ideally a template can be created in the electronic medical record that will import existing information into required fields to streamline data entry. However, it is important to verify all data elements with the patient to ensure that the information is accurate. Consultants have varying styles, but the bottom line is that the report includes all pertinent information, addresses the question being asked, assesses medical optimization and surgical risk, and makes recommendations for perioperative management. Table 1-3 is a checklist for items to be included in the consultation report.

TABLE 1-2. My Ten Commandments for How to Answer the Question

QUESTIONS TO BE ADDRESSED	ANSWERS
1) What's wrong?	List all relevant medical conditions.
2) How bad is it?	Describe the severity of the disease.
3) Is it adequately controlled?	Ensure stability of the disease as well as appropriate medical therapy.
4) Does it affect surgical risk?	Decide if this disease has an important impact on risk and whether it requires treatment now.
5) Are additional tests indicated to improve risk estimation or change management?	Ascertain what other information, if any, will affect clinical decision making.
6) Are there treatments that will reduce risk?	Determine what treatments are available that might lower risk of perioperative complications without potential for harm.
7) How urgent is the surgery?	Decide if there is enough time to do something if necessary.
8) Should surgery be postponed for further workup and treatment?	Assess whether the patient is medically optimized or would benefit in terms of lower risk by additional workup or therapy now as opposed to after surgery.
9) What do the surgeon and anesthesiologist think?	Communicate with your colleagues and get their input.
10) What do the patient and family want?	Discuss risks/benefits with the patient/family to involve them in shared decision making.

TABLE 1-3. "Checklist" for the Consultation Report

Demographics	Patient information (name, DOB, MR#) Reason for consult Referring physician/service/contact info Surgery: planned procedure/date Anesthesia: type, if known
Past medical history (pertinent medical problems—positive or negative)	Cardiopulmonary disease, HTN, DM, thyroid disease, liver disease, bleeding disorder, stroke, seizures
Past surgical history	Operations, type of anesthesia, date, complications Anesthesia issues—difficult airway, IV access, pain
Social history	Tobacco, alcohol, drug use—amount, duration, last use
Medications—Rx and OTC (home and hospital)	Name, dose, frequency, compliance (in-hospital—note when last dose was taken)
Allergies	Description of allergic reaction
Pertinent family history	Genetically related diseases: malignant hyperthermia, bleeding disorders
Review of systems (focused)	Cardiopulmonary (chest pain, dyspnea, cough), functional capacity/METs/ADLs, bleeding/bruising
Physical exam	Vital signs (including height/weight/BMI), usual exam with focus on airway, dentition, murmur/gallop, adventitious sounds, organomegaly, neurologic deficit, mental status/cognitive dysfunction/evidence of frailty
Lab tests	Patient and surgery directed testing (pertinent basic blood tests, ECG) and any specific results of relevant recent/past cardiac tests (stress test, echocardiogram, coronary angiography, pacemaker interrogation), PFTs, CT/MRI/X-rays, carotid Dopplers, etc.
Impression	Patient is/is not in his/her optimal medical condition (or is medically optimized) for the planned procedure
Recommendations	Current meds (continue, stop, resume, change dose), new meds, prophylaxis (SSI, VTE, IE), postop monitoring (ECG, troponin, pulse oximetry, telemetry, ICU)
Assessment & discussion	Discuss specifics of pertinent problems (severity, stability, degree of control), assess level of risk and ASA, and summarize; can include results of various risk calculators (cardiac, OSA, pulmonary, frailty, delirium, bleeding/thrombotic) in terms of increased risk rather than quoting a percent. Note DNR status if applicable.
Consultant information	Name, contact info (cellphone/beeper); date/time consult report was written

DOB, date of birth; MR, medical record; HTN, hypertension; DM, diabetes mellitus; Rx, prescription; OTC, over the counter; ADL, activities of daily living; ECG, electrocardiogram; PFT, pulmonary function test; CT, computerized tomography; MRI, magnetic resonance imaging; SSI, surgical site infection; VTE, venous thromboembolism; IE, infective endocarditis; OSA, obstructive sleep apnea; ASA, American Society of Anesthesiology; DNR, do not resuscitate.

IMPROVING COMPLIANCE WITH RECOMMENDATIONS

Although the consultant evaluates the patient, renders an opinion, and makes recommendations, it is important to understand that these recommendations may not be followed in 10–40% of cases. Missed recommendations may be unintentional or intentional (Figure 1-1).[3] Studies have found various factors that are associated with improving compliance (Table 1-4).[4] In following Goldman's Ten Commandments, determining the question and answering it in an appropriate manner is paramount. Establish the urgency and respond in a timely fashion. Elective consultations should be answered within 24 hours (ideally the same day) and sooner if deemed urgent (within several hours) or emergent (immediate phone contact followed by in-person evaluation within 10–30 minutes or less). Be concise, prioritize crucial recommendations, and limit the number of recommendations. The longer the list, the less likely all recommendations will be addressed. The more severely ill the patient, the more likely recommendations will be implemented. Recommendations regarding therapy are somewhat more likely to be followed than those for diagnostic tests. Use definitive language and be specific, particularly when recommending medications. Specify the drug (not class), dose, frequency, route of administration, and duration of therapy as the surgeon may not be familiar with the medication. Although some electronic medical records may automatically notify the requesting physician when a consult has been completed, and the current generation of clinicians tends to rely on text messaging rather than talking, *direct verbal communication* with the surgeon is the most effective means of discussing your thoughts and recommendations. A preliminary text can be sent, but it should be quickly

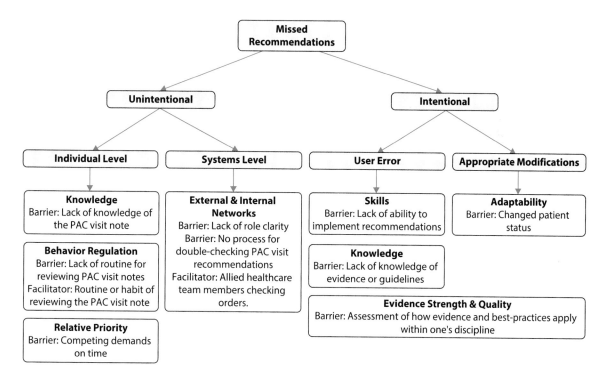

FIGURE 1-1. Framework for understanding missed perioperative recommendations. (Reproduced from Flemons Kristin, Bosch Michael, Coakeley Sarah, Muzammal Bushra, Kachra Rahim, Ruzycki Shannon M. Barriers and facilitators of following perioperative internal medicine recommendations by surgical teams: a sequential, explanatory mixed-methods study. *Perioper Medicine.* 2022;11(1):2.)

TABLE 1-4. Factors That Influence or Improve Compliance with Consultant Recommendations

Prompt response (within 24 hours)
Limit number of recommendations (≤5)
Identify and prioritize crucial or critical recommendations (vs. routine)
Focus on central issues
Make specific relevant recommendations
Use definitive language
Specify drug dosage, route, frequency, duration
Frequent follow-up including progress notes
Direct verbal contact
Therapeutic (vs. diagnostic) recommendations
Severity of illness

followed by a phone call to ensure that the message was received and that there are no questions regarding patient management. Make appropriate follow-up visits to ensure that recommendations were followed, reassess the patient, and document your findings in a progress note. Depending on the situation, follow-up may be as short as a single postoperative visit, or in the case of a severely ill patient or comanagement, may be daily until improvement or discharge. When signing off, document this in the medical record and inform the surgical team. Also, indicate if the patient requires any specific follow-up after discharge. Training in the 5Cs of Consultation model (Contact, Communicate, Core Question, Collaborate, and Close the Loop) may improve communication and increase effectiveness of physician consultations.[5]

SUMMARY

Perioperative medical consultation is a combination of art, science, and politics. The ideal medical consultant is someone who will "render a report that informs without patronizing, educates without lecturing, directs without ordering, and solves the problem without making the referring physician appear to be stupid."[6] By following the principles outlined by Goldman and colleagues, the medical consultant will provide information and advice that will be helpful to the requesting physician who will then implement the recommendations with the goal being improved patient outcomes.

Clinical pearls

- A good consultant follows the 3As of medicine—availability, affability, and ability.
- Obey Goldman's "Ten Commandments"—understand the question, respond to it in a timely fashion with appropriate recommendations, and communicate with the requesting physician and surgical team to ensure compliance.
- Don't "*clear*" patients for surgery—**medically optimize** them.

REFERENCES

1. Goldman L, Lee T, Rudd P. Ten commandments for effective consultations. *Arch Intern Med.* 1983;143(9):1753-1755. PMID: 6615097
2. Salerno SM, Hurst FP, Halvorson S, Mercado DL. Principles of effective consultation: an update for the 21st-century consultant. *Arch Intern Med.* 2007;167(3):271-275. PMID: 17296883
3. Flemons K, Bosch M, Coakeley S, et al. Barriers and facilitators of following perioperative internal medicine recommendations by surgical teams: a sequential, explanatory mixed-methods study. *Perioper Med* (Lond). 2022;11(1):2. PMID: 35101113
4. Cohn SL. Overview of the principles of medical consultation and perioperative medicine. *UpToDate.* Waltham, MA: UpToDate Inc. Available at https://www.uptodate.com. Accessed on January 15, 2024
5. Kessler CS, Afshar Y, Sardar G, et al. A prospective, randomized, controlled study demonstrating a novel, effective model of transfer of care between physicians: the 5 Cs of consultation. *Acad Emerg Med.* 2012;19(8):968-974. PMID: 22905961
6. Bates R. The two sides of every successful consultation. *Med Econ.* 1979;7:173-180. PMID: 22469350

Preoperative Testing

Steven L. Cohn, MD, MACP, SFHM, FRCP and Gerald W. Smetana, MD, MACP

COMMON CLINICAL QUESTIONS

1. In which patients does preoperative testing change management?
2. Which tests are indicated before high-risk surgery?
3. How do I consider the impact of patient comorbidities when deciding which tests to order?
4. Do I need to perform an ECG to estimate risk of postoperative cardiac complications?

INTRODUCTION

Preoperative evaluation of apparently healthy patients is a common activity for internists and other medical specialists. In general, the most important test is a careful medical history to seek elements that may increase perioperative risk above baseline. Individual laboratory and other tests should be ordered selectively based on patient and procedure-related characteristics, and in general, should not be done routinely without a clinical indication. Despite decades of evidence arguing against routine testing, medical culture is such that some of this testing persists. General rationales for ordering preoperative tests are to identify patients at higher risk for particular postoperative complications, to guide anesthetic management, to predict which patients require particular monitoring after surgery, and for medicolegal reasons. In fact, in most instances, testing for any of these indications rarely achieves the desired goals. In this chapter, we discuss the recommended selective indications for testing.

If enough routine tests are ordered, it is likely that one or more tests may be abnormal due to the typical definition of normal as within 2 standard deviations from the mean. This means, by definition, that in 5% of patients without underlying disease, a test will be abnormal. If tests are done routinely, an abnormal test result may cause an unnecessary delay of surgery, patient worry, and additional testing, which may be costly, and in some cases, carry risk for the patient. A selective approach to preoperative test ordering avoids this trap.

An optimal test would be one that accurately identifies patients at risk of postoperative complications who would otherwise be characterized as low risk based on their history and physical examination, is inexpensive, carries little risk, and has a high sensitivity and specificity. Few tests have these qualities.

Increasingly, surgeons, anesthesiologists, and hospital standards committees have recognized this fact and are requiring fewer routine tests than had been the case historically. For example, in the Choosing Wisely guidelines, national societies were given the chance to list five things that we should question or not do. Many of the relevant surgery and anesthesiology guidelines made a recommendation to avoiding unnecessary preoperative testing.[1] At least 13 different societies chose recommendations to limit preoperative testing. Table 2-1 summarizes these recommendations. In 2012, the American Society of Anesthesiologists stated in a practice advisory that

TABLE 2-1. Choosing Wisely Campaign. Society Recommendations to Limit Preoperative Testing

SOCIETY	RECOMMENDATION
American Society of Hematology American Society of Pediatric Hematology/Oncology	Don't perform routine preoperative hemostatic testing (PT, aPTT) in an otherwise healthy child with no prior personal or family history of bleeding.
American Society of Anesthesiologists	Don't obtain baseline laboratory studies in patients without significant systemic disease (ASA I or II) undergoing low-risk surgery—specifically complete blood count, basic or comprehensive metabolic panel, coagulation studies when blood loss (or fluid shifts) is/are expected to be minimal.
Society of General Internal Medicine	Don't perform routine preoperative testing before low-risk surgical procedures.
American College of Surgeons	Avoid admission or preoperative chest x-rays for ambulatory patients with unremarkable history and physical exam.
American Academy of Ophthalmology	Don't perform preoperative medical tests for eye surgery unless there are specific medical indications.
The Society of Thoracic Surgeons	Prior to cardiac surgery, there is no need for pulmonary function testing in the absence of respiratory symptoms.
The Society of Thoracic Surgeons	Patients who have no cardiac history and good functional status do not require preoperative stress testing prior to noncardiac thoracic surgery.
Society of Cardiovascular Computed Tomography	Don't order coronary artery calcium scoring for preoperative evaluation for any surgery, irrespective of patient risk.
American Society for Clinical Pathology	Avoid routine preoperative testing for low-risk surgeries without a clinical indication.
American Society of Echocardiography	Avoid echocardiograms for preoperative/perioperative assessment of patients with no history or symptoms of heart disease.
American College of Radiology	Avoid admission or preoperative chest x-rays for ambulatory patients with unremarkable history and physical exam.
American College of Physicians	Don't obtain preoperative chest radiography in the absence of a clinical suspicion for intrathoracic pathology.

Adapted with permission from Choosing Wisely Clinician Lists. (Accessed on July 13, 2020.) Copyright © 2020 the ABIM Foundation. For more information visit https://www.choosingwisely.org/clinician-lists/#keyword=preoperative.

"preoperative tests should not be ordered routinely … tests may be ordered, required, or performed on a selective basis for purposes of guiding or optimizing perioperative management."[2] In 2016, the National Institute for Health and Care Excellence (NICE) guidelines[3] from the United Kingdom considered both patient- and procedure-related factors when recommending selective testing as well.

As an example of the unnecessary overuse of preoperative tests, in a study of patients undergoing low-risk surgery (elective hernia repair), 34% of patients had no comorbidities (according to National Surgical Quality Improvement Program [NSQIP] definitions), and therefore no indication for preoperative testing.[4] Yet 52% received a preoperative complete blood count (or at least one component) and 15% received a coagulation test. Neither the decision to order routine tests nor the test results predicted rates of postoperative complications.

Routinely obtained preoperative testing without a clinical indication is rarely abnormal. When it is abnormal, the results often do not change preoperative risk assessment or perioperative care. In an early summary of the literature, preoperative testing only modestly influenced the likelihood of postoperative complications. Most patients who were at risk of specific complications could be identified through a careful history and physical examination. The incidence of abnormalities that changed management ranged from 0% to 3%, depending on the test (Table 2-2).

SPECIFIC TESTS

Complete Blood Count

For patients undergoing surgery with a large amount of anticipated blood loss, it is reasonable to perform a CBC, which includes measurement of hemoglobin and hematocrit, before surgery. This will guide discussions with the patient about a potential need for perioperative transfusions. For low-risk surgery, or high-risk surgery with little anticipated blood loss, a preoperative CBC

is not necessary. It is also reasonable for patients over 65 years old who are undergoing major surgery. While preoperative anemia confers a higher risk of postoperative mortality than for patients with normal hemoglobin and hematocrit, it is unknown if the anemia itself increases mortality, or if it is a marker for underlying comorbidities (see Chapter 22) (Table 2-3).

In general, a platelet count adds little if there is no clinical history of bleeding tendency. It is rare for clinically significant thrombocytopenia (<50,000) to exist in the absence of a clinical history of bleeding tendency or a chronic medical condition that can cause thrombocytopenia. We suggest this test for patients undergoing neuraxial anesthesia and those undergoing intracranial neurosurgery. A white blood cell count does not predict infectious or other perioperative complications. However, since both are elements of a CBC, which is an inexpensive test, it is reasonable to perform a full CBC if there is an indication for measuring hemoglobin or hematocrit before surgery.

TABLE 2-2. Incidence of Abnormal Preoperative Tests That Change Management and Change in the Likelihood of Postoperative Complications Based on Test Results

TEST	INCIDENCE OF ABNORMALITIES THAT INFLUENCE MANAGEMENT (%)	LR+	LR−
Hemoglobin	0.1	3.3	0.90
White blood cell count	0.0	0.0	1.00
Platelet count	0.0	0.0	1.00
Prothrombin time (PT)	0.0	0.0	1.01
Partial thromboplastin time (PTT)	0.1	1.7	0.86
Electrolytes	1.8	4.3	0.80
Renal function	2.6	3.3	0.81
Glucose	0.5	1.6	0.85
Liver function tests	0.1		
Urinalysis	1.4	1.7	0.97
Electrocardiogram	2.6	1.6	0.96
Chest radiograph	3.0	2.5	0.72

LR+, positive likelihood ratio; LR−, negative likelihood ratio.

Reproduced with permission from Smetana GW, Macpherson DS. The case against routine preoperative laboratory testing. *Med Clin Am.* 2003;87(1):7-40.

TABLE 2-3. Indications for Commonly Ordered Preoperative Tests

TEST	INDICATIONS
Hemoglobin	Symptoms of anemia, major blood loss surgery
WBC	Infection, myeloproliferative disease, myelotoxic meds
Platelets	Abnormal hemostasis, chemotherapy, or medications associated with thrombocytopenia
PT/INR	History of bleeding diathesis, liver disease, malnutrition, antibiotics, warfarin
PTT	History of bleeding diathesis
Electrolytes	CKD, HF, diarrhea, medications that increase the risk of electrolyte abnormalities (ACEI/ARB, diuretic)
BUN/creatinine	CKD, HTN, cardiac disease, elderly, meds
Glucose	DM (history or suspected); obesity, steroids
LFTs	Hepatitis (acute); cirrhosis
U/A	GU instrumentation
Pregnancy test	Woman of childbearing age, particularly if the possibility of pregnancy cannot be excluded by history
ECG	Known/suspected cardiac disease, intermediate-high risk surgery (+age > 65 as per ESC)
CXR	Active/suspected pulmonary disease

WBC, white blood cell; PT, prothrombin time; INR, international normalized ratio; PTT, partial thromboplastin time; BUN, blood urea nitrogen; LFT, liver function tests; U/A, urinalysis; ECG, electrocardiogram; CXR, chest x-ray; CKD, chronic kidney disease; HF, heart failure; ACEI/ARB, angiotensin converting enzyme inhibitor/angiotensin receptor blocker; HTN, hypertension; DM, diabetes mellitus; GU, genitourinary; ESC, European Society of Cardiology.

Measurement of Renal Function and Electrolytes

Perioperative chronic kidney disease may influence anesthetic management and prompt more careful or frequent monitoring of renal function after surgery. Preoperative chronic kidney disease (serum creatinine >2.0 mg/dL) is also one of six independent risk factors for postoperative cardiac complications in the widely used revised cardiac risk index (RCRI).[5] Preoperative measurement of renal function (primarily serum creatinine) should be performed selectively, rather than in all patients undergoing surgery. Abnormalities are uncommon in patients with no medical conditions or medication use for which chronic kidney disease is possible. For example, it is appropriate to check renal function before major surgery in patients with diabetes, heart failure (HF), or known chronic kidney disease. It is reasonable to measure in patients over 50 years old undergoing major surgery, as the prevalence of chronic kidney disease increases with age. Preoperative renal function testing is also recommended for patients who are taking medications that may affect renal function. This would include angiotensin-converting enzyme (ACE) inhibitors, angiotensin receptor blocker (ARBs), diuretics, and nonsteroidal anti-inflammatory drugs (NSAIDs).

A theoretical reason for measuring electrolytes would be to identify patients who may require potassium supplementation after surgery or to predict the potential for arrhythmia. The indication for measuring preoperative electrolytes is like those noted above for measurement of renal function. In particular, preoperative measurement of electrolytes is appropriate for patients undergoing major surgery who are taking one of the above medications. Neither preoperative renal function nor electrolytes should be measured routinely.

Glucose

Hyperglycemia has been associated with an increase in postoperative complications. While routine screening for all patients is not recommended, a serum glucose is indicated for patients with known diabetes (DM) to assess current control, and those with signs and symptoms suggestive of DM for diagnostic purposes. Other potential indications include corticosteroid use and obesity, both of which may be associated with hyperglycemia.

Although perioperative glucose levels correlate better than A1C levels for perioperative complications, the ADA recommends obtaining A1C in hospitalized patients with DM and those with hyperglycemia (glucose >140 mg/dL) if not done in the past 3 months.[6] Because the A1C level correlates with the average glucose during the past 3 months, serum fructosamine level may be a better measure of recent glucose control as it reflects the average over the past 2–3 weeks (see Chapter 19).

Liver Function Tests

In general, liver function tests should only be obtained in patients with suspected acute hepatitis (viral, alcoholic, or drug-induced), as elective surgery is contraindicated in this setting, or as needed to evaluate patients with cirrhosis. Commonly used tools to estimate perioperative risk for patients with cirrhosis—VOCAL-Penn, Child Pugh, or MELD scores—all require some tests of liver function to predict risk of postoperative complications. Otherwise, liver function tests should not be performed routinely before surgery (see Chapter 26).

Coagulation Tests

Standard coagulation tests such as the prothrombin time/international normalized ratio (PT/INR) and partial thromboplastin time (PTT) are frequently obtained preoperatively to assess coagulopathy and guide therapy. However, the preponderance of evidence from multiple studies suggests that these screening tests are not useful in predicting perioperative bleeding in patients without known bleeding risk factors. Furthermore, abnormal results often lead to additional testing and possible delays in planned surgery. The PT/INR and PTT were designed to monitor the anticoagulant effects of warfarin and heparin and to assess coagulation factor deficiencies—not to predict bleeding or guide hemostatic therapy.

Taking an accurate bleeding history, which includes medications that might affect hemostasis and the patient's personal and family bleeding history, will detect most significant bleeding disorders and is more important than unselected blood testing (see Chapter 23). Most adult patients with hemophilia will have already been diagnosed, and patients with von Willebrand's disease may also be more likely to be identified by history as PTT alone will not necessarily be abnormal. Although bleeding in certain situations like neurosurgery could be catastrophic, a large study in this patient population also found that bleeding history was more predictive of bleeding complications (need for transfusion, return to the operating room, or 30-day mortality) than routine blood tests.[7]

The ASA Task Force on Preanesthesia Evaluation Practice Advisory recommends against routine testing and suggests selective ordering of coagulation tests based on history of bleeding disorders, renal dysfunction, liver dysfunction, type and invasiveness of procedure, and medications.[2] The NICE guidelines also recommend against routine preoperative hemostasis tests but to consider them in people with chronic liver disease undergoing intermediate, major, or complex surgery or in those taking anticoagulants.[3]

Urinalysis

The theory behind ordering a routine urinalysis before surgery is to identify and treat asymptomatic bacteriuria (urinary tract infection or colonization), thereby reducing the risk of perioperative infections. Most studies on routine urinalyses have involved orthopedic patients undergoing total joint arthroplasty with the objective being to prevent a prosthetic joint infection. However, the evidence has not shown a benefit for these patients. Although patients with asymptomatic bacteriuria may have a higher incidence of prosthetic joint infection, there was no difference between those treated with antibiotics and those who were not treated, suggesting that asymptomatic bacteriuria may be a marker for risk of infection rather than the cause. Furthermore, the pathogens in the joint infections did not match those organisms isolated in the urine culture. The International Consensus Meeting on Periprosthetic Joint Infection recommended not to order routine urinalyses before total joint replacements, although this is still a commonly encountered practice.[8] In addition, guidelines from the Infectious Disease Society of America recommend against screening for or treating asymptomatic bacteriuria in patients undergoing elective nonurologic procedures (*strong recommendation, low-quality evidence*).[9] On the other hand, in patients who will undergo endoscopic urologic procedures associated with mucosal trauma, we recommend screening for and treating asymptomatic bacteriuria prior to surgery (*strong recommendation, moderate-quality evidence*).

Urine Pregnancy Test

Routine preoperative pregnancy testing is controversial, although it is commonly required for all women of reproductive age before anesthesia. Pregnancy can be excluded either by history, using a WHO checklist,[10] or by testing. The provider can be reasonably certain that the woman is not pregnant (>99% negative predictive value) if she has no symptoms or signs of pregnancy and meets any of the following criteria: (1) She has not had intercourse since last normal menses. (2) She has been correctly and consistently using a reliable method of contraception. (3) She is within the first 7 days after normal menses. (4) She is within 4 weeks postpartum (for nonlactating women). (5) She is within the first 7 days postabortion or miscarriage. (6) She is fully or nearly fully breastfeeding, amenorrhoeic, and less than 6 months postpartum.

The ASA guidelines recommend offering pregnancy testing to women in whom pregnancy is possible.[2] In some institutions, rather than being a true requirement, women have the option to refuse testing after having a discussion regarding the risks associated with anesthesia, surgery, and pregnancy. If she refuses, it is important to document this process in the medical record. Although the incidence of a positive test is low, it typically results in cancellation of surgery. Since most preoperative testing is done days to weeks prior to surgery, routine screening for pregnancy is typically done on the day of surgery.

Electrocardiogram

Although electrocardiographic abnormalities are often associated with postoperative cardiac complications, they typically do not provide additional information beyond that obtained from the history and physical exam. Multiple abnormalities identified to have prognostic significance, although with poor concordance across various studies, include arrhythmias, pathological Q-waves, left ventricular hypertrophy, ST depression, QTc prolongation, and bundle branch blocks. Some of these are detectable on physical exam, and most do not usually result in any change in management and almost never alter outcomes. The most important ECG finding which is rarely encountered

would be evidence of a recent silent myocardial infarction (pathological Q waves) that was not present on a previous ECG done in the past 2 months. Another reason given for obtaining a preoperative ECG is to have a baseline for comparison postoperatively if needed. However, this is not as helpful as troponin in making the diagnosis of a postoperative myocardial infarction.

Electrocardiographic abnormalities increase with age; therefore, this has often been used as a criterion to obtain a baseline preoperative electrocardiogram. The 2022 ESC guidelines[11] recommend an ECG for patients aged ≥65 years, and those with known cardiovascular disease (CVD), risk factors, or symptoms suggestive of cardiac disease before intermediate or high-risk surgery. They advise against routine preoperative ECG testing for low-risk patients undergoing low- or intermediate-risk surgery. The NICE Guideline Development Group (GDG) also recommends considering a resting ECG in ASA 1 patients over 65 undergoing major or complex surgery if there were no previous ECG results available from the past year.[3] The 2007 ACC/AHA guidelines did not recommend a preoperative ECG based on age alone, required at least one clinical risk factor (except for vascular surgery), and recommended against an ECG in asymptomatic patients for low-risk surgeries.[12] The 2014 ACC/AHA guidelines changed to a more liberal position, basically suggesting that an ECG could be obtained in any asymptomatic patient even without heart disease except for those undergoing low-risk surgery, but did note that a standard age or risk factor cutoff for use of preoperative testing has not been defined.[13] The 2024 ACC/AHA guidelines state that for patients with known cardiac or vascular disease or symptoms of CVD (COR 2a/LOE B) or even asymptomatic patients (COR 2b/LOE B) without specifying any age cutoff undergoing elevated-risk surgery, a preoperative ECG is reasonable to establish a preoperative baseline and guide perioperative management.[14] The CCS guidelines do not discuss preoperative ECGs but suggest performing a postoperative ECG in the postanesthetic care unit in patients with an elevated NT-proBNP/BNP measurement before surgery or, if there is no NT-proBNP/BNP measurement before surgery, in those who have an RCRI score >1, age 45–64 years with significant CVD, or age >65 (Conditional Recommendation; Low-Quality Evidence).[15] The ASA Task Force recognized that age alone may not be an indication for an ECG and stated that cardiovascular risk factors may be an indication for ECG.[2]

We recommend obtaining a preoperative ECG if the history suggests cardiac disease or if the patient is undergoing vascular and possibly other high-risk surgery. It is not indicated for patients undergoing low-risk surgery or based purely on age.

Cardiac Biomarkers

Both B-type natriuretic peptide (BNP or NTproBNP) and troponin values have been evaluated as potential tests to stratify the risk of postoperative cardiac complications. BNP values, more commonly used to diagnose heart failure, also identify patients at risk for postoperative cardiac complications, and in a large prospective cohort study actually outperformed the commonly used RCRI. Similarly, high-sensitivity troponin values identify patients at risk for cardiac complications. The 2022 ESC guidelines[11] recommend measurement of high sensitivity troponin T or I, and to consider BNP testing, in the same patients for whom they recommend preoperative ECG testing, whereas the CCS guidelines[15] only recommend BNP. The 2024 ACC guidelines state it is reasonable to measure natriuretic peptides and may be reasonable to measure preoperative troponin[14] (see Chapter 10).

Chest X-Rays

Abnormal findings on a preoperative chest x-ray are rarely unexpected. For example, x-ray findings of chronic obstructive pulmonary disease (COPD) or CHF would not usually escape detection by a careful history and physical examination. Studies have suggested that approximately 1% of preoperative chest x-rays yield results that are unexpected, and even fewer change management. In addition, these findings do not necessarily predict postoperative pulmonary complication rates more accurately than clinical evaluation. So once again, this test should be performed selectively.

Certain incidental findings may occasionally prompt further elective outpatient evaluation, such as a solitary nodule. However, the recommendations for screening for such conditions do not differ in the perioperative period. Another rationale is to provide a baseline in the event that a postoperative chest x-ray is required for a clinical indication. However, potential findings of pneumonia or CHF can easily be diagnosed without the benefit of a preoperative baseline.

The American College of Physicians[16] recommended a preoperative chest x-ray for patients over 50 years old undergoing major surgery, and those with underlying cardiopulmonary disease. This is largely expert opinion as opposed to strongly evidence-based and is now considered outdated. The American Society of Anesthesiologists observes similar risk factors but does not feel that these are unequivocal indications for a preoperative chest x-ray.[2] These risk factors include smoking, recent upper respiratory tract infection, COPD, cardiac disease, and advanced age. We do not recommend preoperative chest x-rays in the absence of active cardiopulmonary symptoms.

SARS-CoV-2 (COVID-19) Testing

Most institutions have local protocols regarding preoperative COVID-19 testing that must be followed. In the absence of protocols, the recommendations for testing have relaxed given the end of the declared public health emergency in 2023, the impact of vaccinations and prior COVID-19 illness on immunity, and lower morbidity from COVID-19 than in the beginning of the pandemic in 2020. As a result, in 2022, the American Society of Anesthesiologists recommended against universal preoperative screening for patients with no symptoms suggestive of COVID-19[17] (see Chapter 24).

Clinical pearls

- Preoperative testing is NOT indicated when used as screening/routine testing or for minimally invasive surgeries or procedures.
- Do not repeat tests when recent studies were done within the past 6 months, and results are unlikely to have changed.
- Preoperative testing IS indicated when done selectively based on a targeted history and physical or for higher-risk surgical procedures in higher-risk patients.
- Age alone should generally not be a criteria to order a test.
- Do NOT order preoperative tests IF the results will NOT influence management.

REFERENCES

1. Choosing Wisely Campaign. "Search on: preoperative." Available at https://www.choosingwisely.org/. Accessed January 27, 2020.

2. Committee on Standards and Practice Parameters, Apfelbaum JL, Connis RT, et al. Practice advisory for preanesthesia evaluation: an updated report by the American Society of Anesthesiologists Task Force on Preanesthesia Evaluation. *Anesthesiology*. 2012;116(3):522-538. PMID: 22273990

3. O'Neill F, Carter E, Pink N, Smith I. Routine preoperative tests for elective surgery: summary of updated NICE guidance. *BMJ*. 2016;354:i3292. Available at https://www.nice.org.uk/guidance/ng45/chapter/Recommendations. PMID: 27418436

4. Benarroch-Gumpel J, Sheffield KM, Duncan CB, et al. Preoperative laboratory testing in patients undergoing low-risk ambulatory surgery. *Ann Surg*. 2012;256:518-522. PMID: 228683625

5. Lee TH, Marcantonio E, Mangione CM, et al. Derivation and prospective validation of a simple index for prediction of cardiac risk of major noncardiac surgery. *Circulation*. 1999;100:1043-1049. PMID: 10477528

6. American Diabetes Association. 15. Diabetes Care in the Hospital: Standards of Medical Care in Diabetes-2020. *Diabetes Care*. 2020;43(suppl 1):S193-S202. PMID: 31862758

7. Seicean A, Schiltz NK, Seicean S, et al. Use and utility of preoperative hemostatic screening and patient history in adult neurosurgical patients. *J Neurosurg*. 2012;116:1097-1105. PMID: 22339164

8. Gehrke T, Parvizi J. Proceedings of the International Consensus Meeting on Periprosthetic Joint Infection. 2013. Available at https://rothmanortho.com/stories/blog/rothman-jefferson-philadelphia-international-joint-consensus. Accessed June 4, 2020.

9. Nicolle LE, Gupta K, Bradley SF, et al. Clinical Practice Guideline for the Management of Asymptomatic Bacteriuria: 2019 Update by the Infectious Diseases Society of America. *Clinical Infectious Diseases*. 2019;68:e83-e110. doi: 10.1093/cid/ciy1121. PMID: 30895288

10. World Health Organization. *Selected Practice Recommendations for Contraceptive Use*. 3rd ed. World Health Organization; 2016. Available at https://apps.who.int/iris/handle/10665/252267.

11. Halvorsen S, Mehilli J, Cassese S, et al. 2022 ESC guidelines on cardiovascular assessment and management of patients undergoing non-cardiac surgery. Developed by the task force for cardiovascular assessment and management of patients undergoing non-cardiac surgery of the European Society of Cardiology (ESC). *Eur Heart J*. 2022;43:3826-3924. PMID: 36017553

12. Fleisher LA, Beckman JA, Brown KA, et al. ACC/AHA 2007 guidelines on perioperative cardiovascular evaluation and care for noncardiac surgery: a report of the American College of Cardiology/American Heart Association Task Force on Practice Guidelines (Writing Committee to Revise the 2002 Guidelines on Perioperative Cardiovascular Evaluation for Noncardiac Surgery) developed in collaboration with the American Society of Echocardiography, American Society of Nuclear Cardiology, Heart Rhythm Society, Society of Cardiovascular Anesthesiologists, Society for Cardiovascular Angiography and Interventions, Society for Vascular Medicine and Biology, and Society for Vascular Surgery. *J Am Coll Cardiol*. 2007;50(17):e159-e241.

13. Fleisher LA, Fleischmann KE, Auerbach AD, et al. 2014 ACC/AHA guideline on perioperative cardiovascular evaluation and management of patients undergoing noncardiac surgery: a report of the American College of Cardiology/American Heart Association Task Force on practice guidelines. *J Am Coll Cardiol*. 2014;64(22):e77-e137. PMID: 17950140

14. Thompson A, Fleischmann KE, Smilowitz NR, et al. 2024 AHA/ACC/ACS/ASNC/HRS/SCA/SCCT/SCMR/SVM guideline for perioperative cardiovascular management for noncardiac surgery: a report of the American College of Cardiology/American Heart Association Joint Committee on Clinical Practice guidelines. *J Am Coll Cardiol*. 2024;84(19):1869-1969. doi: 10.1016/j.jacc.2024.06.013. PMID 39320289

15. Duceppe E, Parlow J, MacDonald P, et al. Canadian Cardiovascular Society Guidelines on perioperative cardiac risk assessment and management for patients who undergo noncardiac surgery. *Can J Cardiol*. 2017;33(1):17-32. PMID: 27865641

16. Smetana GW, Lawrence VA, Cornell JE. Preoperative pulmonary risk stratification for noncardiothoracic surgery: systematic review for the American College of Physicians. *Ann Intern Med*. 2006;144:581-595. PMID: 16618956

17. ASA and APSF updated statement on perioperative testing for SARS-CoV-2 in the asymptomatic patient. December 20, 2022. Available at https://www.asahq.org/about-asa/newsroom/news-releases/2022/12/asa-and-apsf-updated-statement-on-perioperative-testing-for-sars-cov-2-in-the-asymptomatic-patient. Accessed April 8, 2024.

Anesthesia for Nonanesthesiologists

Jeffrey W. Simmons, MD, MSHQS, FASA

COMMON CLINICAL QUESTIONS

1. How does the ASA Patient Severity Score group patients?
2. What factors contribute to the possibility of a difficult-to-intubate airway?
3. What is MAC anesthesia?
4. What is meant by opioid-sparing technique or multimodal technique?

INTRODUCTION: BEYOND PHARMACOLOGY AND PHYSIOLOGY

Anesthesia is an interplay between pharmacology and physiology. Medications used during anesthesia provide a specific function of a balanced anesthetic technique comprised of amnesia, analgesia, akinesia, hypnosis, and control of autonomic responses. The anesthesiologist directs this biological interaction while also playing a vital leadership role in the perioperative team. This physician leads a team of nurse anesthetists, anesthesia assistants, or residents, engages with hospital consults to develop a safe anesthetic plan, communicates risks and plans with the surgery team, and directs intraoperative and perioperative care. Most importantly, the anesthesiologist will explain the anesthesia-related risks, benefits, and alternatives with the patient with the goal of shared decision making.

PREOPERATIVE EVALUATION

The overall goal of preoperative evaluation for anesthesiologists is threefold. One, identify modifiable risks that are amenable to optimization before surgery and create a plan of action to address or improve the comorbidity in an attempt to improve overall patient outcomes. Two, risk stratify the patient based on a thorough assessment to determine the need for additional cardiopulmonary testing, delay in the procedure, or move to an appropriate surgical location. Ideally, the first two goals are accomplished in the weeks before surgery to allow for intervention. Optimization for surgery includes patient education on the risks, benefits, and alternatives to surgery and anesthetic options. Three, develop a patient-specific anesthetic plan based on the type of surgery and comorbidities. On the day of surgery, anesthesia care team determines the final anesthetic plan, including drug choice and dosing sequence, level of sedation required, definitive airway management, and communication with the surgery team.

The anesthesia and surgical teams often solicit input from primary care or specialty medicine services, such as cardiology or pulmonology, to aid in preoperative risk stratification. The purpose of this consultation is to assess the opportunity for optimization of chronic medical conditions that have a direct bearing on surgical and anesthetic outcomes.

Surgical clearance is an older term that implies a degree of certainty of outcome. It does not address perioperative care, risk factor modification, or coordination of care issues, and is not focused on longitudinal health improvement and management. Clearance often leaves patients feeling as though there is "zero risk" to them from their anesthetic and surgical procedure. Writing "cleared for surgery" has no meaning to the surgery and anesthesia teams as there is no indication of the basis of the clearance. Equally less useful are the common recommendations to "avoid hypoxia, hypotension, and hypothermia," since avoidance of these factors is fundamental to all anesthetics.

All surgical procedures carry an element of risk, where total risk is the sum of intrinsic and modifiable factors.[1] Optimization focuses on the preemptive reduction of elements of modifiable risk, such as preoperative smoking cessation. Optimization purposely does not imply outcome certainty and sets the stage for coordinated perioperative care among a multitude of providers, such as primary and specialty care, physical and occupational therapy, and social workers, to name a few. Furthermore, optimization focuses on longitudinal healthcare improvement. High-quality, risk-factor-modifying recommendations, such as increasing preoperative exercise tolerance, nutrition, smoking cessation, and anemia management, significantly improve anesthetic and surgical outcomes (Table 3-1).

ASA Scoring

The American Society of Anesthesiologists (ASA) patient severity scoring scale groups patients into one of six different categories based on comorbidities and functional impairment (Table 3-2). Interrater reliability is paramount when using the ASA patient severity scoring system and can be improved when specific examples are provided related to each score. The ASA scoring system demonstrates excellent risk prediction in multiple studies and is often a component of combined risk scoring systems.

Airway Evaluation

Airway management is a critical skill for anesthesia providers and is a primary focus of the preoperative evaluation. Numerous factors on the preanesthesia assessment suggest difficulties in airway management (Table 3-3). Numerous scoring systems predict difficult intubation. The Mallampati score identifies patients with poorly visualized pharyngeal structures and is the most widely used (Figure 3-1). No scoring system is perfectly predictive, and anesthesia providers must anticipate the unexpected difficult airway. Proper utilization of airway scoring systems coupled with a physical examination is essential to executing a safe anesthetic and minimizing unexpected difficulty. Equally crucial to assessing for difficult intubation is anticipating and planning for airway difficulty at extubation.

MANAGEMENT OF THE DIFFICULT AIRWAY

The incidence of difficult-to-ventilate airway and difficult-to-intubate airway are each approximately 5–10%.[2,3] Several factors predict the possibility of a difficult-to-ventilate or intubate airway, and all factors should be considered additive (Table 3-3). A single test evaluating retrognathia called the upper lip bite test seems to have excellent predictive value for difficult intubation with a sensitivity of 60%.[3] Once the intubating provider has determined the risk of difficulty, it is imperative to prepare by ensuring patient preoxygenation, proper equipment, and emergency backup are available. Anesthesiologists routinely have surgical backup ready if a surgical airway is needed due to a failed intubation/ventilation. Two arms of

| TABLE 3-1. Surgical Clearance Versus Optimization ||
CLEARANCE	OPTIMIZATION
• Implies a degree of certainty of outcome • Usually does not address coordination of care issues • Does not usually address perioperative care specifically • Not focused on longitudinal healthcare improvement and management	• Purposefully does not imply certainty of outcome • Recommends perioperative management • Integrates care of medical issues with other involved care providers • Establishes ownership for patient care initiatives • Focuses on longitudinal healthcare improvement and management

TABLE 3-2. American Society of Anesthesiologists Patient Classifications

ASA PS CLASSIFICATION*	DEFINITION	EXAMPLES, INCLUDING, BUT NOT LIMITED TO:
ASA I	A normal healthy patient	Healthy, nonsmoking, no or minimal alcohol use
ASA II	A patient with mild systemic disease	Mild diseases only without substantive functional limitations. Examples include (but not limited to): current smoker, social alcohol drinker, pregnancy, obesity (30 < BMI < 40), well-controlled DM/HTN, mild lung disease
ASA III	A patient with severe systemic disease	Substantive functional limitations; one or more moderate to severe diseases. Examples include (but not limited to): poorly controlled DM or HTN, COPD, morbid obesity (BMI ≥40), active hepatitis, alcohol dependence or abuse, implanted pacemaker, moderate reduction of ejection fraction, ESRD undergoing regularly scheduled dialysis, premature infant PCA <60 weeks, history (>3 months) of MI, CVA, TIA, or CAD/stents.
ASA IV	A patient with severe systemic disease that is a constant threat to life	Examples include (but not limited to): recent (<3 months) MI, CVA, TIA, or CAD/stents, ongoing cardiac ischemia or severe valve dysfunction, severe reduction of ejection fraction, sepsis, DIC, ARD, or ESRD not undergoing regularly scheduled dialysis
ASA V	A moribund patient who is not expected to survive without the operation	Examples include (but not limited to): ruptured abdominal/thoracic aneurysm, massive trauma, intracranial bleed with mass effect, ischemic bowel in the face of significant cardiac pathology or multiple organs/system dysfunction
ASA VI	A declared brain-dead patient whose organs are being removed for donor purposes	

*The addition of "E" denotes Emergency surgery: (An emergency is defined as existing when delay in treatment of the patient would lead to a significant increase in the threat to life or body part)

the American Society of Anesthesiologists Difficult Airway Algorithm are described for adult patients: Intubation Attempt in an Awake Patient and Intubation After Induction of General Anesthesia.[4] Awake intubation implies that the patient will undergo tracheal intubation in an awake state but with the airway anesthetized by any number of strategies such as airway topical numbing agents, selective airway nerve blocks, or nebulized numbing agents. Extreme caution should be taken if considering sedating the patient during the awake intubation, as loss of spontaneous ventilation could result in failed intubation/ventilation and cardiovascular collapse. When intubation fails in an awake and spontaneously breathing patient, the case is postponed, and considerations are made for alternative, safe ways to perform the surgery. Intubation after general anesthesia is induced is separated into two arms on the algorithm: Able to Ventilate or Unable to Ventilate. If the intubating provider can ventilate, the situation is considered non-emergent, as oxygenation and ventilation can be maintained. Options for failed intubation in a patient able to be mask-ventilated are supraglottic airways or awakening and consideration of other options. If the intubating provider cannot intubate after induction of general anesthesia and subsequently cannot ventilate, the provider should

TABLE 3-3. Anatomic and Physiologic Predictors of Difficulty with Airway Management

ANATOMIC	
Predictors of difficult direct laryngoscopy	Limited mouth opening; blood or emesis in the oropharynx; narrow dental arch; limited mandibular protrusion; short thyromental distance; poor submandibular compliance; modified Mallampati class III or IV; limited head and upper neck extension; increased neck circumference; obesity; adverse dentition; difficult face-mask ventilation; operator inexperience with direct laryngoscopy
Predictors of difficult video laryngoscopy	Limited mouth opening; blood or emesis in the oropharynx; limited mandibular protrusion; short thyromental distance; history of neck irradiation or neck surgery, neck disease, limited neck mobility; thick neck; obesity; known Cormack–Lehane grade 3 or 4 during direct laryngoscopy; operator inexperience with video laryngoscopy
Predictors of difficult face-mask ventilation	Beard or other factor affecting mask seal; male sex; lack of teeth; age >50 y; limited mandibular protrusion; modified Mallampati class III or IV; BMI >26; history of snoring or obstructive sleep apnea; history of neck irradiation; difficult intubation
Predictors of difficult SGA insertion or use	Limited mouth opening; obstructing or distorting lesion in the upper airway; fixed neck-flexion deformity; applied cricoid pressure; BMI >29
Predictors of difficult front-of-neck airway access	Female sex; age <8 y; thick neck; obesity; displaced trachea; overlying disorder (e.g., irradiation damage or other tissue induration); fixed neck-flexion deformity
PHYSIOLOGIC	
Full stomach; rapid oxygen desaturation and the onset of apnea due to reduced functional residual capacity or increased oxygen consumption (e.g., obese, septic, or pregnant patients); large minute ventilation (e.g., compensatory for metabolic acidosis); hemodynamic instability: shock states, including hypovolemia and right ventricular failure	

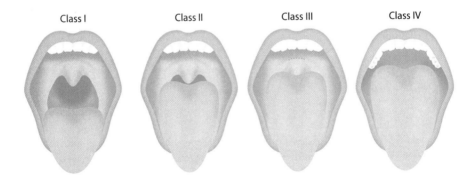

Class I Class II Class III Class IV

FIGURE 3-1. Mallampati diagram. (Modified with permission from Ouchi K, Hosokawa R, Yamanaka H, et al. Mallampati test with phonation, tongue protrusion and supine position is most correlated with Cormack-Lehane test. *Odontology.* 2020;108(4):617-625 and Reproduced with permission from Grippi MA, Antin-Ozerkis DE, Dela Cruz CS, Kotloff RM, Kotton C, Pack AI. Fishman's Pulmonary Diseases and Disorders, 6e. New York: McGraw-Hill Education; 2023.)

transition quickly to a supraglottic airway, call for emergency backup, and prepare for invasive emergency airway such as cricothyrotomy.

Contextual issues affect the success of patient intubation. Intubation may be required in a hospital ward where proper patient positioning and equipment are challenging to obtain. Ideal intubating circumstances may not be achievable due to urgency or situation. The use of video laryngoscopy should be considered to increase the chances of first-attempt success.

The rate for tracheal intubation with video laryngoscopy is between 97.1% and 99.6%.[5] Non-anesthesiologists performing intubations should become skilled in recognizing predictors of difficult airway, mask ventilation, supraglottic airway insertion, and video laryngoscopy.

ANESTHESIA MEDICATIONS

General anesthesia is a medication-induced state of unconsciousness, resulting in amnesia and analgesia with or without reversible skeletal muscle paralysis. The concept of "balanced anesthesia" refers to the use of two or more medications to produce a comparable effect as that of a larger dose of a single medication (Table 3-4). Balanced anesthesia minimizes patient risk and maximizes patient comfort and safety. The objectives are to relieve patient anxiety, minimize pain, and reduce the potential for adverse effects inherent in larger doses of analgesic and anesthetic medications.

Common Induction Agents

Etomidate. Etomidate is an induction medication selected for its hemodynamic stability. While etomidate does provide hemodynamic stability, it is associated with considerably higher rates of nausea and vomiting when compared with propofol. Induction doses are associated with transient adrenal suppression, the clinical significance of which remains debated.

Propofol. Propofol is the most commonly used induction agent due to its rapid onset and recovery. It has beneficial antiemetic properties and relatively benign side effects. In addition to antiemetic properties, propofol has antipruritic and bronchodilatory properties. In the hypovolemic patient, propofol can

TABLE 3-4. Hemodynamic Changes with Common Anesthetic Medications						
AGENT	CLASS	DOSE	CO	SVR	CBF/CMRO2	SIDE EFFECTS
Propofol	Hypnotic/Induction	1–2 mg/kg	↓↓	↓	↓↓/↓	Hypotension/injection pain
Etomidate	Hypnotic/Induction	0.2–0.4 mg/kg	↔	↔	↓/↓	Myoclonus, nausea, adrenal suppression
Ketamine	Hypnotic/Induction/Analgesic	1–3 mg/kg	↑	↔	↑/↓	Psychotropic effects/hypertension
Midazolam	Hypnotic/Induction	0.05–0.1 mg/kg	↔	↔	↓/↓	Ventilatory depression
Fentanyl	Analgesic	0.5–1.5 mcg/kg	↔	↔	↔	Ventilatory depression
Morphine	Analgesic	0.05–0.1 mg/kg	↔	↓	↔	Ventilatory depression
Lidocaine	Analgesic/Anti-inflammatory	0.5–1 mg/kg	↔	↔	↔	Tinnitus
Rocuronium	Muscle relaxant	0.5–1.2 mg/kg	↔	↔	↔	Histamine release
Succinylcholine	Muscle relaxant	1–2 mg/kg	↔	↔	↔	Myoclonus and myalgias
Volatile gases	Hypnotic/Analgesic/Muscle relaxant	Varies by gas	↓	↓↓	↓↓/↓	Nausea

cause profound hypotension due to reduced cardiac output and systemic vascular resistance.

Ketamine. Ketamine is a rapidly acting anesthetic agent administered intravenously or intramuscularly. In addition to its hypnotic and analgesic effects, ketamine has minimal cardiovascular depressant effects. In situ, ketamine may increase heart rate and cardiac output, making it an ideal medication in trauma anesthesia and has been used as a battlefield anesthetic by the military for many years. Ketamine's hypnotic action works through blocking NMDA receptors, while its analgesic actions may have cholinergic, aminergic, and opioid system properties.

Analgesia

Opioid medications such as fentanyl, hydromorphone, or morphine are often used as part of a balanced anesthetic plan and generally have minimal hemodynamic effects. Opioid administration is associated with postoperative and post-discharge nausea and vomiting. Opioid-sparing techniques of pain management, standard in enhanced recovery pathways, employ regional techniques (nerve blockade), or multimodal adjuncts (acetaminophen, NSAIDs, GABA inhibitors) *to reduce the overall need for opioids, thereby reducing their adverse postoperative side effects.*

Amnesia

Amnesia in anesthesiology is a medication-induced short-term loss of memory surrounding the surgical experience. Depending on medication selection, amnesia can be anterograde or retrograde. Benzodiazepine medications and volatile anesthetic agents reliably produce amnesia. Benzodiazepines administered in low doses (midazolam 1–2 mg IV or diazepam 5–10 mg orally) have minimal respiratory depressant effects and are used in preprocedural sedation for regional nerve blocks or to reduce patient anxiety.

Neuromuscular Blocking

There are two classes of neuromuscular blocking agents: depolarizing or nondepolarizing. Depolarizing agents such as succinylcholine activate the motor endplate on skeletal muscle causing visual fasciculations followed by a period of flaccid paralysis lasting 6–12 minutes. Nondepolarizing medications (NDMR) such

as rocuronium or vecuronium are used during the induction of anesthesia or for maintenance muscle relaxation during surgery. Acetylcholinesterase inhibitors, such as neostigmine, or binding agents such as sugammadex, reverse the effects of NDMRs. Volatile gases administered during anesthesia provide some muscle relaxation, but also cause significant systemic vascular vasodilation. Intravenous NDMR is hemodynamically stable and allows for a reduction in volatile gas concentration (balanced anesthetic approach).

Vasopressors

The use of vasopressor medications is common during anesthesia to reverse the vasodilatory and myocardial depressant effects of anesthetic agents. Phenylephrine and ephedrine are commonly used for their vasoconstrictive and contractility augmenting effects, respectively. Temporary use of vasopressors during periods of surgical bleeding or restoration of intravascular volume is standard practice.

Antiemetics

Volatile anesthetic medications are known risk factors for postoperative nausea and vomiting (PONV). Other risk factors include being female, receiving concomitant opioids, being a nonsmoker, and having a history of PONV. The incidence of PONV can be reduced by administering at least two antiemetics from different classes. In modern anesthesia, this is commonly accomplished with 5-HT3 antagonist (ondansetron) and glucocorticoids (dexamethasone). Other agents, such as transdermal scopolamine, should be placed the night before surgery or a minimum of 3 hours before the procedure. Newer agents, such as aprepitant, have very high success rates in reducing PONV. Aprepitant 40 mg capsule should be taken within 3 hours of induction of anesthesia to prevent anesthesia-related postoperative vomiting (see Chapter 43).

INDUCTION OF ANESTHESIA

The induction of anesthesia is the process of administering medications to produce unconsciousness. Preparation for induction of general anesthesia requires optimal patient positioning for intubation as well as placement of monitors such as pulse oximetry, blood pressure cuff, EKG electrodes, end-tidal carbon dioxide monitor, and temperature probe. Once optimally positioned, the patient breathes 100% oxygen for several tidal volume breaths to denitrogenate the lungs (often referred to as preoxygenation). Preoxygenation is a critical step in the induction of anesthesia as a patient will become apneic after anesthetic medication administration and may rapidly desaturate and become hypoxic. After preoxygenation, medication administration occurs in either a "rapid sequence" fashion or "normal/routine sequence." Rapid sequence intubation describes administering medications to produce unconsciousness and muscle relaxation and then immediately placing an endotracheal tube (without proving the ability to mask ventilate). Selection of rapid sequence intubation occurs when a patient is having an urgent procedure and has been NPO (*nil per os* [nothing by mouth]) for less than 6 hours, or where mask ventilation may increase the chance of aspiration of stomach contents. A routine intubation sequence occurs with mask ventilation following the administration of anesthetic medications and loss of consciousness. A combination of anesthetic medications is given, depending on the level of anesthesia required. Once the endotracheal tube is confirmed by auscultating the lungs for bilateral breath sounds, verifying equal chest rise, and visualizing persistent end-tidal CO_2 on the monitor, the operating room nursing staff begins skin preparation and final positioning for surgery.

Hemodynamic Concerns

Following induction and intubation, patients display hemodynamic changes consistent with the medications delivered and airway management. Patients often manifest a period of hypertension and tachycardia following intubation and tracheal stimulation, followed by a period of hypotension as they are "prepped and draped," during which minimal stimulation occurs. The induction of anesthesia is a tumultuous period of the anesthetic experience and requires the vigilance and finesse of the anesthesia team. Seasoned and vigilant anesthesia providers predict these hemodynamic changes based on the comorbidities of the patient and alter the amounts of medications given on induction or have the proper medications available to counteract periods of low stimulation. The overall goal of induction is to safely and efficiently produce a state of unconsciousness and analgesia sufficient for the procedure while maintaining the patient's hemodynamics comparable to their baseline values.

MAINTENANCE OF ANESTHESIA

The maintenance phase of anesthesia maintains a level of patient unresponsiveness and relaxation that allows the performance of the surgical procedure (Table 3-5). Maintenance involves the use of volatile inhalational anesthetic gases and intravenous narcotic medications.

TABLE 3-5. Stages of Anesthesia		
STAGE OF ANESTHESIA	**DESCRIPTION**	**EFFECTS**
1	Analgesia	Analgesia without amnesia; disorientation; consciousness maintained
2	Excitation	Excitation and delirium with struggling; coughing and vomiting possible; rapid, irregular respirations; rapid eye movements; pupillary dilation; divergent pupils; amnesia
3	Surgical anesthesia	Loss of consciousness; loss of touch sensation; amnesia; divided into four planes of increasing depth: • Plane 1: decreased eye movement and pupillary constriction • Plane 2: loss of corneal reflex; increased tearing • Plane 3: loss of laryngeal reflexes, pupillary dilation; loss of light reflex • Plane 4: progressive loss of breathing and muscle tone
4	Medullary depression	Apnea; cardiovascular instability; necessitate cardiac and respiratory support; amnesia

TABLE 3-6. ASA Standard Monitors
Oxygenation: inspired oxygen-gas concentrations, including a low oxygen concentration alarm
Continuous end-tidal carbon dioxide
Noninvasive blood pressure at least every 5 minutes
Continuous electrocardiogram
Body temperature
Pulse oximetry
Breathing circuit disconnection alarm in cases involving mechanical ventilation

Monitoring

Patient monitoring during the maintenance of general anesthesia includes standard monitors recommended by the ASA and neuromuscular blockade monitoring (Table 3-6). Selective employment of anesthetic depth and invasive cardiovascular monitors, such as bispectral index, arterial lines, central venous catheters, and transesophageal echocardiography, is based on patient and procedural risk assessment.

Mechanical Ventilation

Lung protective ventilation strategies are individualized mechanical ventilation plans that advocate for lower tidal volumes, a reduced fraction of inspired oxygen, and the use of positive end-expiratory pressure (PEEP). Mechanical ventilation begins with tidal volumes of 6–8 mL/kg ideal body weight (IBW) and 4–5 cm H_2O PEEP and individualized adjustments after that. When compared with patients receiving large-tidal-volume ventilation, lung-protective ventilation improves outcomes by reducing the incidence of supraventricular cardiac arrhythmias, atelectasis, ventilator-induced lung inflammation, and postoperative pulmonary complications, as well as reducing hospital length-of-stay and healthcare resource utilization.[6]

Fluid Management

Excessive fluid administration increases the potential for acute lung injury and contributes to the high incidence of postoperative pulmonary complications. Goal-directed fluid management guided by noninvasive cardiac output monitors results in reduced hospital length-of-stay, decreased PONV, and earlier return of gastrointestinal function.[3] Liberal fluid management using crystalloid infusion volumes up to 20–30 mL/kg/h reduces postoperative dizziness, drowsiness, pain, nausea and vomiting, and length-of-stay in the ambulatory surgery setting. Liberal fluid management is associated with worsened outcomes in more complex patients and procedures, such as colon resection. Restrictive or zero-balance fluid management seeks to replace only fluid loss during surgery as well as a maintenance crystalloid infusion of 1–3 mL/kg/h to replace sensible and insensible fluid loss. Restrictive fluid management has a higher association with postoperative acute kidney injury than liberal or goal-directed strategies.[7]

TYPES AND LOCATIONS OF ANESTHESIA

The prescription of general versus regional anesthesia is a balance of multiple factors weighed by the anesthesia team on the day of surgery, particularly focusing on provision of the safest anesthetic for the patient. There are two theoretical reasons why regional anesthesia should be safer than general anesthesia: a total regional technique may provide less cardiovascular stress, which is significant since most perioperative complications and adverse outcomes result from the stress response to surgery, particularly in patients with chronic disease, and a regional anesthetic provides preemptive analgesia.[8] Medical consultants should refrain from recommending a certain anesthetic technique but should discuss with an anesthesia provider when concerns exist.

The debate between superiority of regional versus general anesthesia is timeless. Each modality has advantages and disadvantages. While general anesthesia is the most commonly prescribed anesthetic technique, it is increasingly common to see both general and regional anesthesia used adjunctively. Enhanced recovery protocols rely on general and regional anesthetic techniques. The use of the two together improves postoperative pain management, reduces postoperative and post-discharge nausea and vomiting, opioid consumption, blood transfusions, complications, healthcare costs, and length of stay, and improves patient satisfaction across multiple surgical specialties.[9-11] Regardless of the technique or combination chosen, the anesthetic plan is individually formulated after a detailed assessment of patient risks and benefits in conjunction with the patient and surgical care teams. The selected anesthetic plan maximizes quality, safety, and satisfaction while reducing the risk of adverse outcomes.

Monitored Anesthesia Care

Monitored anesthesia care (MAC) is a type of anesthesia service where an anesthesia provider continuously monitors the patient's hemodynamics and vital signs while providing a level of sedation appropriate for the procedure (light to heavy sedation) with conversion to general anesthesia if needed. MAC does not describe a level of anesthesia. It denotes the presence of an anesthesia provider capable of performing all levels of anesthesia. MAC is often provided for lower-intensity procedures such as endoscopy or superficial skin procedures. MAC accounts for 30–35% of all cases performed in the ambulatory setting.[12]

Regional Anesthesia and Neuraxial Anesthesia

Regional and neuraxial anesthesia may be appropriate for many surgical procedures as the sole anesthetic or combined with intravenous sedation (Table 3-7). The

TABLE 3-7. Regional Nerve Blocks		
TECHNIQUE	BLOCK AREA	MOTOR/SENSORY
Interscalene	Upper extremity	+/+
Supraclavicular		
Infraclavicular		
Axillary		
PECS/serratus	Breast	−/+
Quadratus lumborum	Unilateral or bilateral truncal	−/+
Transversus abdominis plane		
Erector spinae	Unilateral or bilateral truncal	+/+
Paravertebral		
Rectus sheath	Front of abdomen	−/+
Ilioinguinal and iliohypogastric	Groin and genitals	+/+
Femoral	Anterior lower extremity	+/+
Adductor canal	Anterior lower extremity	−/+
Sciatic	Posterior lower extremity	+/+
Popliteal	Posterior lower extremity	+/+
Ankle	Posterior lower extremity	−/+
Spinal	Below T6	+/+
Epidural		
Combined spinal epidural		

potential for regional or neuraxial anesthetic failure necessitates preoperative optimization in the same way as a general anesthesia patient.

Nonoperating Room Anesthesia

Nonoperating room anesthesia (NORA) refers to anesthesia services performed outside of the typical theater of the operating room. Service lines requesting NORA are electrophysiology, cardiac catheterization, electroconvulsive therapy, gastrointestinal endoscopy, MRI and CT scans, or radiation oncology. Services performed outside of the operating room must comply with standards set by the ASA and local hospital policies.

NORA services provided to medically complex patients with ancillary staff unfamiliar with anesthesia support and where supplies, space, and traditional resources are limited lead to significant and potentially preventable patient complications. Closed claims analysis demonstrates increased complications with oversedation, respiratory compromise, and inadequate patient monitoring. Protocols and interdisciplinary teamwork can facilitate safe, efficient, and cost-effective procedural care in the NORA suite.[13]

PATIENT SAFETY AND CONTINUOUS QUALITY IMPROVEMENT IN ANESTHESIA

Advancements in medications, monitoring technology, safety systems, and employment of the Anesthesia Care Team Model, including highly educated anesthesia providers, allow for a significant reduction in the risk of severe anesthesia-related patient harm. The patient risk of harm attributable to anesthesia is exceptionally remote, with mortality occurring at rates of less than 1 in 100,000 provided anesthetics.[14] Minor adverse events, such as PONV or sore throat, occur more frequently and are self-limiting in duration and severity.

Anesthesiology has long been involved in continuous quality improvement initiatives to reduce risk and healthcare costs while maximizing patient safety and improved surgical outcomes. Entities such as the Anesthesia Patient Safety Foundation, the ASA Closed Claims Project, and the Anesthesia Quality Institute work collaboratively to analyze critical events and minimize the risk of recurrence.

Clinical pearls

- The term "cleared for surgery" has fallen out of favor, as the patient may still have a considerable risk for unavoidable injury or complication.
- Evaluating the ease of mask ventilation is equally important in overall airway evaluation. The ability to mask ventilate the patient after induction of anesthesia provides a measure of safety if intubation becomes difficult. Beards, obesity, mandibular protrusion, history of snoring, advanced age, and high Mallampati class are all associated with difficult mask ventilation.
- Ketamine is associated with vivid psychotropic effects that can be mitigated by preadministering benzodiazepines.
- The continued use of vasopressors after induction of anesthesia should prompt evaluation of the patient's volume status as well as possible iatrogenic causes such as too much intravenous sedation.
- Nonemergent induction of anesthesia should always be proceeded with a time-out to ensure all providers understand the planned procedure, possibility of difficult airway, and additional equipment needed in case of emergency.
- Calculate ventilator tidal volumes based on the patient's ideal body weight.
- When planning for regional or neuraxial anesthesia, the anesthesia provider must plan for possible failure and the need for general anesthesia.

REFERENCES

1. Riggs K, Segal J. What is the rationale for preoperative medical evaluations? A closer look at surgical risk and common terminology. *Br J Anaesth*. 2016;117(6):681-684. PMID: 27956664
2. Heidegger T. Management of the difficult airway. *N Engl J Med*. 2021;384(19):1836-1847. PMID: 33979490
3. Detsky ME, Jivraj N, Adhikari NK, et al. Will this patient be difficult to intubate?: the rational clinical examination

systematic review. *JAMA*. 2019;321(5):493-503. PMID: 30721300

4. Apfelbaum JL, Hagberg CA, Connis RT, et al. 2022 American Society of Anesthesiologists Practice guidelines for management of the difficult airway. *Anesthesiology*. 2022;136(1):31-81. PMID: 34762729

5. Aziz MF, Abrons RO, Cattano D, et al. First-attempt intubation success of video laryngoscopy in patients with anticipated difficult direct laryngoscopy: a multicenter randomized controlled trial comparing the C-MAC D-blade versus the GlideScope in a mixed provider and diverse patient population. *Anesth Analg*. 2016;122(3):740-750. PMID: 26579847

6. Young CC, Harris EM, Vacchiano C, et al. Lung-protective ventilation for the surgical patient: international expert panel-based consensus recommendations. *Br J Anaesth*. 2019;123(6):898-913. PMID: 31587835

7. Simmons JW, Dobyns JB, Paiste J. Enhanced recovery after surgery: intraoperative fluid management strategies. *Surgical Clinics*. 2018;98(6):1185-1200. PMID: 30390851

8. Roy RC. Choosing general versus regional anesthesia for the elderly. *Anesthesiol Clin North Am*. 2000;18(1):91-104. PMID: 10935002

9. Pędziwiatr M, Mavrikis J, Witowski J, et al. Current status of enhanced recovery after surgery (ERAS) protocol in gastrointestinal surgery. *Med Oncol*. 2018;35(6):95. PMID: 29744679

10. Patel SY, Getting REG, Alford B, et al. Improved outcomes of enhanced recovery after surgery (ERAS) protocol for radical cystectomy with addition of a multidisciplinary care process in a US comprehensive cancer care center. *World J Surg*. 2018;42(9):2701-2707. PMID: 29750321

11. Hopkins P. Does regional anaesthesia improve outcome? *Br J Anaesth*. 2015;115(suppl_2):ii26-ii33. PMID: 26658198

12. Bayman EO, Dexter F, Laur JJ, Wachtel RE. National incidence of use of monitored anesthesia care. *Anesth Analge*. 2011;113(1):165-169. PMID: 21596866

13. Walls JD, Weiss MS. Safety in non-operating room anesthesia (NORA). 2019. Available at https://www.apsf.org/article/safety-in-non-operating-room-anesthesia-nora/. Accessed November 11, 2019. PMID: 32628402

14. Dutton RP. Quality improvement and patient safety organizations in anesthesiology. *AMA Ethics*. 2015;17(3):248-252. PMID: 25813592

4

Perioperative Medication Management

Paul J. Grant, MD, SFHM, FACP, Karen F. Mauck, MD, MSc, FACP, and Steven L. Cohn, MD, MACP, SFHM, FRCP

COMMON CLINICAL QUESTIONS

1. Which medications are essential and need to be continued?

2. Which medications are potentially harmful and should be withheld or have their dose adjusted?

3. How do you manage medications where there is no consensus?

INTRODUCTION

The majority of patients undergoing surgery take one or more prescription or over-the-counter medications, and this number increases with age. Clinicians must decide whether or not to continue each medication in the perioperative period. Unfortunately, there are no randomized controlled trials (RCTs) for perioperative management of most medications, and as a result, there is significant variation in clinical practice. The recommendations in this chapter are based on information from literature reviews, theoretical considerations, expert opinion, and our clinical experience.

PREOPERATIVE EVALUATION— GENERAL PRINCIPLES (SEE ALGORITHM IN FIGURE 4-1)

Obtain a complete medication history from the patient including prescription and over-the-counter medications, supplements, and substance use. Confirm the dose, frequency, and compliance with the regimen. In deciding whether or not to continue a medication preoperatively, consider the following issues: (1) indication for the drug; (2) effect on the primary disease if the drug is stopped (clinical deterioration, withdrawal symptoms, rebound effect); (3) drug pharmacokinetics (half-life, metabolism, and elimination) and potential changes in the perioperative setting (absorption, route of administration); (4) potential adverse effects on perioperative risk (bleeding, hypoglycemia) or drug interaction with anesthetic agents. Using these principles in a risk-benefit analysis, decide whether to continue, discontinue, or modify the current regimen for each medication.

Certain medications are essential and need to be continued. Many other medications can be safely continued but may not be necessary and are therefore considered optional. Finally, a few medications are potentially harmful and therefore should be discontinued or dose adjusted. Medications taken orally that must be continued should be given with a small amount of water on the morning of surgery. For hospitalized patients who may be "NPO" (*nil per os*) before surgery, it is important to add "except for medications." Additionally, for medications that would normally be administered later in the morning, it is important to specify that the patient receives them on call to the operating room if the procedure is scheduled earlier.

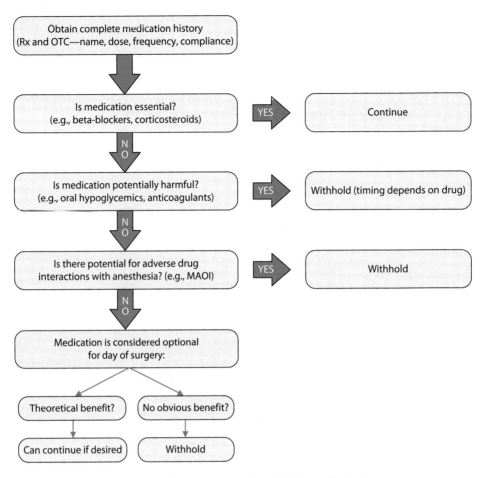

FIGURE 4-1. Algorithm for perioperative medication management (see table for specific drugs).

It is beyond the scope of this chapter to discuss all medications, so we have chosen the medications and drug classes that are most common or important in our opinion. For additional information, the reader is referred to other online sources (UpToDate.com, pre-opevalguide.com, Dynamed.com).

PERIOPERATIVE MANAGEMENT— RECOMMENDATIONS BY DRUG CATEGORY (SEE TABLE)

Cardiovascular Medications[1]

Most cardiovascular drugs should be continued on the morning of surgery with the possible exceptions of diuretics, angiotensin converting enzyme inhibitors (ACEIs), angiotensin receptor blockers (ARBs), anticoagulants, and antiplatelet drugs. The latter two classes will be discussed separately. Recently, the POISE-3 trial compared a hypotension avoidance strategy with a hypertension avoidance strategy finding no significant difference in postoperative adverse events.[2] While this study questions how antihypertensive medications should be managed perioperatively, the following recommendations represent current practice.

Diuretics can cause hypovolemia and hypokalemia. However, with chronic administration, a steady state is achieved so that giving a single dose on the morning of surgery should not cause hypokalemia or significant volume depletion. A small RCT of patients on chronic furosemide found no difference between taking or holding the drug on the morning of surgery with respect to hypotension, use of vasopressors, or adverse cardiac outcomes. However, in general, diuretics are typically held on the morning of surgery but may be given to some patients with heart failure on a case-by-case basis.

ACEIs/ARBs have been associated with increased risk of hypotension particularly with induction of anesthesia, but there is no increase in "hard outcomes" such as myocardial infarction or death. Since one study noted increased risk when given within 10 hours before surgery, the drug can be taken the night before rather than on the morning of surgery. Because the hypotension is sometimes refractory to standard treatment, these drugs are typically held on the morning of surgery. However, a subgroup analysis of patients on these medications in POISE-3 did not demonstrate any differences in adverse events whether the medication was taken on the morning of surgery or withheld.[2] Although the STOP (discontinue 3 days preoperatively) or NOT trial found an increase in intraoperative hypotensive episodes in the group continuing the drug, there was no difference in postoperative complications or mortality between groups.[3] The SPACE trial found no increase in the incidence of perioperative hypotension if the medications were continued but noted an increase in hypertension if they were discontinued.[4] It is reasonable to continue them in patients with heart failure or poorly controlled blood pressure, but if they are withheld, it is important to restart them within several days of surgery.

Beta-blockers should be continued in patients already taking them, assuming there is no profound bradycardia, as they have been associated with decreased risk of ischemia, myocardial infarction, and supraventricular arrhythmias. Furthermore, abrupt withdrawal may cause rebound hypertension and ischemia. They should not be started on the day of or within 24 hours of surgery as this was associated with increased risk of bradycardia, hypotension, death, and stroke in the POISE study[5] (see Chapter 11).

Alpha-2 agonists like clonidine should be continued in patients already on them as withdrawal is associated with rebound hypertension and tachycardia due to increased peripheral sympathetic activity. Continuation may also have perioperative benefits in that they may decrease blood pressure lability, preoperative anxiety, and the amount of anesthesia required for maintenance. Alpha-2 agonists should not be started preoperatively as a cardiac risk reduction strategy as they were associated with an increase in hypotension, bradycardia, and nonfatal cardiac arrest in the POISE-2 study.[6]

Alpha blockers in general should be continued, but they are rarely used today to treat hypertension except in patients with pheochromocytoma (doxazosin, prazosin). Tamsulosin is not used for hypertension (see genitourinary medications) but has been associated with floppy iris syndrome in patients undergoing cataract surgery. Stopping it before surgery does not seem to change the outcome, but the ophthalmologist should be notified in advance that the patient is taking it as the surgical technique may change.

Alpha-beta blockers should be continued perioperatively. Labetalol is used in patients with hypertension, pheochromocytoma, and heart failure and is often given IV to treat hypertensive emergencies and perioperative hypertension.

Calcium channel blockers (CCBs) were evaluated in a meta-analysis which found them to be associated with decreased ischemia, supraventricular tachycardia, and major morbid events in the perioperative setting, primarily related to the use of diltiazem. CCBs should be continued perioperatively.

Nitrates should be continued on the morning of surgery in patients taking them chronically, but they were not associated with improved mortality and cardiac complications in a Cochrane systematic review of patients undergoing noncardiac surgery. Prophylactic IV doses given intraoperatively did not significantly reduce ischemia but decreased mean blood pressure. Transdermal nitrates should be removed or transitioned to oral preoperatively as transdermal absorption is not predictable during anesthesia.

Antiarrhythmics (digoxin, amiodarone, sotalol) should be continued on the morning of surgery. If there is any question of toxicity, a drug level can be obtained.

MEDICATIONS BY SYSTEM	EXAMPLES	PERIOPERATIVE MANAGEMENT	SPECIAL CONSIDERATIONS
Cardiovascular			
Diuretics	Hydrochlorothiazide, furosemide	Usually hold on day of surgery	May continue for patients with HF
ACEIs/ARBs	Lisinopril, enalapril, losartan, valsartan	May hold on day of surgery	May continue for patients with HF or uncontrolled HTN
Neprilysin inhibitor/ARB	Sacubitril/valsartan	May hold on day of surgery	May continue for patients with HF—consult cardiology
Beta-blockers	Metoprolol, atenolol, bisoprolol, propranolol	Continue	May develop rebound HTN and ischemia if discontinued abruptly May reduce perioperative cardiovascular risk if continued in higher-risk patients
Alpha-2 agonists	Clonidine	Continue	May develop rebound HTN if discontinued abruptly
Alpha blockers and direct vasodilators	Doxazosin, prazosin, tamsulosin; hydralazine	Continue	Inform ophthalmologist if patient is on tamsulosin (floppy-iris syndrome)
Alpha-beta blockers	Labetalol, carvedilol	Continue	
Calcium channel blockers	Amlodipine, nifedipine, diltiazem, verapamil	Continue	
Nitrates	Isosorbide dinitrate, nitroglycerin	Continue	Remove transdermal nitrates; consider transition to oral formulation
Antiarrhythmics	Amiodarone, digoxin, sotalol	Continue	
Lipid-lowering			
Statins	Atorvastatin, rosuvastatin, simvastatin	Continue Continue	May reduce perioperative cardiovascular risk
PCSK9 inhibitors	Evolocumab, alirocumab		

(*Continued*)

MEDICATIONS BY SYSTEM	EXAMPLES	PERIOPERATIVE MANAGEMENT	SPECIAL CONSIDERATIONS
Bile acid sequestrants	Cholestyramine	Hold on day of surgery	
Fibric acid derivatives	Gemfibrozil	Hold on day of surgery	
Ezetimibe		Hold on day of surgery (unless combined with statin)	
Niacin		Hold on day of surgery	
Anticoagulants (full-dose; not prophylaxis)		Stop before surgery unless low bleeding risk procedure	
Warfarin		Stop 5 days before	Consider bridging in high-risk settings
Heparin (IV)		Stop 4–6 hours before	
Low molecular weight heparin (LMWH)	Enoxaparin, dalteparin	Stop 24 hours before for full-dose anticoagulation	Consider holding prophylactic dose for 12 hours before surgery
Indirect parenteral Xa inhibitor	Fondaparinux	Stop at least 2 days before	
Direct oral Xa inhibitors	Apixaban, rivaroxaban, edoxaban	Stop 1–2 days before (3 days before neuraxial anesthesia) depending on bleeding risk of procedure and renal function	No need for bridging
Oral direct thrombin inhibitors	Dabigatran	Stop 1–4 days before depending on bleeding risk of procedure and renal function	No need for bridging
Antiplatelet agents			
Aspirin		Continue low-dose aspirin for patients on aspirin for secondary prevention Otherwise stop 5–7 days before	Consider indication and bleeding risk (see text)
P2Y12 inhibitors	Clopidogrel Prasugrel Ticagrelor	Stop 5–7 days before Stop 7 days before Stop 3–5 days before	
Dipyridamole		Stop 2 days before	
Cilostazol		Stop 2–5 days before	
Nonsteroidal anti-inflammatory drugs (NSAIDs)	Ibuprofen Naproxen, diclofenac Celecoxib (COX-2) inhibitor	Stop 1 day before Stop 1–3 days before Stop 1–3 days before	May continue if part of multimodal pain management

(Continued)

MEDICATIONS BY SYSTEM	EXAMPLES	PERIOPERATIVE MANAGEMENT	SPECIAL CONSIDERATIONS
Pulmonary			
Inhaled beta-agonists anticholinergics	Albuterol, salmeterol Ipratropium, tiotropium	Continue Continue	
Methylxanthines	Theophylline	Hold	Consider checking level if suspicion of toxicity
Glucocorticoids	Fluticasone, budesonide (inhaled) Prednisone (oral/systemic)	Continue	May consider stress dose steroids depending on current dose and duration
Leukotriene inhibitors Phosphodiesterase (PDE) inhibitors Antihistamines (H1 receptor antagonists) Decongestants	Zafirlukast, montelukast Roflumilast Diphenhydramine, loratadine, cetirizine Oxymetazoline, phenylephrine, pseudoephedrine	Continue Continue Hold on day of surgery Hold on day of surgery	May have unwanted anticholinergic side effects
Gastrointestinal			
Proton pump inhibitors	Omeprazole, lansoprazole, pantoprazole, esomeprazole	Continue	Holding may cause rebound acid reflux
H2-receptor antagonists	Famotidine, ranitidine	Continue	
Stool softeners, laxatives	Docusate, sennosides, osmotic laxatives (polyethylene glycol)	Hold on day of surgery	Restart postoperatively, particularly if using opioids for pain control
Antidiarrheals	Diphenoxylate/atropine, loperamide	Hold on day of surgery	
Antiemetics	Ondansetron, prochlorperazine, promethazine	Continue as needed	
Aminosalicylates	Sulfasalazine, mesalamine	Continue	

(Continued)

MEDICATIONS BY SYSTEM	EXAMPLES	PERIOPERATIVE MANAGEMENT	SPECIAL CONSIDERATIONS
TNF-α inhibitors	Adalimumab, infliximab	Inflammatory bowel disease (IBD): May consider continuation (discuss with surgeon) Rheum: Hold for 1 dosing cycle prior to surgery to reduce perioperative infection risk	Associated with increased risk of infection and delayed wound healing. For patients with IBD, it may be safe to perform bowel surgery without interruption of TNF-α inhibitors, (see text)
Genitourinary			
Antispasmodics	Oxybutynin, tolterodine	Hold on day of surgery	May reduce catheter-related bladder discomfort but anticholinergic effects may increase risk of delirium
Benign prostatic hyperplasia	Finasteride, tamsulosin, doxazosin	Continue	Continuation may avoid postoperative urinary retention
Endocrine			
Long-acting insulins	Glargine, detemir	Continue full dose or partial dose (~80%) based on glycemic control and history of hypoglycemia	
Intermediate-acting insulins	NPH	Continue partial dose (50–65%) on morning of surgery	
Short-acting insulins	Aspart, lispro, glulisine	Hold on day of surgery	
Noninsulin injectables	Dulaglutide, exenatide, liraglutide	Hold on day of surgery	
Oral diabetes medications	Metformin Sulfonylureas (glipizide, glimepiride) Thiazolidinediones (pioglitazone) SGLT2 inhibitors (empagliflozin) GLP-1 agonists (exenatide) DPP-4 inhibitors (sitagliptin)	Hold on day of surgery for most	Hold SGLT2 inhibitors for 3–4 days prior to surgery due to risk of euglycemic DKA. DPP-4 agonists may be safe to continue on the day of surgery. Consider holding long-acting injectable GLP-1 agonists 1 week before surgery

(Continued)

MEDICATIONS BY SYSTEM	EXAMPLES	PERIOPERATIVE MANAGEMENT	SPECIAL CONSIDERATIONS
Hypothyroidism	Levothyroxine, liothyronine	Continue	Intravenous formulations are available if patient cannot take orally
Hyperthyroidism	Methimazole, propylthiouracil	Continue	
Obesity	Glucagon-like peptide-1 (GLP-1) agonists (liraglutide, semaglutide)	Hold on day of surgery for daily dosing; hold for 1 week before surgery for weekly dosing	Increased risk of regurgitation and aspiration; full-stomach precautions
Osteoporosis	Bisphosphonates (alendronate, ibandronate)	Hold on day of surgery	Oral formulations are held during hospitalization as patients need to be sitting upright and drink plenty of water to avoid esophagitis
Corticosteroids	Prednisone	Continue	Adrenal insufficiency or crisis may develop with abruptly stopping. Administering higher doses of steroids perioperatively ("stress dosing") may be reasonable but there is little evidence to support this practice except for Addison's disease
Rheumatologic			
Folate antagonist	Methotrexate	Typically safe to continue	Mostly studied in elective orthopedic surgery, continuing methotrexate does not appear to increase risk of infection Reasonable to hold if severe renal or hepatic impairment

(Continued)

MEDICATIONS BY SYSTEM	EXAMPLES	PERIOPERATIVE MANAGEMENT	SPECIAL CONSIDERATIONS
TNF-α inhibitors	Adalimumab, etanercept, infliximab, golimumab	Hold for one dosing cycle prior to surgery to reduce perioperative infection risk	Typically held before joint replacement surgery but must weigh the risks and benefits of holding vs. continuing perioperatively. See Chapter 29 for more information
JAK inhibitors	Tofacitinib	Hold 3 days before surgery	
Monoclonal antibody (B-cell depletion)	Rituximab	Schedule elective surgeries 6–7 months after last dose	Half-life is 76 hours, but effect lasts >6 months Has a lower risk of bacterial infections compared to TNF-α inhibitors
Other DMARDs	Hydroxychloroquine Azathioprine	Continue	
	Leflunomide	Continue for elective surgeries (i.e., joint arthroplasty)	Consider stopping 2–4 weeks before surgery in patients with higher infection risk and/or large surgical wounds
	Cyclosporine Mycophenolate Tacrolimus	If severe rheumatologic disease: continue perioperatively If nonsevere disease: hold 1 week before surgery	
Gout medications	Allopurinol Colchicine	Continue Continue	The perioperative period increases risk for a gouty flare. Colchicine can be resumed postoperatively once patient is tolerating a diet

(*Continued*)

MEDICATIONS BY SYSTEM	EXAMPLES	PERIOPERATIVE MANAGEMENT	SPECIAL CONSIDERATIONS
Neurologic			
Parkinson's disease	Carbidopa/levodopa Rivastigmine Selegiline	Continue Continue Hold on day of surgery	For selegiline, discuss with neurologist and anesthesiology. If not deemed necessary, may wean off over 2 weeks prior to surgery as life-threatening interactions are possible with meperidine, anticholinergics, and sympathomimetic agents
Dementia	Donepezil, memantine	Continue	
Seizure disorders	Phenytoin, carbamazepine, levetiracetam, lamotrigine, lacosamide, phenobarbital, topiramate, divalproex sodium, valproic acid	Continue	Parenteral alternatives may be needed postoperatively for patients with prolonged NPO status
Myasthenia gravis	Pyridostigmine	Typically continue	Discuss with anesthesiologist as patients are highly resistant to depolarizing muscle relaxants and highly sensitive to non-depolarizing agents
Multiple sclerosis	Interferon beta 1a/1b, glatiramer	Typically continue with possible exceptions	The interferons cause immunosuppression and may be held 1–2 weeks before surgery in patients with higher infection risk and/or large surgical wounds
Neuropathic pain	Gabapentin, pregabalin, duloxetine, amitriptyline	Continue	

(Continued)

MEDICATIONS BY SYSTEM	EXAMPLES	PERIOPERATIVE MANAGEMENT	SPECIAL CONSIDERATIONS
Psychiatric			
Antidepressants	SSRIs (citalopram, fluoxetine, paroxetine, sertraline) SNRIs (venlafaxine, duloxetine) TCAs (amitriptyline, nortriptyline, mirtazapine)	Continue	The rarely used MAOIs should be weaned off prior to surgery as long as the psychiatric risk is acceptable, especially with the older MAOIs that are nonselective and irreversible (discussion with the patient's psychiatrist is strongly advised)
Anxiolytics	Benzodiazepines (clonazepam, diazepam, lorazepam, alprazolam) Buspirone Antidepressants (see above)	Continue	Patients taking benzodiazepines chronically will need to continue them perioperatively to avoid withdrawal
Bipolar disorder (mood stabilizers)	Lithium Antiepileptics (valproic acid, lamotrigine)	Continue	
Schizophrenia	Antipsychotics (risperidone, olanzapine, quetiapine, aripiprazole, ziprasidone)	Continue	
Attention deficit hyperactivity disorder (ADHD)	Dextroamphetamine/amphetamine, methylphenidate, atomoxetine	Hold on day of surgery	
Opioids			
Short-acting	Morphine, hydromorphone, oxycodone, tramadol	Continue	Although data are limited, reducing preoperative opioid usage may improve postoperative pain control

(Continued)

MEDICATIONS BY SYSTEM	EXAMPLES	PERIOPERATIVE MANAGEMENT	SPECIAL CONSIDERATIONS
Long-acting	Morphine, oxycodone, methadone, fentanyl (transdermal)	Continue	Although data are limited, reducing preoperative opioid usage may improve postoperative pain control
HIV medications			
Multiple drug classes	Nucleoside reverse transcriptase inhibitors (NRTIs) Non-nucleoside reverse transcriptase inhibitors (NNRTIs) Protease inhibitors (PIs) Integrase strand transfer inhibitors (INSTIs) Fusion inhibitors (FIs) Chemokine receptor antagonists (CCR5 antagonists)	Full regimen is generally continued perioperatively	If needed, holding antiretroviral therapy for a few days is unlikely to cause viral resistance
Alternative medications			
Vitamins, herbals, supplements	Ginkgo, ginseng, ephedra, garlic, kava, valerian, echinacea, St John's wort, fish oil	Hold 1–2 weeks before surgery	These agents have the potential to be harmful in the perioperative setting. Exception may include water-soluble vitamins (B, C), vitamin D, and calcium that can be continued until surgery

ACEIs, angiotensin converting enzyme inhibitors; ACS, acute coronary syndrome; ARBs, angiotensin II receptor blockers; CEA, carcinoembryonic antigen; DKA, diabetic ketoacidosis; DMARDs, disease-modifying antirheumatic drugs; HF, heart failure; HTN, hypertension.

Lipid-Lowering Agents

Statins (HMG-CoA Reductase Inhibitors). Perioperative use of statins has been associated with improved cardiac outcomes and decreased mortality in numerous observational studies and a few RCTs. This appears to be a class effect and is most likely due to their pleiotropic, anti-inflammatory effects rather than cholesterol-lowering ability. There are suggestions that a more potent statin (rosuvastatin, atorvastatin) and a moderate to high dose are more beneficial. There are no significant safety issues (rhabdomyolysis, elevated liver enzymes) with starting or continuing a statin perioperatively. In view of the potential benefit with little or no harm, statins should be continued perioperatively and started prophylactically in patients undergoing vascular surgery as well as those with independent indications for them (see Chapter 11).

Other Agents for Lipid Control. Bile acid sequestrants (cholestyramine, colestipol), fibric acid derivatives (gemfibrozil), ezetimibe, and niacin are used for various aspects of lipid control but are not usually continued on the morning of surgery. Bile acid sequestrants may interfere with absorption of other medications. There is little evidence to inform perioperative management of proprotein convertase subtilisin/kexin type 9 (PCSK9) inhibitors. They are administered subcutaneously, have a long half-life, and there is no compelling reason to hold them prior to surgery.

Medications Affecting Hemostasis (Anticoagulant, Antiplatelet, NSAID)[7]

The potential increased risk of bleeding with continuation of these drugs must be balanced against the potential risks of discontinuing them preoperatively. This risk-benefit analysis considers the specific drug, its indication, the timing of surgery, and the patient's bleeding risk.

Anticoagulants (Warfarin, Heparins, Fondaparinux, Direct Oral Anticoagulants (DOACs)). These medications are typically discontinued before surgery unless the bleeding risk of the procedure is low. When they are stopped depends on the individual drug, bleeding risk of the surgery, renal function, and indication for anticoagulation. In certain cases where the risk of thrombosis is high if the drug is stopped, "bridging therapy" may be indicated. For a detailed discussion and recommendations, see Chapter 5.

Antiplatelet Medications (Aspirin, P2Y12 Inhibitors)

Aspirin irreversibly inhibits cyclooxygenase, rendering a patient's circulating platelets ineffective for the rest of their lifespan. If continued perioperatively, aspirin is associated with an increased risk of bleeding; however, this is offset by its potential benefits in reducing risk of stent thrombosis and myocardial infarction in patients with coronary stents in whom it should be continued. Aspirin is also continued in patients undergoing carotid endarterectomy and

those with recent acute coronary syndrome or stroke. The POISE-2 trial found no benefit of perioperative aspirin in other subgroups for either continuing or starting aspirin prophylactically, but it was associated with increased bleeding in the aspirin initiation subgroup.[8] The decision to continue aspirin preoperatively should take this information into account along with the bleeding risk of the surgical procedure. Approximately 10–15% of the platelet pool is generated every day, so if aspirin is to be stopped, it should be done 5–7 days before surgery to allow time for the patient to produce new platelets not exposed to aspirin. There is no need to stop aspirin 10–14 days before surgery which may be harmful. In general, the minimum platelet count for most surgery is 50,000, but it is 100,000 for spine and neurosurgical procedures. Any management plan should involve discussion with the patient, surgeon, cardiologist, and anesthesiologist. See Chapter 11 for more details.

Thienopyridines (clopidogrel, prasugrel, ticagrelor) inhibit P2Y12 ADP-induced platelet aggregation, and their effect is more potent than aspirin. Either alone or in combination with aspirin, they are associated with an increased bleeding risk. Clopidogrel and prasugrel are irreversible platelet inhibitors, whereas ticagrelor's effect is reversible, which means the patient's platelets will recover function once the drug is metabolized. These medications are typically used in patients with cerebrovascular events, acute coronary syndromes, and coronary or vascular stents. As part of dual antiplatelet therapy (DAPT) with aspirin, premature discontinuation of these drugs is associated with stent thrombosis and myocardial infarction. In general, these medications tend to be stopped before surgery, but again it depends on the indication and procedure. The timeframe for when to stop these drugs varies—clopidogrel is stopped 5–7 days before surgery, prasugrel 7 days before, and ticagrelor 3–5 days before. If they are stopped as part of DAPT, aspirin should be continued. See Chapter 11 for more information about dual antiplatelet recommendations.

Dipyridamole is a reversible platelet adhesion inhibitor with a 10-hour half-life. It is typically used for patients with a TIA or stroke. There are no specific guidelines for its perioperative management, but if it is stopped, it should probably be at least 2 days before surgery.

Cilostazol is a reversible cAMP PDE-3 inhibitor with a 12-hour half-life. It is used for patients with claudication and is usually stopped 2–5 days before surgery.

Nonsteroidal Anti-Inflammatory Drugs (NSAIDs)[9]

These medications are reversible inhibitors of cyclo-oxygenase (COX-1) and may increase the risk of perioperative bleeding and AKI, but they also decrease postoperative pain and use of opioids. Elimination half-life correlates poorly with COX inhibition and effects upon platelet aggregation, and the relationship between timing of NSAID discontinuation and perioperative bleeding is poorly defined. If not part of a multimodal pain regimen, NSAIDs are typically discontinued 1–3 days before surgery. Platelet function normalizes within 3 days of discontinuation for most NSAIDs, but ibuprofen can be stopped 24 hours before surgery. The selective COX-2 inhibitors (celecoxib) have no adverse effect on platelet function at the usual doses. However, because of theoretical concerns for renal insufficiency and controversy regarding earlier reports of possible risk of myocardial infarction, these drugs are also often stopped 1–3 days before surgery.

Pulmonary Medications[10]

Inhaled Beta-Agonists and Anticholinergics.
These medications are used to control obstructive lung disease and may reduce postoperative pulmonary complications in patients with asthma and COPD. They should be continued via metered-dose inhalers or nebulizers.

Theophylline.
The use of theophylline is infrequent due to its narrow therapeutic window, cardiotoxic side effects, and multiple drug interactions. This drug should be held on the morning of surgery.

Glucocorticoids.
Inhaled and/or systemic glucocorticoids should be continued to optimize pulmonary function and minimize risk of adrenal insufficiency. In certain cases, stress-dose steroids may be considered although supporting evidence is lacking. The American College of Rheumatology/American Association of Hip and Knee Surgeons Guidelines recommend trying to reduce the dose of corticosteroids to <15 mg

prednisone (or its equivalent) and do not recommend stress-dose steroids[11] (see Chapter 21). Despite concerns about poor wound healing and hyperglycemia, the risk of infection and postoperative complications related to glucocorticoids is low.

Leukotriene Inhibitors.
Montelukast and zafirlukast are used as maintenance agents for treating asthma and allergic rhinitis. They also have been reported to help with postoperative pain after otorhinolaryngologic surgical procedures. These may be continued on the morning of surgery.

Phosphodiesterase (PDE) Inhibitors.
Roflumilast is an inhaled PDE 4 inhibitor that reduces inflammatory mediators in the lung to help decrease exacerbations in patients with chronic obstructive pulmonary disease. It can be continued on the morning of surgery.

Antihistamines and Decongestants.
First-generation antihistamines penetrate the blood-brain barrier and have both central and peripheral anticholinergic side effects, which can contribute to somnolence and neurocognitive dysfunction in elderly patients, as well as increase the risk of urinary retention, constipation, and delirium in the perioperative period. Second-generation antihistamines do not have central anticholinergic effects, with the exception of cetirizine, because they do not penetrate the blood-brain barrier, but they still have some unwanted peripheral anticholinergic effects. Consider holding first-generation antihistamines and cetirizine on the morning of surgery. Decongestants are sympathomimetic agents and can cause elevated blood pressure and tachycardia. Because their use is noncritical for disease treatment and they may potentiate hypertension, they should be held on the morning of surgery.

Gastrointestinal Medications[10]

Some of the most common medications in the United States include those used to treat gastroesophageal reflux disease (GERD), constipation, diarrhea, and nausea. Continuing proton pump inhibitors (PPIs) and H2 blockers throughout the perioperative period may have advantages including a decreased risk of stress-related GI mucosal damage, a decreased risk of GERD rebound symptoms, and a decreased risk of aspiration pneumonia. While these agents are generally continued on the day of surgery, medications to treat constipation, diarrhea, and nausea are often held on the morning of surgery unless patients are symptomatic.

Patients with inflammatory bowel disease (IBD), such as Crohn's disease and ulcerative colitis, may be taking a variety of medications including aminosalicylates (i.e., sulfasalazine and mesalamine), immunomodulators (i.e., azathioprine, 6-mercaptopurine, methotrexate, mycophenolate mofetil, tacrolimus), corticosteroids, and tumor necrosis factor alpha (TNF-α) inhibitors (i.e., adalimumab and infliximab) and various other biologic agents and small molecules (i.e., ustekinumab, natalizumab, vedolizumab, tofacitinib, ozanimod). While aminosalicylates and immunomodulators are likely safe to continue perioperatively, systemic corticosteroids, TNF-α inhibitors and other biologics require careful attention in the perioperative period. Recent data suggest that patients taking TNF-α inhibitors had similar rates of postoperative infectious complications after intra-abdominal surgery as those who were not taking them; however, the postoperative infection rates were fairly high in both groups (18–20%).[12] Limited retrospective data available for the other biologic agents suggest that there is no significant difference in the rate of overall or infectious complications compared to patients taking TNF-α inhibitors. More recently, some experts have suggested that most of the biologic agents can be continued in the perioperative period, with the exception of small-molecule drugs such as tofacitinib which is associated with increased risk of perioperative venous thrombosis and should be held for 3–7 days prior to surgery. Perioperative corticosteroid use in this patient population is associated with an increase in postoperative infections and complications, and their use should be minimized or avoided in patients with IBD undergoing abdominal surgery. Controversy still exists regarding this issue, and it is important to discuss the perioperative management of biologic agents with the surgeon and gastroenterologist). The SPAQI consensus statement has suggested following a more conservative recommendation of holding the TNF-α inhibitors for one dosing cycle prior to surgery.[10]

Genitourinary Medications[13]

Antispasmodic medications (i.e., tolterodine and oxybutynin) are commonly used for overactive bladder syndromes, and although they may decrease catheter-related bladder discomfort, they should be held on the day of surgery given their anticholinergic effects that may increase the risk for postoperative delirium. Medications used to treat benign prostatic hyperplasia (i.e., finasteride, tamsulosin, and doxazosin) should be continued perioperatively. This is important due to the high incidence of postoperative urinary retention, particularly in men. Phosphodiesterase type 5 (PDE-5) inhibitors, used for erectile dysfunction and benign prostatic hyperplasia (i.e., avanafil, sildenafil, tadalafil, and vardenafil), cause relaxation of endothelial smooth muscle and vasodilation and can potentiate perioperative hypotension. Safety studies of PDE-5 inhibitors during anesthesia have been reported in patients with pulmonary hypertension, but not in patients taking them for erectile dysfunction or prostate symptoms. PDE-5 inhibitors used for GU symptoms should be held on the morning of surgery and if time allows, for 3 days prior to surgery.

Endocrine Medications[13]

Diabetes mellitus is a common disease with many medication treatment options with different mechanisms of actions. In general, oral medications are held on the morning of surgery as well as all short-acting (mealtime) insulins to avoid hypoglycemia as patients are typically NPO status. SGLT-2 inhibitors should be held 3–4 days before surgery to minimize the risk of euglycemic ketoacidosis. Long-acting (basal) insulins are continued prior to surgery at either full dosing or at a reduced dose (approximately 80% of the patient's home dose depending on their baseline glycemic control). Noninsulin injectables are usually continued the day before surgery but held on the day of surgery. For more information on the perioperative management of diabetes, please refer to Chapter 19.

Hypothyroidism represents a common endocrine disorder with thyroid replacement therapy (i.e., levothyroxine) being the mainstay of treatment. Medications for both hypo- and hyperthyroidism are continued perioperatively.

Patients with adrenal insufficiency may be at increased risk for perioperative adrenal crisis. Although there are many causes of adrenal insufficiency, prolonged exposure to exogenous corticosteroids (i.e., prednisone) is the most common.

Suppression of the hypothalamic-pituitary-adrenal (HPA) axis can occur with variable doses of steroids and can take up to 1 year to resolve. Although HPA-axis activation occurs with most surgical procedures, the incidence of significant perioperative adrenal insufficiency is rare (<1%). In certain cases, stress-dose steroids may be considered although supporting evidence is lacking. For patients with primary adrenal insufficiency (Addison's disease) who cannot produce corticosteroids in response to stress, supplemental or stress-dose steroids are required. However, for patients on exogenous steroids, the need for stress-dose steroids is controversial (see Chapter 21).

Estrogen exposure, whether in the form of oral contraceptives or postmenopausal hormone therapy, is known to increase the risk for venous thromboembolism (VTE). Perioperative management of these agents requires careful consideration as this risk may be compounded in the surgical setting. It is generally advised to continue oral contraceptives to minimize risk of unplanned pregnancy. Postmenopausal hormone replacement therapy can be held unless patients have significant postmenopausal symptoms with discontinuation of hormone therapy. For patients at high risk for VTE, it is reasonable to hold these agents 4 weeks prior to surgery, but this is rarely practical. Appropriate VTE prophylaxis should be provided for all patients on estrogen therapy throughout the perioperative period.

Selective estrogen receptor modulators (SERMs) including tamoxifen and raloxifene also increase the risk for VTE. For patients taking a SERM for breast cancer prevention, it is reasonable to discontinue the medication 2 weeks prior to surgery, especially for procedures associated with a higher risk for VTE. For SERMs prescribed for breast cancer treatment, continuation of the drug is generally advised while ensuring adequate perioperative VTE prophylaxis. In these cases, a discussion with the patient's oncologist is recommended.

Glucagon-like peptide-1 (GLP-1) receptor agonists (i.e., semaglutide, liraglutide) are increasingly being used to treat obesity and are associated with delayed gastric emptying. A number of case reports have described patients with retention of gastric contents despite several hours of fasting which can increase the risk of perioperative regurgitation and pulmonary aspiration. This risk is greater in the escalation phase, with higher doses, weekly dosing, presence of gastrointestinal symptoms, and other conditions which may delay gastric emptying. The American Society of Anesthesiologists along with several other societies has provided consensus-based guidance for patients at elevated risk to hold weekly dosed medications for the week prior to elective surgery and to hold daily dosed GLP-1 agonists on the day of surgery (although this latter recommendation does not take into account the half-life of the drugs).[14] Other considerations include diet modification (liquid diet the day before surgery) and possible gastric ultrasound on the day of surgery if concern for retained gastric contents. For patients requiring urgent or emergent surgery, it is advised that "full stomach" precautions be taken.

Rheumatologic Medications[9]

Disease-modifying antirheumatic drugs (DMARDs) represent an expanding category of medications used to treat a variety of rheumatologic disorders. Broadly speaking, these therapies suppress the immune system in order to slow disease progression. Due to their mechanism of action, the decision to continue or hold these agents prior to surgery has the potential for risk. Continuing these medications may increase the risk for infection and impair wound healing, while holding them may lead to disease flare, which can compromise postoperative recovery and rehabilitation. Although published data are limited, guidelines by the American College of Rheumatology provide recommendations for the perioperative management of DMARDs in patients undergoing hip or knee arthroplasty,[11] which are often extrapolated to nonorthopedic surgery. The Society for Perioperative Assessment and Quality Improvement (SPAQI) also published a consensus statement on the perioperative management of immunosuppressant and biologic drugs.[9] When possible, consultation with the patient's rheumatologist is advised. For more information on the perioperative management of rheumatologic medications, please refer to Chapter 29.

Neurologic Medications[15]

Essentially all medications used to treat common neurologic disorders are continued perioperatively. This includes medical therapies prescribed for dementia, seizure disorders, Parkinson's disease, tremors, myasthenia gravis, fibromyalgia, and neuropathies including neuropathic pain. It is worth noting that the standard treatment for Parkinson's disease, carbidopa/levodopa, is particularly important to continue perioperatively with the last dose administered as close to the time of surgery as possible. Abrupt discontinuation of levodopa can cause disease flare, hyperpyrexia syndrome, and, in some cases, neuroleptic malignant syndrome.

In patients with multiple sclerosis, it is recommended to discuss medication management with the prescribing neurologist as some therapies cause immunosuppression (i.e., interferons). In cases with high infection risk or complicated wound healing, the decision to hold these medications 1–2 weeks before surgery may be advised.

Psychiatric Medications[16]

With rare exceptions, medications prescribed for psychiatric disorders are continued perioperatively. This includes medications used to treat depression, bipolar disorder, anxiety, schizophrenia, and attention deficit hyperactivity disorder. The most common class of antidepressant medications, selective serotonin reuptake inhibitors (SSRIs), have been associated with an increased risk of perioperative bleeding in some studies. Although studies have been inconsistent, an increased bleeding risk may be more common in orthopedic surgeries but have the potential to be more dangerous in cardiac and neurosurgical procedures. However, most experts feel any increase in bleeding risk is unlikely to be clinically relevant, making the risk of discontinuing SSRIs greater than any potential benefit.

Although now rarely used for treating depression, the monoamine oxidase inhibitors (MAOIs) should be weaned off 2 weeks prior to surgery unless the psychiatric risk of discontinuation is deemed too high, and the anesthesiologist is agreeable with drug continuation. This is particularly true for the older MAOIs that are nonselective and irreversible. Nonselective MAOIs can have life-threatening interactions with meperidine, anticholinergics, and sympathomimetic agents. A discussion with the patient's psychiatrist and anesthesiologist is advised for patients taking these agents.

Opioids[17]

Short- and long-acting opioids should be continued prior to surgery. Although abrupt cessation of opioids can lead to profound withdrawal and is never advised, the preoperative period often provides an opportunity to gradually reduce opioid usage. Although data are limited, a reduction in preoperative opioid exposure may improve postoperative pain management when opioids are often needed.

Buprenorphine is an opioid agonist-antagonist that is used for the treatment of opioid use disorders such as addiction. It is available in different formulations including sublingual, buccal, and transdermal (intravenous and intramuscular preparations are also available for inpatient use). Discussions regarding the perioperative management of buprenorphine with the outpatient prescriber, anesthesiologist, and surgeon are strongly recommended. In most cases, buprenorphine is continued perioperatively including on the morning of surgery. Preoperative buprenorphine dosing may be decreased, however, for patients prescribed larger doses and/or if significant postoperative pain is anticipated (see Chapter 45).

Herbal Supplements and Cannabis[18]

Approximately one-third of adults in the United States take some form of herbals, supplements, or alternative medications. It is important for the perioperative provider to inquire about these agents as patients often do not consider them to be medications but rather "natural" agents and thus harmless. In fact, herbal supplements have been poorly studied and are largely unregulated yet are known to be potentially harmful in the perioperative setting. Adverse effects may include bleeding, CNS depression, blood sugar derangement, and drug–drug interactions among others. With rare exceptions, all herbal supplements should be held 1–2 weeks prior to surgery.

Cannabis use has drastically increased over recent years, particularly with the legalization of recreational use in many parts of the United States. Although there is very little information pertaining to the perioperative effects of cannabis exposure, a recent retrospective population-based cohort study assessed the perioperative risk of over 13,000 patients with an active cannabis use disorder undergoing a variety of surgical procedures. Although no difference was found in perioperative respiratory failure, patients with an active cannabis use disorder had an increased risk of perioperative myocardial infarction. A recent consensus statement recognized the potential need for increased postoperative analgesia and nausea/vomiting prophylaxis in patients who use cannabis.[19] Although more data are needed, it seems appropriate for providers to ask patients about cannabis exposure, counsel them on the potential risks and unknowns of perioperative use, and consider monitoring for cannabis withdrawal (see Chapter 30).

Clinical pearls

- Always continue medications with potential rebound or withdrawal effects, such as beta-blockers, clonidine, benzodiazepines, opioids, and corticosteroids.
- Continue medications deemed essential, including most cardiopulmonary drugs.
- Withhold drugs with potential for adverse effects perioperatively, such as anticoagulants and oral hypoglycemics.
- Individualize preoperative management of drugs with potential for benefit and harm, such as antiplatelet drugs, based on clinical practice guidelines, risk-benefit analysis, and discussion with all involved parties.
- Continue the patient's home dose of corticosteroids on the day of surgery. While prednisone doses of 5 mg daily or less certainly do not require perioperative stress dosing, there is limited evidence to support administering stress-dose steroids for patients taking higher doses.
- Always ask about vitamins, supplements, and herbals and advise stopping them 1–2 weeks prior to surgery.

REFERENCES

1. Sahai SK, Balonov K, Bentov N, et al. Preoperative management of cardiovascular medications: a Society for Perioperative Assessment and Quality Improvement (SPAQI) consensus statement. *Mayo Clin Proc.* 2022;97(9):1734-1751. PMID: 36058586
2. Marcucci M, Painter TW, Conen D, et al. POISE-3 trial investigators and study groups. Hypotension-avoidance versus hypertension-avoidance strategies in noncardiac surgery: an international randomized controlled trial. *Ann Intern Med.* 2023 May;176(5):605-614. PMID: 37094336
3. Legrand M, Falcone J, Cholley B, et al. Stop-or-not trial group. Continuation vs discontinuation of renin-angiotensin system inhibitors before major noncardiac surgery: the stop-or-not randomized clinical trial. *JAMA.* 2024;332(12):970-978. PMID: 39212270
4. Ackland GL, Patel A, Abbott TEF, et al. Stopping perioperative ACE-inhibitors or angiotensin-II receptor blockers (SPACE) trial investigators. Discontinuation vs. continuation of renin-angiotensin system inhibition before non-cardiac surgery: the SPACE trial. *Eur Heart J.* 2024 Apr 1;45(13):1146-1155. PMID: 37935833
5. POISE Study Group, Devereaux PJ, Yang H, et al. Effects of extended-release metoprolol succinate in patients undergoing non-cardiac surgery (POISE trial): a randomised controlled trial. *Lancet.* 2008;371(9627):1839-1847. PMID: 18479744
6. Devereaux PJ, Sessler DI, Leslie K, et al. Clonidine in patients undergoing noncardiac surgery. *N Engl J Med.* 2014;370(16):1504-1513. PMID: 24679061
7. Douketis JD, Spyropoulos AC, Murad MH, et al. Perioperative management of antithrombotic therapy: an American College of Chest Physicians clinical practice guideline. *Chest.* 2022 Nov;162(5):e207-e243. PMID: 35964704
8. Devereaux PJ, Mrkobrada M, Sessler DI, et al. Aspirin in patients undergoing noncardiac surgery. *N Engl J Med.* 370(16):1494-1503. PMID: 24679062
9. Russell, LA., Chad C, Eva KF, et al. Preoperative management of medications for rheumatologic and HIV diseases: Society for Perioperative Assessment and Quality Improvement (SPAQI) consensus statement. *Mayo Clin Proc.* 2022;97(8):1551-1571. PMID: 35933139
10. Pfeifer KJ, SelzerA, Whinney CM. Preoperative management of gastrointestinal and pulmonary medications: Society for Perioperative Assessment and Quality Improvement (SPAQI) consensus statement. *Mayo Clin Proc.* 2021;96(12):3158-3177. PMID: 34736777
11. Goodman SM, Springer B, Chen AF, et al. 2022 American College of Rheumatology/American Association of Hip and Knee Surgeons guideline for the perioperative management of antirheumatic medication in patients with rheumatic diseases undergoing elective total hip or total knee arthroplasty. *Arthritis Rheumatol.* 2022 Sep;74(9):1464-1473. PMID: 35722708
12. Cohen BL, Fleshner P, Kane SV, et al. Prospective cohort study to investigate the safety of preoperative tumor necrosis factor inhibitor exposure in patients with inflammatory bowel disease undergoing intra-abdominal

surgery. *Gastroenterology.* 2022;163(1):204-221. PMID: 35413359

13. Pfeifer KJ, Selzer A, Mendez CE, et al. Preoperative management of endocrine, hormonal, and urologic medications: Society for Perioperative Assessment and Quality Improvement (SPAQI) consensus statement. *Mayo Clin Proc.* 2021;96(6):1655-1669. PMID: 33714600

14. Kindel TL, Wang AY, Wadhwa A, et al. Representing the American Gastroenterological Association, American Society for Metabolic and Bariatric Surgery, American Society of Anesthesiologists, International Society of Perioperative Care of Patients with Obesity, and the Society of American Gastrointestinal and Endoscopic Surgeons. Multi-society clinical practice guidance for the safe use of glucagon-like peptide-1 receptor agonists in the perioperative period. *Surg Endosc.* 2024;Oct 29. doi: 10.1007/s00464-024-11263-2. Epub ahead of print. PMID: 39370500

15. Oprea AD, Keshock MC, O'Glasser AY, et al. Preoperative management of medications for neurologic diseases: Society for Perioperative Assessment and Quality Improvement (SPAQI) consensus statement. *Mayo Clin Proc.* 2022;97(2):375-396. PMID: 35120701

16. Oprea AD, Keshock MC, O'Glasser AY, et al. Preoperative management of medications for psychiatric diseases: Society for Perioperative Assessment and Quality Improvement consensus statement. *Mayo Clinic Proceedings.* 2022;97(2):397-416. PMID: 35120702

17. O'Rourke MJ, Keshock C, Boxhorn CE, et al. Preoperative management of opioid and nonopioid analgesics: Society for Perioperative Assessment and Quality Improvement (SPAQI) consensus statement. *Mayo Clin Proc.* 2021;96(5):1325-1341. PMID: 33618850

18. Cummings KC, Keshock M, Ganesh R, et al. Preoperative management of surgical patients using dietary supplements: herbal and alternative medications: recommendations from the Society for Perioperative Assessment and Quality Improvement (SPAQI) consensus statement. *Mayo Clin Proc.* 2021;96(5):1342-1355. PMID: 33741131

19. Ladha KS, McLaren-Blades A, Goel A, et al. Perioperative Pain and Addiction Interdisciplinary Network (PAIN): consensus recommendations for perioperative management of cannabis and cannabinoid-based medicine users by a modified Delphi process. *British J Anaesth.* 2021;126(1):304-318. PMID: 33129489

## 5

Perioperative Management of Anticoagulants

Scott Kaatz, DO, MSc, FACP, SFHM and James D. Douketis, MD, FRCPC

COMMON CLINICAL QUESTIONS

1. How long should I interrupt a direct oral anticoagulant (DOAC) for an invasive procedure or surgery?

2. Should I use bridging parenteral anticoagulation when interrupting warfarin for an invasive procedure or surgery in patients with mechanical heart valves?

3. What should I use to reverse oral anticoagulants for emergent/urgent surgery or an invasive procedure?

INTRODUCTION

It is estimated that 6 million patients with atrial fibrillation worldwide will require perioperative anticoagulant management per year for an invasive procedure, or about 1 in 6 patients annually,[1] and the number is increased when also including anticoagulated patients with a mechanical valve or venous thromboembolism (VTE). Periprocedural anticoagulant management is anchored on the following components: (a) need for interruption; (b) pre-procedure interruption timing; (c) post-procedure resumption timing; (d) need for heparin bridging anticoagulation; and (e) urgent reversal for emergent procedures. Four primary guidelines help inform periprocedural anticoagulation interruption: the 2022 American College of Chest Physicians (ACCP) guidelines,[2] the 2017 American College of Cardiology (ACC) Expert Consensus Decision Pathway, which offers guidance for patients with atrial fibrillation only,[3] the 2018 American Society of Regional Anesthesia (ASRA) and Pain Medicine guidelines,[4] and the 2022 American College of Gastroenterology-Canadian Association of Gastroenterology (ACG-CAG) Clinical Practice Guideline: Management of Anticoagulants and Antiplatelets During Acute Gastrointestinal Bleeding and the Periendoscopic Period.[5]

LOW-RISK PROCEDURES THAT CAN CONTINUE UNINTERRUPTED ORAL ANTICOAGULATION

Warfarin

The ACCP guidelines suggest patients undergoing minor dental procedures (e.g., uncomplicated extractions, cleaning), minor dermatologic procedures (e.g., skin biopsies, small cancer removal), and cataract surgery (with topical, not retrobulbar, anesthesia) do not require interruption of warfarin.[2] Although these guidelines do not address direct oral anticoagulant (DOAC) management for these procedures, due to lack of relevant data, expert opinion suggests DOACs can be continued with the caveat that on the procedure day, the DOAC dose is delayed for 4–6 hours post-procedure or omitted altogether for that day alone. The ACC consensus pathway recommends not interrupting warfarin for patients with no clinically important or low bleeding risk and includes a series of tables in the appendix listing procedural bleeding risks from multiple specialty societies.[3]

ACCP guidelines *recommend* continuation of vitamin K antagonist (VKA) over VKA interruption with heparin bringing in patients having pacemaker or implanted cardiac defibrillator (ICD) implantation based on a study reporting an increased risk of pocket hematomas in the bridging group with no difference in thromboembolic complications.

The 2022 ACG-CAG Clinical Practice Guideline *suggests* that warfarin be continued for patients undergoing elective/planned endoscopy and emphasizes the very low certainty of the evidence and includes a table categorizing procedures and high and low bleeding risk that may guide the decision.

Direct Oral Anticoagulants

The ACCP guidelines do not specifically address continuation of DOACs for dental, ophthalmologic, and minor dermatologic procedures as they do for warfarin. The PAUSE management study, which assessed the periprocedural management of DOAC-treated patients, only assessed procedures that required anticoagulant interruption.[1]

Based on expert opinion, in DOAC-treated patients who require a minor dental, skin, or cataract procedure, it is likely safe to continue DOACs without interruption or hold one dose just before the procedure to avoid a peak anticoagulant effect around the time of the procedure.

PRE-PROCEDURE INTERRUPTION TIMING

Warfarin

We suggest measuring the international normalized ratio (INR) about 7 days prior to invasive procedures, and warfarin should be held 5 days before if the INR is between 2.0 and 3.0 with longer and shorter hold times for higher and lower INRs, respectively.[2] For patients undergoing neuraxial (spinal/epidural) anesthesia or deep nerve blocks, ASRA recommends holding warfarin for 5 days, and having the INR normalized prior to the procedure.[4]

Direct Oral Anticoagulants (DOAC)

The 2022 ACCP guideline and the 2017 ACC consensus pathway recommend DOAC interruption timing based on creatinine clearance (CrCl) and surgery/procedure-associated bleeding risk. In general, we suggest withholding DOACs for 1 day before and 1 day after a low/moderate-bleeding-risk procedure (2 days total DOAC interruption) and for 2 days before and 2 days after a high-bleed-risk procedure (4 days total DOAC interruption). The exception to this approach is for dabigatran-treated patients with a CrCl <50 mL/min in whom an additional 1–2 days of pre-procedure interruption is recommended.

The ASRA guidelines recommend holding apixaban, edoxaban, and rivaroxaban for 72 hours and holding dabigatran for 72–120 hours based on CrCl before insertion of neuraxial catheters and recommend waiting at least 6 hours after their removal before postoperative resumption of apixaban, edoxaban, and rivaroxaban.[4] Of note, the ACC and ASRA recommendations were published before the publication of the PAUSE study.[1]

The ACCP 2022 guidelines anchor their suggestions on the PAUSE study, which was conducted in patients with atrial fibrillation. No similar management study has been done in patients with VTE but extrapolating the interruptions schedule to these patients is reasonable. Of note, ACCP guidelines point out that longer pre-procedure hold times are sensible in patients with decreased renal function (CrCl, 30 mL/min), impaired liver function, and those receiving medications that inhibit CYP3A4 or P-glycoprotein pathways.[2]

The PAUSE management study prospectively quantified rates of bleeding and thromboembolic complications in patients with atrial fibrillation who needed DOAC interruption for an invasive procedure using a simple standardized protocol based on the procedure-related bleeding risk and renal function (only for patients taking dabigatran). The study included 3,007 patients from 23 sites in Canada, the United States, and Europe who were on a DOAC (apixaban, dabigatran, or rivaroxaban) and had a CrCl ≥25 mL/min for apixaban and 30 mL/min for dabigatran and rivaroxaban. The standardized perioperative DOAC management approach in PAUSE (Figure 5-1)

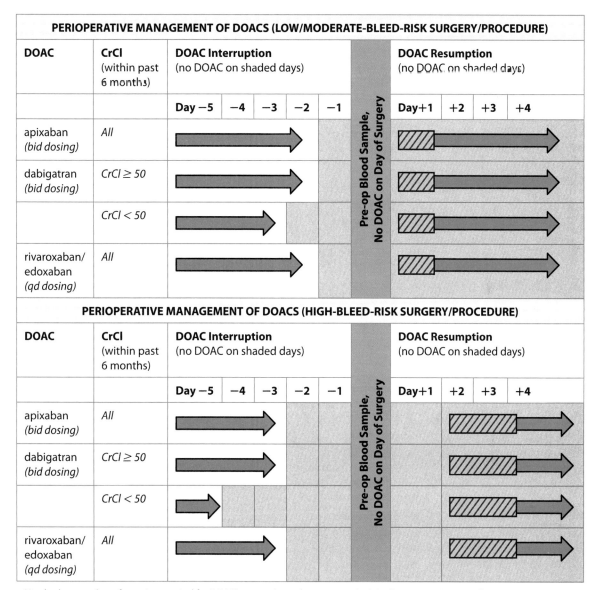

Hatched rectangles refer to time period for DOAC resumption, whenever surgical site hemostasis is secured.

FIGURE 5-1. PAUSE–DOAC interruption protocol.[1]

was associated with low 30-day postoperative rates of major bleeding (0.9–1.8%) and thromboembolism (0.3–0.6%), depending on the DOAC.[1] Moreover, >90% of patients had minimal-to-no residual DOAC effect (<50 ng/mL) at the time of the surgery/procedure (although we do not recommend routine use of drug levels in usual clinical practice).

TIMING OF POST-PROCEDURE RESUMPTION

Warfarin

The full therapeutic effect of warfarin after resumption usually takes 5–7 days, and the ACC recommends and the ACCP suggests restarting warfarin within

24 hours. For most patients, this would be the evening of the procedure at the usual dose with the caveat from both organizations that hemostasis is secured. The issue of whether to resume post-procedure warfarin by doubling the dose is not resolved. Although it may reduce the time needed to reach a therapeutic INR by about 1 day, there are concerns about how to operationalize such practice and the potential for patients to misunderstand warfarin dose instructions.

Direct Oral Anticoagulants (DOAC)

For low-bleeding-risk procedures, the ACC recommends beginning full dose DOACs the next day and waiting 48–72 hours for high-bleeding-risk procedures[3]; the PAUSE study used the same timing in its protocol.[1] The ACCP suggests resuming DOAC at least 24 hours after surgery/procedure.

BRIDGING ANTICOAGULATION (SEE TABLE 5-1)

Warfarin

ACCP guidelines categorize risk of thromboembolic events for mechanical heart valves, VTE, and atrial fibrillation as high, moderate, or low risk and suggest no bridging for low-to-moderate risk, and limiting bridging to high-risk patients. This suggested approach may be modified based on individual patient characteristics and clinical judgment. For example, patients in a low- or moderate-risk category may be deemed high risk and considered for heparin bridging, if they had a prior thromboembolism that occurred perioperatively. Both the ACCP and ACC discuss atrial fibrillation only—ACC bases their recommendations on the CHA_2DS_2-VASc score whereas the ACCP guidelines use either the CHA_2DS_2-VASc or $CHADS_2$ score. The 2022 ACG-CAG Clinical Practice Guideline suggests against bridging anticoagulation if warfarin is interrupted for elective/planned endoscopy.[5]

The BRIDGE trial randomized 1,813 atrial fibrillation patients who required warfarin interruption for an invasive procedure to placebo or low-molecular-weight heparin (LMWH) bridging with an intention to show similar (noninferior) rates of arterial thromboembolism and less (superiority) bleeding 30 days post-procedure. Rates of thromboembolism were noninferior for placebo and LMWH (0.4% vs. 0.3%) and significantly less for major bleeding (1.3% vs. 3.2%).[6] Table 5-2 is a sample bridging protocol similar to that used in the BRIDGE trial.

The 2022 ACCP guidelines suggest against bridging for patients with mechanical heart valves, a change from the 2012 guidelines, that was informed by the 2021 PERIOP2 randomized trial.[7] However, in the guideline implementation considerations, for select patients at high risk, pre- and post-procedure bridging is suggested, and this includes older-generation valves like ball-cage and tilting disk; mitral valves with >1 additional stroke risk factors (which encompasses most patients with a mitral valve); recent (<3 months) stroke since valve implantation; or other high-risk events like prior post-procedure thromboembolism.[2]

The PERIOP2 trial randomized 1,471 patients with atrial fibrillation or mechanical heart valves to LMWH bridging or placebo.[7] Of note, all patients received pre-procedure LMWH bridging with therapeutic dose dalteparin (200 IU/kg) pre-procedure days −3 and −2 and half dose (100 IU/kg) on day −1. Randomization was done post-procedure, and the bridging arm received therapeutic dose dalteparin at least 12 hours post low bleeding risk procedures or prophylactic dose (dalteparin 5,000 IU) for high bleeding risk procedures; the no bridging group received placebo. In the 304 patients with mechanical valves, there was no difference in major thromboembolism (0 with no bridging, 1 with bridging) or major bleeding (3 with no bridging, 1 with bridging).[7]

A systematic review of observational cohort studies in VTE showed no difference in recurrent VTE with bridging versus no bridging (0.7% vs. 0.5%) and an increase in major bleeding for bridging versus no bridging (1.8% vs. 0.4%).[8]

Direct Oral Anticoagulants

Bridging parenteral anticoagulation is generally *not* required per ACC guidelines with the possible exception in patients with prolonged postoperative inability to take oral medications in whom a low-dose prophylactic LMWH regimen (not considered therapeutic-dose bridging *per se*) may be used.[3] Rivaroxaban and apixaban can be crushed and given via a nasogastric tube whereas dabigatran cannot.[3] In

TABLE 5-1. Bridging Guidelines[2,3]			
AMERICAN COLLEGE OF CHEST PHYSICIAN GUIDELINES			
RISK CATEGORY	HIGH	MODERATE	LOW
Mechanical heart valves	Mitral valve with major stroke risk factors: • Atrial fibrillation • Prior stroke/TIA • Prior valve thrombosis • Rheumatic heart disease • Hypertension • Diabetes • Congestive heart failure • Age >75 years	Mitral valve *without* major stroke risk factors Aortic valve *with* major stroke risk factors	Bileaflet aortic valve and no major stroke risk factors
Venous thromboembolism	Acute VTE within 3 months Severe thrombophilia Antiphospholipid antibodies High VTE risk active cancer	Acute VTE within 3–12 months Nonsevere thrombophilia Recurrent VTE Active cancer or recent history of cancer	Acute VTE more than 1 year ago
Atrial fibrillation	CHA_2DS_2VASC score >7 CHADS$_2$ score 5 or 6 Stroke or TIA within 3 months Rheumatic valvular heart disease	CHA_2DS_2VASC score 5 or 6 CHADS$_2$ score 3 or 4	CHA_2DS_2VASC score 1–4 CHADS$_2$ score 0, 1, or 2 and no prior stroke or TIA
Bridging	*Suggest bridging*	*Case by case decision*	*Suggest no bridging*
AMERICAN COLLEGE OF CARDIOLOGY			
Atrial fibrillation	CHA_2DS_2-VASc score ≥7 or Stroke, TIA, or systemic embolism within 3 months	CHA_2DS_2-VASc score 5 or 6 or Stroke or TIA within 3 months	CHA_2DS_2-VASc score ≤4 and no previous stroke, TIA, or systemic embolism
Bridging	*Bridging should be considered*	*Increase bleeding risk: no bridging* *Previous stroke, TIA, or systemic embolism: likely bridge* *No prior stroke, TIA, or systemic embolism: bridging not advised*	*No*

TIA, transient ischemic attack; VTE, venous thromboembolism.

TABLE 5-2. Sample Bridging Protocol

	INR	WARFARIN	PARENTERAL BRIDGING
Pre-procedure day 7	Check	If supra or subtherapeutic, adjust warfarin stop date accordingly	
Pre-procedure day 5		Stop warfarin in most cases	
Pre-procedure day 3			Begin bridging for most cases
Pre-procedure day 1	Check	If INR elevated, consider 1 mg of vitamin K and repeat on day of procedure	Last dose on morning prior to procedure
Day of procedure		Begin warfarin evening of procedure if hemostasis secure	
Post-procedure day 1	Check	Continue warfarin at pre-procedure dose	Reinitiate bridging for *low* bleeding risk procedures at approximately *24* hours
Post-procedure day 2	Check	Continue warfarin at pre-procedure dose	Reinitiate bridging for *high* bleeding risk procedures at approximately *48–72* hours
Post-procedure day 3	Check	Continue warfarin at pre-procedure dose	Reinitiate bridging for *high* bleeding risk procedures at approximately *48–72* hours
Post-procedure day 4 onward	Check	Continue warfarin at pre-procedure dose	Stop bridging when INR is therapeutic (no need for 2 days of overlap at therapeutic INR)

INR, international normalized ratio.

the PAUSE study, perioperative DOAC management did not include heparin bridging, but patients who had major surgery and were unable to take oral medications postoperatively were allowed to receive low-dose LMWH for 2–3 days after surgery, mainly to prevent VTE, until DOACs could be resumed. ACCP guidelines also suggest against bridging with DOAC interruption.

EMERGENT AND URGENT ORAL ANTICOAGULATION REVERSAL

In general, preprocedural anticoagulation reversal should be considered for procedures that need to be done within 24 hours. In patients taking warfarin, whose offset of action usually takes about 5 days, it is usually not possible to delay an urgent surgery/

procedure to allow the anticoagulant effect to recede unless the INR at presentation is already subtherapeutic (<2.0). In patients taking a DOAC, which have half-lives of approximately 9–14 hours (with normal renal function), delaying an urgent surgery/procedure for longer than 24 hours (longer than 48 hours if high bleeding risk), as was done in the PAUSE study for an elective surgery/procedure, may not be clinically acceptable.[2] Consequently, reversal agents for warfarin and DOACs should only be considered in such circumstances where delaying a procedure is not possible.[9]

Warfarin

In a randomized trial, patients on warfarin with an INR >2.0 who needed surgery or an invasive procedure within 24 hours were allocated to 4-factor prothrombin complex concentrate (4F-PCC) or fresh frozen plasma (FFP), and all patients received vitamin K. Doses of 4F-PCC ranged from 25 to 50 IU/kg (maximum 100 kg) and FFP from 10 to 15 mL/kg (maximum 100 kg) based on the INR. For an 80 kg patient, the dose of FFP was approximately 4–6 units. Effective hemostasis was better with 4F-PCC compared to FFP (90% vs. 75%, P = 0.01); superior for the proportion of patients with INR correction to <1.3 half an hour after infusion (55% vs. 10%, *P* < 0.01), and there was a trend toward earlier mean time to start of surgery after randomization for 4F-PCC (3.6 hours) compared to FFP (8.5 hours).[10]

Dabigatran

The Anticoagulation Forum suggests use of idarucizumab 5 g intravenously, and if not available, 50 units/kg of activated PCC.[9] Idarucizumab is a humanized monoclonal antibody to dabigatran approved by the U.S. Food and Drug Administration and was studied in the REVERSE-AD study.[11] Of the 503 patients studied, 202 needed an urgent procedure (others had bleeding). All patients were treated with 5 g of idarucizumab, and the mean time to procedure was 1.6 hours; 93.4% were assessed as normal and none with severally abnormal hemostasis. Thirty-day mortality was 12.6%.

Oral Factor Xa Inhibitors

The Anticoagulation Forum suggests andexanet alfa at the same dose used for major bleeding and, if not available, 2,000 units of 4F-PCC.[9] Andexanet alfa is a modified recombinant inactive form of factor Xa that acts as a decoy that binds to the anticoagulant and is U.S. Food and Drug Administration approved for reversal of bleeding. The ANNEXA 4 study included 352 patients with major bleeding on factor Xa inhibitor, and of note, no patients in need of urgent procedures were in the study. Hemostatic efficacy was judged to be excellent or good in 82% of patients.[12]

Reinitiation of Anticoagulation

An important caveat, thromboembolic complications were relatively high after reversal in the studies above, and anticoagulation should be resumed once hemostasis is secured post-procedure.

LABORATORY TESTS TO MEASURE DOAC LEVELS TO DETERMINE THE SAFETY OF PROCEEDING WITH A SURGERY OR INVASIVE PROCEDURE

A DOAC level of <30 ng/mL has traditionally been used to indicate non-important drug levels, but DOAC-specific assays are not widely available. ACCP suggests against routine DOAC testing to guide periprocedural management. Eight-five percent of patients in the PAUSE study had pre-procedure DOAC levels performed as well as the prothrombin time (PT) and activated partial thromboplastin time (aPTT). The traditional coagulation test of PT and aPTT had poor sensitivity and approximately 25% of apixaban patients and 10% of rivaroxaban patients had normal PT and aPTT when DOAC levels were above 30 ng/mL suggesting these tests are not valuable in ruling out important DOAC levels.[13]

Dabigatran (Direct Thrombin Inhibitor)

Although the aPTT has been considered to measure dabigatran levels, some aPTT assays are not sufficiently sensitive to detect dabigatran levels, and test results may be falsely normal. The thrombin time appears to be a reliable test to measure dabigatran levels. A normal thrombin time rules out clinically important levels of dabigatran, but it is exquisitely sensitive and may be elevated even in the presence of minimal, clinically unimportant dabigatran levels.[14]

Apixaban, Edoxaban, and Rivaroxaban (Factor Xa Inhibitors)

Although the PT or INR has been assessed for the measurement of rivaroxaban and apixaban levels, it is unreliable and not recommended for clinical use. Antifactor Xa assays, when calibrated for each oral factor Xa inhibitor, appear to be reliable tests but are not widely available and are not FDA approved. However, a normal anti-Xa assay that is used to titrate unfractionated heparin and to measure LMWH levels excludes clinically important drug levels.[14]

Clinical pearls

- Continue warfarin for most low-bleeding-risk procedures without interruption. In DOAC-treated patients, avoid taking the DOAC before the procedure to avoid a peak anticoagulant effect occurring at the time of the procedure; instead, delay that day's dose (once-daily DOACs) or skip the morning dose (twice-daily DOACs).

- For warfarin patients, check an INR 7 days before a procedure and hold 5 days prior for most patients. INRs higher than what the surgeon or proceduralist desire the day before can usually be corrected with 1 mg of oral vitamin K. Most patients with CrCl >25–30 mL/min on a DOAC should follow the PAUSE protocol.

- For most patients, restart warfarin the evening of an invasive procedure once hemostasis is secured and restart DOACs the next day for low and 48–72 hours later for high bleeding risk procedures.

- Parenteral anticoagulation bridging should be reserved for high thromboembolic risk patients with mechanical valves based primarily on the position, type, and additional stroke risk factors; atrial fibrillation patients with high CHA_2DS_2-VASc (≥ 7) scores, and VTE with a recent event. Bridging is not needed for DOAC interruption.

- PCC is superior to FFP for warfarin reversal, idarucizumab should be used to reverse dabigatran, and there are little data to guide Xa inhibitors, although andexanet alfa or PCC may be useful. Reinitiation of anticoagulation post-procedure should be addressed in all patients.

- A normal thrombin time for dabigatran and a normal anti-Xa assay for apixaban, edoxaban, and rivaroxaban exclude clinically important drug levels.

REFERENCES

1. Douketis JD, Spyropoulos AC, Duncan J, et al. Perioperative management of patients with atrial fibrillation receiving a direct oral anticoagulant. *JAMA Intern Med.* 2019;179:1469-1478. PMID: 31380891

2. Douketis JD, Spyropoulos AC, Murad MH, et al. Perioperative management of antithrombotic therapy: an American College of Chest Physicians clinical practice guideline. *Chest.* 2022 Nov;162(5):e207-e243. PMID: 35964704

3. Doherty JU, Gluckman TJ, Hucker WJ, et al. 2017 ACC expert consensus decision pathway for periprocedural management of anticoagulation in patients with nonvalvular atrial fibrillation: a report of the American College of Cardiology Clinical Expert Consensus Document Task Force. *J Am Coll Cardiol.* 2017;69:871-898. PMID: 28081965

4. Horlocker TT, Vandermeulen E, Kopp SL, et al. Regional anesthesia in the patient receiving antithrombotic or thrombolytic therapy: American Society of Regional Anesthesia and Pain Medicine evidence-based guidelines (fourth edition). *Reg Anesth Pain Med.* 2018;43:263-309. PMID: 29561531

5. Abraham NS, Barkun AN, Sauer BG, et al. American College of Gastroenterology-Canadian Association of Gastroenterology Clinical Practice Guideline: management of anticoagulants and antiplatelets during acute gastrointestinal bleeding and the periendoscopic period. *J Can Assoc Gastroenterol.* 2022 Mar 17;5(2):100-101. PMID: 35368325

6. Douketis JD, Spyropoulos AC, Kaatz S, et al. Perioperative bridging anticoagulation in patients with atrial fibrillation. *N Engl J Med.* 2015;373:823-833. PMID: 26095867

7. Kovacs MJ, Wells PS, Anderson DR, et al; PERIOP2 investigators. Postoperative low molecular weight heparin bridging treatment for patients at high risk of arterial thromboembolism (PERIOP2): double blind randomised controlled trial. *BMJ.* 2021 Jun 9;373:n1205. PMID: 34108229

8. Baumgartner C, de Kouchkovsky I, Whitaker E, et al. Periprocedural bridging in patients with venous thromboembolism: a systematic review. *Am J Med.* 2019 Jun;132(6):722-732.e7. PMID: 30659809

9. Cuker A, Burnett A, Triller D, et al. Reversal of direct oral anticoagulants: guidance from the Anticoagulation Forum. *Am J Hematol.* 2019;94:697-709. PMID: 30916798

10. Goldstein JN, Refaai MA, Milling TJ Jr, et al. Four-factor prothrombin complex concentrate versus plasma for rapid vitamin K antagonist reversal in patients needing urgent surgical or invasive interventions: a phase 3b, open-label, non-inferiority, randomised trial. *Lancet.* 2015;385:2077-2087. PMID: 25728933

11. Pollack CV Jr, Reilly PA, van Ryn J, et al. Idarucizumab for dabigatran reversal—full cohort analysis. *N Engl J Med.* 2017;377:431-441. PMID: 28693366

12. Connolly SJ, Crowther M, Eikelboom JW, et al. Full study report of andexanet alfa for bleeding associated with factor Xa inhibitors. *N Engl J Med.* 2019;380:1326-1335. PMID: 30730782

13. Shaw JR, Li N, Nixon J, Moffat KA, et al. Coagulation assays and direct oral anticoagulant levels among patients having an elective surgery or procedure. *J Thromb Haemost.* 2022 Dec;20(12):2953-2963. PMID: 36200348

14. Samuelson BT, Cuker A, Siegal DM, et al. Laboratory assessment of the anticoagulant activity of direct oral anticoagulants: a systematic review. *Chest.* 2017;151:127-138. PMID: 27637548

PROPHYLAXIS

Prevention of Venous Thromboembolism

Smita K. Kalra, MD, FACP, SFHM

COMMON CLINICAL QUESTIONS

1. What are the common risk factors for venous thromboembolism (VTE)?
2. Is aspirin a reasonable choice for VTE prophylaxis?
3. What do the guidelines suggest for VTE prevention after major surgery?
4. When should extended VTE prophylaxis be considered?

INTRODUCTION

Venous thromboembolism (VTE), which includes pulmonary embolism (PE) and deep venous thrombosis (DVT), is a serious and costly complication after surgery. It affects an estimated 300,000–600,000 individuals in the United States each year, causing considerable morbidity and mortality.[1] Approximately 25% of VTE occur in patients who have been hospitalized for surgery, and this number will likely be higher if silent VTE is included. Sudden death may be the initial presentation in a quarter of the patients with PE; therefore, prevention is the key.[1] Other potential consequences of VTE include recurrence, post-thrombotic syndrome, pulmonary hypertension, and right heart failure. Despite the availability of effective VTE prophylaxis, it remains underutilized in patients undergoing major surgical procedures.

All major surgeries increase the risk for the development of VTE, but the extent of that risk varies greatly across different types of surgeries. Careful preoperative assessment of patients, focusing on their risk for VTE, can help guide postoperative prophylaxis. Evidence-based guidelines from different societies provide support in relation to the timing of initiation, duration, and choice of prophylaxis. This chapter will focus on risk assessment and prevention of VTE based on recent guidelines.

PATIENT-RELATED RISK FACTORS

Virchow's triad describes three underlying mechanisms for the development of VTE—venous stasis, endothelial injury, and hypercoagulability. Patients undergoing surgery typically have several risk factors, such as immobility, malignancy, or prior VTE, that reflect these underlying processes. Table 6-1 provides a more extensive list of patient-related risk factors for VTE.

SURGERY-RELATED RISK FACTORS

Although the risk for postoperative VTE increases with an increasing number of patient-related risk factors, healthy patients are also at significant risk for VTE after certain surgical procedures. Major orthopedic surgeries are among the highest risk procedures for VTE. In general, major surgery refers to surgery

TABLE 6-1. Patient and Surgery-Specific Risk Factors for VTE

PATIENT-SPECIFIC RISK FACTORS	SURGERY-SPECIFIC RISK FACTORS
Increasing age	Hip and leg fracture
Obesity	Hip and knee arthroplasty
Prolonged immobility	Major trauma or polytrauma
Malignancy	Emergency surgery
Congestive heart failure (CHF)	Cancer-related major surgery
Personal history of VTE	Spinal surgery with >4-day immobilization
Family history of VTE	Arthroscopic surgery
Varicose veins	Major abdominal surgery
History of thrombophilia	
Presence of central line	
Stroke	
Pregnancy	
Spinal cord injury	

lasting longer than 45 minutes, and prolonged surgery refers to operative time of 2 hours or more. Many surgery-related factors contribute to the risk of VTE in non-orthopedic patients, including the extent and duration of surgery, intraoperative positioning, type of anesthesia, site of surgery, and postoperative mobility. Table 6-1 outlines these surgery-specific risk factors.

TOOLS TO ASSESS PERIOPERATIVE VTE RISK

There are a variety of score-based tools to assess the risk of VTE in hospitalized patients. The Caprini model classifies surgical patients into low, moderate, and high-risk groups based on a score from 20 risk factors obtained from the patient history (Tables 6-2 and 6-3). The 2012 American College of Chest Physicians (ACCP) guidelines for VTE prevention recommended using this tool for risk assessment in general surgery patients. A meta-analysis of over 14,000 patients in 2017 found that VTE risk varied from 0.7% to 10.7% among surgical patients who did or did not receive chemoprophylaxis, respectively.[2] Patients with higher Caprini scores had higher risk, and those with a score >7 had significant reduction in VTE risk after surgery with chemoprophylaxis.

The Rogers score was derived using data from the Patient Safety in Surgery (PSS) study and included patients undergoing general and vascular surgeries.[3] It uses type of surgery, ASA classification, cancer history, hematocrit, and need for transfusion among other variables for risk stratification. Other scoring systems available include IMPROVE, IMPROVEDD, and PADUA which are mainly utilized in hospitalized medical patients but have not been specifically evaluated in the surgical population. For patients in whom pharmacologic VTE prophylaxis is indicated, the risk for major bleeding should be assessed using the patient's baseline risk of bleeding and adding surgical risk to determine overall bleeding risk. Tables 6-4 and 6-5 show patient-specific and surgery-specific risk factors for bleeding.

SOCIETY GUIDELINES FOR VTE PROPHYLAXIS

Early mobilization after surgery remains a recommendation from various societal guidelines. Until recently

TABLE 6-2. Modified Caprini Scoring System[2,5]

1 POINT	2 POINTS	3 POINTS	5 POINTS
Age 41–60 years	Age 61–74 years	Age ≥75 years	Stroke (<1 month)
Minor surgery	Arthroscopic surgery	History of VTE	Elective arthroplasty
BMI ≥25 kg/m²	Major open surgery (>45 minutes)	Family history of VTE	Hip, pelvis, or leg fracture
Swollen legs	Laparoscopic surgery (>45 minutes)	Factor V Leiden	Acute spinal cord injury (<1 month)
Varicose veins	Malignancy	Prothrombin 20210A mutation	
Pregnancy or postpartum	Confined to bed rest (>72 hours)	Lupus anticoagulant	
Oral contraceptive or hormone replacement	Immobilizing plaster cast	Anticardiolipin antibodies	
History of recurrent or unexplained spontaneous abortions	Central venous access	Elevated serum homocysteine	
Sepsis (<1 month)		Heparin-induced thrombocytopenia	
Serious lung disease (<1 month)		Other congenital or acquired thrombophilia	
Abnormal pulmonary function			
Acute myocardial infarction			
Congestive heart failure (<1 month)			
History of inflammatory bowel disease			
Medical patient on bed rest			

BMI, body mass index; VTE, venous thromboembolism.

Reproduced with permission from Gould MK et al. Prevention of VTE in nonorthopedic surgical patients: Antithrombotic Therapy and Prevention of Thrombosis, 9th ed: American College of Chest Physicians Evidence-Based Clinical Practice Guidelines. *Chest.* 2012;141(2):e227S-e277S.

the most extensively used guidelines have been from the ACCP in 2012 making separate recommendations for VTE prevention in orthopedic surgery[4] and nonorthopedic surgery patients.[5] These guidelines are still useful but have been criticized for being too complex and lacking consensus on VTE risk assessment. In 2018, the National Institute for Health and Care Excellence (NICE) of the United Kingdom (UK) released their guideline for VTE prevention in hospitalized patients, and these were updated in 2019.[6] In the same year, the American Society of Hematology (ASH) released their guidelines on prevention of VTE in surgical hospitalized patients.[7] These guidelines largely align with the ACCP guidelines and are based on updated and original systematic reviews conducted by the authors. Broadly speaking, these guidelines

TABLE 6-3. Caprini Risk Score and Estimated VTE Events in Absence of Pharmacological or Mechanical Prophylaxis

SCORE	RISK	ESTIMATED VTE RISK IN ABSENCE OF PROPHYLAXIS (%)
0	Very low	
1–2	Low	1.5
3–4	Moderate	3.0
≥5	High	6.0

Reproduced with permission from Gould MK et al. Prevention of VTE in nonorthopedic surgical patients: antithrombotic therapy and prevention of thrombosis, 9th ed: American College of Chest Physicians Evidence-Based Clinical Practice Guidelines. *Chest.* 2012;141(2 Suppl):e227S-e277S.

TABLE 6-4. Patient and Procedure-Specific Bleeding Risk[5,16]

RISK FACTORS FOR MAJOR BLEEDING		
	PROCEDURE-SPECIFIC RISK FACTORS	
PATIENT-SPECIFIC RISK FACTORS	HIGH BLEEDING RISK (30-D RISK OF MAJOR BLEED >2%)	MINOR OR LOW BLEEDING RISK (30-D RISK OF MAJOR BLEED 0–2%)
Active bleeding	Major surgery with extensive tissue injury	Arthroscopy
Previous major bleeding (intracranial, gastrointestinal, or others requiring transfusion)	Cancer-related surgery, especially solid tumor resection	Cutaneous or lymph node biopsy
Recent use of antiplatelets, NSAIDs, or anticoagulants	Major orthopedic surgery including shoulder replacement surgery	Foot/hand surgery
Bleeding disorder	Urologic or gastrointestinal surgery especially anastomotic surgery	Coronary angiography
Thrombocytopenia (<50,000)	Transurethral prostate resection, bladder resection, or tumor ablation	Upper or lower GI endoscopy +/− biopsy
Severe hepatic or renal failure	Colonic polyp and bowel resection	Abdominal hysterectomy
Acute stroke	Endoscopic retrograde cholangiopancreatography (ERCP)	Laparoscopic cholecystectomy
Uncontrolled hypertension (BP >180 systolic and/or >120 diastolic)	Surgery or biopsy in highly vascular organs (kidney, liver, spleen)	Abdominal hernia repair
	Cardiac, intracranial, or spinal surgery	Epidural injections
	Reconstructive plastic surgery	Most ophthalmologic procedures
	Neuraxial anesthesia	Minor dental procedures
	Any major surgery (procedure duration >45 min)	Cardiac pacemaker/defibrillator device implantation
		Hemorrhoidal surgery
		Bronchoscopy +/− biopsy

TABLE 6-5. Summary of VTE Prophylaxis for Select Surgery Patients (based on ASH guidelines 2019)[7]

SURGICAL CATEGORY		RECOMMENDED PROPHYLAXIS
Orthopedic Surgery		
For THR and TKR		Aspirin or anticoagulants Add IPCs during hospitalization DOAC preferred over LMWH
Hip fracture repair		Anticoagulants (LMWH or UFH) Aspirin (as per ACCP guidelines 2012) Add IPCs during hospitalization
Major General Surgery		
Laparoscopic cholecystectomy	No VTE risk factors	No pharmacologic prophylaxis
	VTE risk factors*	Pharmacological prophylaxis (LMWH or UFH)
Major trauma	Low to moderate bleeding risk (see Table 6-4)	Anticoagulants (LMWH preferred over UFH) Add IPCs during hospitalization
	High bleeding risk (see Table 6-4)	IPCs alone
Other non-outpatient surgeries	No cancer, trauma, or HIT	UFH or LMWH Add IPCs during hospitalization
	Surgery for abdominopelvic cancer	UFH or LMWH Add IPCs during hospitalization. Extended prophylaxis with LMWH at discharge
	History of HIT	Fondaparinux
Neurosurgery		
Craniotomy, major spine surgery	Prolonged immobility with additional VTE risk factors	Pharmacological prophylaxis (LMWH preferred over UFH) Add IPCs during hospitalization
	No additional VTE risk factors	IPCs alone
Urological Surgery		
TURP	No additional VTE risk factors	IPCs alone
	VTE risk factors	LMWH or UFH Add IPCs during hospitalization
Radical prostatectomy	Laparoscopic or without lymph node dissection or no additional VTE risk factors	IPCs alone
	Extended lymph node dissection, open, or additional VTE risk factors	LMWH or UFH All IPCs during hospitalization
Cardiac or Major Vascular Surgery		LMWH or UFH with IPCs during hospitalization or IPCs alone
Major Gynecological Surgery		LMWH or UFH Add IPCs during hospitalization

*VTE risk factors, thrombophilia, previous VTE, or malignancy.

VTE, venous thromboembolism; THR, total hip replacement; TKR, total knee replacement; DOAC, direct oral anticoagulants; LMWH, low-molecular-weight heparin; UFH, unfractionated heparin; IPC, intermittent pneumatic compression; HIT, heparin induced thrombocytopenia.

Recommendations based on Anderson DR, et al. American Society of Hematology 2019 guidelines for management of venous thromboembolism: prevention of venous thromboembolism in surgical hospitalized patients. *Blood Adv.* 2019;3(23):3898-3944.

recommend using prophylaxis over no prophylaxis in patients undergoing major surgery. These guidelines also support a collaborative approach between clinicians and patients in choosing recommendations based on individual risk, values, and preferences. For patients undergoing major surgery, the guideline panel suggests using pharmacologic or mechanical prophylaxis. If pharmacologic prophylaxis cannot be administered, then mechanical prophylaxis is preferred over no prophylaxis. Depending on the risk of VTE and bleeding based on individual patient and type of surgery, the ASH guidelines favor combined pharmacologic and mechanical prophylaxis over pharmacologic or mechanical prophylaxis alone. For mechanical prophylaxis, they suggest using intermittent pneumatic compression (IPC) over graduated compression stockings. As in the ACCP guidelines, the ASH guidelines are further based on the type of surgery (Table 6-5).

An algorithm for assessing risk and choosing appropriate prophylaxis is shown in Figure 6-1.

Both the ACCP and ASH guidelines recommend against using inferior vena cava (IVC) filters for prophylaxis purposes. The ACCP guidelines separated orthopedic surgeries from other surgeries when making recommendations, whereas the ASH guidelines do not. Regarding the timing of prophylaxis initiation, there was no suggestion in the ACCP guidelines. The ASH panel arbitrarily chose 12 hours following surgery as the cut-off point between early and delayed postoperative administration of prophylaxis. There is no recommended preference between early versus delayed prophylaxis. One of the criticisms of the ASH guidelines is that the recommendations for mechanical prophylaxis are extrapolated from studies in orthopedic patients and may not be applicable to all other surgeries.

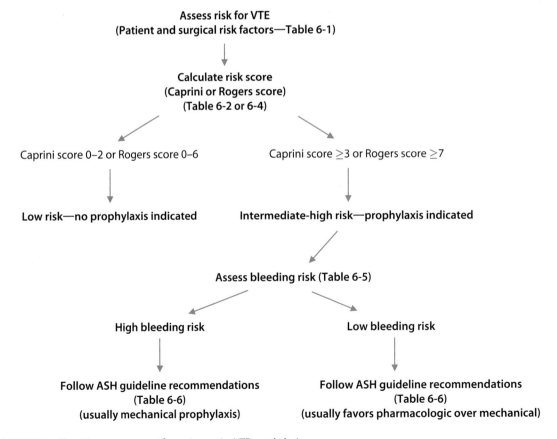

Assess risk for VTE
(Patient and surgical risk factors—Table 6-1)

Calculate risk score
(Caprini or Rogers score)
(Table 6-2 or 6-4)

Caprini score 0–2 or Rogers score 0–6

Caprini score ≥3 or Rogers score ≥7

Low risk—no prophylaxis indicated

Intermediate-high risk—prophylaxis indicated

Assess bleeding risk (Table 6-5)

High bleeding risk

Low bleeding risk

Follow ASH guideline recommendations
(Table 6-6)
(usually mechanical prophylaxis)

Follow ASH guideline recommendations
(Table 6-6)
(usually favors pharmacologic over mechanical)

FIGURE 6-1. Algorithm—assessment for perioperative VTE prophylaxis.

Pharmacological Options for VTE Prophylaxis in Surgical Patients

Choices for pharmacologic prophylaxis include the following.

Aspirin (ASA). Aspirin use has been validated mainly in the orthopedic surgical population and is recommended for use after hip and knee arthroplasty for VTE prophylaxis in the ASH guidelines.[7] The typical dosage prescribed in the United States is 81–162 mg daily. In patients with additional VTE risk factors or contraindications to ASA, use of an anticoagulant is recommended. It should, however, be noted that in major trials comparing ASA with low-molecular-weight heparin (LMWH)[8] or DOAC,[9] both groups received an initial period of anticoagulation for 5 or 10 days.[8,9] In contrast to ASH guidelines, NICE guidelines do not recommend aspirin for VTE prevention in hip fracture and recommend aspirin in elective hip replacement after 10 days of LMWH. For elective knee replacement, they recommend aspirin as an option for total duration of 14 days. Since publication of these guidelines, the CRISTAL study found that aspirin was associated with significantly more symptomatic VTE but no difference in mortality compared with enoxaparin in patients undergoing TKA or THA. In the PREVENT CLOT study in patients with a fracture, aspirin was found to be noninferior to enoxaparin for preventing death, had a low incidence of VTE, PE, and mortality, and no difference in bleeding.[6,10,11]

Unfractionated Heparin (UFH). Low-dose heparin is an inexpensive and effective thromboprophylaxis agent that works by inactivating thrombin, thereby preventing conversion of fibrinogen to fibrin. It is specifically useful in patients with low creatinine clearance (CrCl). Platelet count should be monitored due to its risk for heparin-induced thrombocytopenia (HIT). Dosing recommendation is 5,000 units subcutaneous (s.c.) two or three times daily. No dosing adjustments are needed for renal patients. Although easier to administer during hospitalization, multiple daily injections at home are not practical leading to preferential use of LMWH at discharge.

Low-Molecular-Weight Heparin. LMWHs work by binding to antithrombin which then inhibits Factor Xa. Unlike heparin, LMWH inhibits thrombin (Factor IIa) to a much lesser degree; therefore the ratio of Factor Xa:Factor IIa inhibition is variable compared to 1:1 inhibition ratio of UFH. Although LMWH is less likely to cause HIT than UFH, it is contraindicated in patients with HIT. The two commonly available anti coagulants in this class are enoxaparin and dalteparin. Tinzaparin is used infrequently. These drugs are renally excreted, dosing is based on CrCl, and they need dose adjustment and monitoring in patients with CrCl <30 mL/min. Typical dosage for enoxaparin is 30 mg s.c. twice daily if started postoperatively (North American protocol) or 40 mg s.c. once daily if started preoperatively (European protocol) for hip arthroplasty. The usual dose is 40 mg once daily for other surgical patients. Dalteparin dosage is 5,000 units s.c. daily. The safety and efficacy of these agents in patients with high body mass index (BMI) >40 kg/m² remains an area of controversy. Certain practice recommendations have suggested empirically increasing the dose of LMWH prophylaxis by 30% in patients with BMI >40 kg/m². Published literature in high quality bariatric studies lacks consensus on the exact dosing of LMWH in bariatric surgery patients who are at least at moderate risk for VTE. The most updated position statement from the American Society for Metabolic and Bariatric Surgery (ASMBS) in 2022 recommends either fixed LMWH dosing or BMI or weight-tiered dosing based on anti-Factor Xa (AFXa) activity level. However, target AFXa activity levels are also not supported by high level data but peak concentrations of 0.2–0.4 IU/mL for VTE prophylaxis measured 4 hours after administration of the third dose of LMWH have been suggested.[12] A Cochrane analysis of randomized controlled trials of LMWH and UFH in cancer patients undergoing surgery found no benefit or harm of LMWH over UFH in mortality, PE, DVT, or major bleeding,[13] but the ASH guidelines for VTE prevention in cancer patients made a conditional recommendation suggesting using LMWH or fondaparinux over UFH.[14]

Fondaparinux. This is a Factor Xa inhibitor and is an alternative to UFH/LMWH when they are contraindicated due to HIT. The dose is 2.5 mg s.c. once daily, initiated 6–8 hours after skin closure postoperatively. Like LMWH, fondaparinux is also renally excreted and used with caution if CrCl is 30–50 mL/min but contraindicated in patients with CrCl <30 mL/min. There is evidence of superiority of fondaparinux over LMWH but at the cost of increased major bleeding.[15]

Direct Oral Anticoagulants (DOACs). DOACs include direct thrombin inhibitors (dabigatran) and direct Factor Xa inhibitors (apixaban, rivaroxaban, edoxaban). In the ASH guidelines, DOACs are preferred over LMWH for VTE prophylaxis in both hip and knee arthroplasty patients. Apixaban, rivaroxaban, and dabigatran are currently the only DOACs FDA-approved for prophylaxis in hip (THA) and knee replacement (TKA) surgery—edoxaban is not. The NICE 2019 guideline also recommends apixaban, rivaroxaban, dabigatran as an option for VTE prevention after THA or TKA but unlike ASH guidelines, they do not have a preferential recommendation of DOACs over LMWH.[6] Taken orally, DOACs have a rapid onset of action and do not need laboratory monitoring. Dabigatran is 85% renally excreted and is contraindicated when CrCl is <30 mL/min. Dose reduction for apixaban, rivaroxaban, and edoxaban is recommended with declining renal function, but they are not contraindicated unless CrCl is <15 mL/min. Dabigatran and rivaroxaban can cross the placenta, but there is limited evidence with apixaban and edoxaban. DOACs should therefore be avoided in pregnant and breastfeeding women. Although DOACs do not have multiple drug interactions like warfarin, hepatic enzyme CYP34 inducers can affect the concentration of rivaroxaban and apixaban. Similarly, all DOACs are substrates for p-glycoprotein transporter, and levels can be affected by medications affecting this pathway. Table 6-6 gives dosing recommendations for currently approved DOACs for VTE prophylaxis. Like LMWH, DOAC use in patients with high BMI (>40 kg/m^2) also remains an area of controversy. Updated position statement from the International Society of Thrombosis and Hemostasis (ISTH) suggests standard dosing of rivaroxaban and apixaban for VTE prevention regardless of weight or BMI, and suggests not to use dabigatran or edoxaban for VTE prevention in patients with BMI >40 kg/m^2 due to lack of convincing data.[16] In a randomized trial of rivaroxaban in bariatric surgery patients with average BMI >40, once-daily VTE prophylaxis with 10 mg of rivaroxaban was effective and safe in the early postoperative phase after in both the short (7 days) and long (28 days) prophylaxis groups.[17]

Additionally, due to their mechanism of absorption, dabigatran and edoxaban are also not recommended with enteral feeding tubes, whereas rivaroxaban and apixaban are recommended with enteral feeding tubes if terminated in the stomach. The ISTH guidelines do not recommend using DOACs for bariatric surgery patients.[16]

Warfarin. This is one of the oldest known oral anticoagulants and works by inhibiting the vitamin K-dependent pathway of synthesis of clotting factors (II, VII, IX, X, as well as proteins C and S). It is inexpensive and widely available, but it has a narrow therapeutic range, requires monitoring with an INR, and has multiple drug and food interactions. With the introduction of DOACs, its use has declined, but it is still useful in patients who cannot afford DOACs or in whom impaired renal function prohibits use of DOACs. It can take up to 5 days for patients to have a therapeutic level, and during this time, they will be at risk for VTE and may need additional prophylaxis with UFH, LMWH, or IPCs.

Indications for Extended VTE Prophylaxis

Based on the type of surgery and underlying disease state, the risk for VTE can last up to 12 weeks postoperatively. The ASH guidelines defined extended

TABLE 6-6. Prophylactic Dosing Recommendation for THA/TKA for Available DOACs

DOAC	BRAND NAME	PROPHYLACTIC DOSE	RENAL DOSE ADJUSTMENT
Dabigatran	Pradaxa	110 mg initially followed by 220 mg daily	Contraindicated with CrCl <30 mL/min
Apixaban	Eliquis	2.5 mg twice daily	Caution with CrCl <15 mL/min
Rivaroxaban	Xarelto	10 mg once daily	Avoid use if CrCl <15 mL/min
Edoxaban	Savaysa, Lixiana	Not FDA-approved for this indication	

prophylaxis as greater than 3 weeks and short-term prophylaxis as less than 2 weeks and suggested using extended prophylaxis over short-term prophylaxis for major surgeries but with low certainty of evidence. Their literature review found no difference in mortality but a small reduction in symptomatic VTE. The panel felt that extended VTE prophylaxis was cost-effective but also acknowledged that most studies are in high-risk patients (those undergoing knee or hip arthroplasty, hip fracture repair, and cancer-related major surgeries).[9] Patients with additional risk factors and previous history of VTE may also benefit from extended prophylaxis, but surgery-specific bleeding risk[18] needs to be considered in a risk-benefit discussion between the patient and care team. Optimal duration of extended VTE prophylaxis remains uncertain. ACCP guidelines from 2012 recommended extended prophylaxis for up to 35 days for hip and knee arthroplasty and hip fracture repair surgeries.[4] The most recent ASH guidelines do not specify duration of extended prophylaxis for major orthopedic surgeries, but the UK NICE guidelines recommend 14 days for TKA and 28 days for THA.[6] Furthermore, a recommendation for up to 30 days of prophylaxis in cancer-related major abdominal and pelvic surgeries is supported in current guidelines.[14]

CONCLUSION

Surgical patients are at high risk for VTE, and the burden of disease remains high in this population. Careful assessment of VTE risk preoperatively can help formulate a plan for the choice and duration of prophylaxis. Patient-specific risk factors and surgery-associated risk factors should be considered when making recommendations for prophylaxis. When initiating pharmacologic prophylaxis, the risk of bleeding should be assessed daily. Combined pharmacologic and mechanical prophylaxis should be used in all major surgeries whenever possible. Assessment for appropriate duration of prophylaxis should be made keeping patient and procedural characteristics in mind. Lastly, effective prophylaxis relies on effective communication and collaboration between the care team members. Therefore, shared decision making between patients and providers can help provide the best prevention method keeping in mind the evidence and patient's preference.

Clinical pearls

- Use the Caprini or Rogers score to assess risk for VTE.

- For patients at moderate to high risk, VTE prophylaxis is indicated. In general, pharmacologic prophylaxis is preferred to mechanical prophylaxis unless bleeding risk is elevated.

- For patients at high risk for VTE, combined pharmacologic and mechanical prophylaxis (IPCs) is favored over mechanical prophylaxis alone.

- In patients undergoing neuraxial (spinal or epidural) anesthesia or with an epidural catheter for analgesia, precautions should be taken to avoid a potential complication of spinal hematoma. The American Society of Regional Anesthesia (ASRA) recommends delaying initiation of LMWH until 4 hours after catheter removal. LMWH (twice-daily dosing), fondaparinux, and DOACs are contraindicated while the catheter is in place.

- Patients undergoing major neurosurgical procedures are expected to receive mechanical prophylaxis (IPCs), but pharmacologic prophylaxis may be warranted after adequate hemostasis in patients with prolonged immobility or additional VTE risk.

- Consider extended-duration prophylaxis for patients after total hip or knee arthroplasty, hip fracture surgery, and major abdominal-pelvic surgery for cancer.

REFERENCES

1. Beckman MG, Hooper WC, Critchley SE, Ortel TL. Venous thromboembolism: a public health concern. *Am J Prev Med*. 2010;38(4 Suppl):S495-S501. PMID: 20331949

2. Pannucci CJ, Swistun L, MacDonald JK, Henke PK, Brooke BS. Individualized venous thromboembolism risk stratification using the 2005 Caprini score to identify the benefits and harms of chemoprophylaxis in surgical patients: a meta-analysis. *Ann Surg*. 2017;265(6):1094-1103. PMID: 28106607

3. Rogers SO Jr, Kilaru RK, Hosokawa P, Henderson WG, Zinner MJ, Khuri SF. Multivariable predictors of

postoperative venous thromboembolic events after general and vascular surgery: results from the patient safety in surgery study. *J Am Coll Surg.* 2007;204(6):1211-1221. PMID: 17544079

4. Falck-Ytter Y, Francis CW, Johanson NA, et al. Prevention of VTE in orthopedic surgery patients: antithrombotic therapy and prevention of thrombosis, 9th ed: American College of Chest Physicians Evidence-Based Clinical Practice Guidelines. *Chest.* 2012;141 (2 Suppl):e278S-e325S. PMID: 22315265

5. Gould MK, Garcia DA, Wren SM, et al. Prevention of VTE in nonorthopedic surgical patients: antithrombotic therapy and prevention of thrombosis, 9th ed: American College of Chest Physicians Evidence-Based Clinical Practice Guidelines. *Chest.* 2012;141(2 Suppl):e227S-e277S. PMID: 22315263

6. (NICE) NIfHaCE. *Venous thromboembolism in over 16s: reducing the risk of hospital-acquired deep vein thrombosis or pulmonary embolism.* Vol Nice Guideline No. 89. London: NICE; 2019.

7. Anderson DR, Morgano GP, Bennett C, et al. American Society of Hematology 2019 guidelines for management of venous thromboembolism: prevention of venous thromboembolism in surgical hospitalized patients. *Blood Adv.* 2019;3(23):3898-3944. PMID: 31794602

8. Anderson DR, Dunbar MJ, Bohm ER, et al. Aspirin versus low-molecular-weight heparin for extended venous thromboembolism prophylaxis after total hip arthroplasty: a randomized trial. *Ann Intern Med.* 2013;158(11):800-806. PMID: 23732713

9. Anderson DR, Dunbar M, Murnaghan J, et al. Aspirin or rivaroxaban for VTE prophylaxis after hip or knee arthroplasty. *N Engl J Med.* 2018;378(8):699-707. PMID: 29466159

10. CRISTAL Study Group; Sidhu VS, Kelly T-L, Pratt N, et al. Effect of Aspirin vs Enoxaparin on 90-Day Mortality in Patients Undergoing Hip or Knee Arthroplasty: A Secondary Analysis of the CRISTAL Cluster Randomized Trial. *JAMA Newn Open.* 2023;1(6):e2317838. PMID: 37294566

11. Major Extremity Trauma Research Consortium (METRC); O'Toole RV, Stein DM, O'Hara NN, et al. Aspirin or Low-Molecular-Weight Heparin for Thromboprophylaxis after a Fracture. *N Engl J Med.* 2023 Jan 19;388(3):203-213. PMID: 36652352

12. Aminian A, Vosburg RW, Altieri MS, et al. The American Society for Metabolic and Bariatric Surgery (ASMBS) updated position statement on perioperative venous thromboembolism prophylaxis in bariatric surgery. *Surg Obes Relat Dis.* 2022;18(2):165-174. PMID: 34896011

13. Matar CF, Kahale LA, Hakoum MB, et al. Anticoagulation for perioperative thromboprophylaxis in people with cancer. *Cochrane Database Syst Rev.* 2018;7(7):CD009447. PMID: 29993117

14. Lyman GH, Carrier M, Ay C, et al. American Society of Hematology 2021 guidelines for management of venous thromboembolism: prevention and treatment in patients with cancer. *Blood Adv.* 2021;5(4):927-974. PMID: 33570602

15. Kumar A, Talwar A, Farley JF, et al. Fondaparinux sodium compared with low-molecular-weight heparins for perioperative surgical thromboprophylaxis: a systematic review and meta-analysis. *J Am Heart Assoc.* 2019;8(10):e012184. PMID: 31070069

16. Martin KA, Beyer-Westendorf J, Davidson BL, et al. Use of direct oral anticoagulants in patients with obesity for treatment and prevention of venous thromboembolism: updated communication from the ISTH SSC Subcommittee on Control of Anticoagulation. *J Thromb Haemost.* 2021;19(8):1874-1882. PMID: 34259389

17. Kroll D, Nett PC, Rommers N, et al. Efficacy and safety of rivaroxaban for postoperative thromboprophylaxis in patients after bariatric surgery: a randomized clinical trial. *JAMA Netw Open.* 2023;6(5):e2315241. PMID: 37227726

18. Spyropoulos AC, Brohi K, Caprini J, et al. Scientific and Standardization Committee Communication: guidance document on the periprocedural management of patients on chronic oral anticoagulant therapy: recommendations for standardized reporting of procedural/surgical bleed risk and patient-specific thromboembolic risk. *J Thromb Haemost.* 2019;17(11):1966-1972. PMID: 31436045

7

Prevention of Surgical Site Infections

J. Njeri Wainaina, MD, FACP, FHM, FIDSA

COMMON CLINICAL QUESTIONS

1. What factors contribute to patients' risk for surgical site infections (SSIs)?
2. What can be done preoperatively to minimize patient-related risk for SSIs?
3. How can procedural SSI risk factors be mitigated?

INTRODUCTION

As recently as the early 20th century, infection after surgery and related mortality was considered nearly inevitable. With increasing acceptance of microbes as the cause of infection, the importance of antisepsis around surgical procedures, and increasing availability of antibiotics to treat postoperative infections and later for prophylaxis, the rate of infections related to surgery has dropped dramatically. However, surgical site infections (SSIs) still contribute substantially to morbidity and mortality. It is estimated that 0.5–3%[1] of hospital inpatients undergoing surgery will suffer a surgical wound infection. The Center for Disease Control's (CDC) National Health Safety Network (NHSN) 2022 Healthcare Acquired Infection (HAI) progress report found a 4% increase across all reported operative procedure categories compared to the previous year.[2]

As the most common category of nosocomial infections, SSIs account for 20% of hospital-acquired infections and confer a 2- to 11-fold increase in mortality with 75% of SSI-related deaths directly attributable to the infection. In addition, SSIs prolong the length of stay by an average of 9.7 days, increase overall cost by over $20,000 per hospitalization, and trigger more than 900,000 readmissions costing another $700 million.[3] To facilitate surveillance of postsurgical infections that allows comparison and benchmarking, the Centers for Disease Control and Prevention's NHSN defines SSI as infection related to an operative procedure that occurs at or deep to the surgical incision (incisional, deep, or organ space) within 30–90 days of the procedure.[2] Clinical criteria are summarized in Table 7-1.

GENERAL CONCEPTS BEHIND PREVENTION OF SURGICAL SITE INFECTIONS

Bacterial contamination through surgical wounds is ubiquitous and is thought to originate from the patient's normal flora. Other sources such as contaminated instruments, airborne organisms, hematogenous spread from other infections, and operating room staff have also been reported but are difficult to trace outside of targeted outbreak investigations. Whether contamination leads to infection or not is influenced by the interplay of host, procedure, and operating environmental factors with microbial virulence and load. Factors that predispose the development of SSIs can be categorized as procedure-related or intrinsic to the patient. Procedural factors can exist during the pre-, intra-, or postoperative phases of care.

TABLE 7-1. Clinical Criteria for Defining Surgical Site Infections

SURGICAL SITE INFECTION (SSI) CLASS	DEFINITION
Superficial incisional SSI	Occurs within 30 days of surgery
AND	Involves only skin and subcutaneous tissues
AND at least one of the following	Purulent drainage from incision
OR	Organism(s) identified from an aseptically collected specimen obtained for diagnosis
OR	Evidence of inflammation at incision site AND
	Incision deliberately opened to evaluate or treat AND
	No microbiological testing performed
OR	Diagnosis by a clinician
Deep incisional SSI	Occurs within 30 or 90 days of surgery
AND	Involves deep soft tissues
AND at least one of the following	Purulent drainage from incision
OR	Spontaneous dehiscence or deliberate aspiration or opening of incision AND
	Organism(s) identified from a specimen obtained for diagnosis AND
	Patient has either localized pain or tenderness or fever (>100.4°F)
OR	Abscess or other evidence of infection at the surgical site detected on clinical examination, imaging or histopathological evaluation
Organ/Space SSI	Occurs within 30 or 90 days of surgery
AND	Involves any part of the body deeper than fascial or muscle layers manipulated during the surgical procedure
AND at least one of the following	Purulent drainage from a drain OR
	Organism(s) identified from a specimen obtained for diagnosis OR
	Abscess or other evidence of infection at the surgical site detected on clinical examination, imaging, or histopathological evaluation
AND	Meets criteria for the specific surgical site

Data from CDC National and State Healthcare-Associated Infections Progress Report, published November 2023. Available from https://www.cdc.gov/hai/data/portal/progress-report.html. Accessed January 27, 2024.

Identification of modifiable risk factors prior to surgery allows for mitigation to reduce the surgical patient's risk of infectious complications (Table 7-2).

Risk modification strategies can be grouped into measures that diminish bacterial wound inoculation and those that augment the patient's ability to contain any invading organisms (Table 7-3).

PREOPERATIVE ANTIBIOTIC PROPHYLAXIS (SEE ALGORITHM IN FIGURE 7-1)

The National Academy of Sciences and National Research Council surgical wound classification system stratifies surgical incisions based on the expected degree of microbial contamination and has been widely adopted as one of the predictors of SSI risk (Table 7-4).

Hundreds of trials conducted by numerous investigators involving multiple kinds of surgery in varying settings around the world have firmly established the effectiveness of antibiotic prophylaxis in clean and clean-contaminated procedures.[4] On this basis, the 2022 update of recommendations for SSI prevention developed collaboratively by the Society of Healthcare Epidemiology of America (SHEA), Infectious Diseases Society of America (IDSA), and Association for Professionals in Infection Control (APIC), with contributions from the American Hospital Association

(AHA), the Joint Commission (JC) along with multiple organizations and societies with content expertise, listed administration of antimicrobial prophylaxis according to evidence-based standards and guidelines as the first of essential practices with high-quality evidence.[5] Antibiotics used for dirty or infected wounds are considered part of treatment, not prophylaxis, and care should be taken to ensure that surgical procedures do not interfere with the prescribed antibiotic schedule.

Selection of Antibiotics for Prophylaxis

Surgical wound contamination is thought to occur predominantly from direct entry of commensals found at the surgical site. The choice of antibiotic for surgical prophylaxis should be based on the expected susceptibility profile of predominant endogenous flora at the surgical site, available data on common wound infection pathogens, the ability of the agent to achieve adequate concentrations at the surgical site, and patient allergies (Table 7-5).

Due to a combination of appropriate antibacterial spectrum, favorable pharmacokinetics, safety, and low cost, first- and second-generation cephalosporins are the most common agents used. However, with the emergence of antibiotic-resistant strains of various bacteria, multidrug-resistant organisms (MDROs) are becoming increasingly prevalent causes of nosocomial infections including SSIs. This makes knowledge

TABLE 7-2. Risk Factors for Surgical Site Infections		
HOST FACTORS	**PROCEDURAL FACTORS**	**ENVIRONMENTAL FACTORS**
Obesity	Unnecessary hair removal	Suboptimal operating room ventilation
Tobacco use	Hair removal using a razor	High operating room traffic
Peripheral vascular disease	Inadequate perioperative skin antisepsis	
Concurrent steroid use of other immunocompromising condition	Incorrect prophylactic antibiotic selection, dosing, and/or timing	
Prior site irradiation	Perioperative hypothermia	
Staphylococcus aureus carriage	Perioperative hypoxia	
ASA class	Breach in sterile technique	
Perioperative hyperglycemia	Prolonged procedure duration	

TABLE 7-3. Essential Practices for Surgical Site Infection Prevention

DIMINISHING BACTERIAL WOUND INOCULATION

PREOPERATIVE	INTRAOPERATIVE AND POSTOPERATIVE
S. aureus decolonization before orthopedic and cardiothoracic surgery. Consider other procedures at high SSI risk	Immediately before incision, prepare skin using combined alcohol-antiseptic agents
Preoperative skin preparation with chlorhexidine	Isolate clean from contaminated surgical fields
Avoid hair removal at the surgical site. If necessary, wait until the day of surgery and use clippers	Minimize immediate use of steam sterilization for surgical instruments and implants
Appropriately selected and timed antibiotics. Add oral antibiotics and vaginal antiseptics for qualifying colorectal and gynecological procedures	Use plastic wound protectors for gastrointestinal and biliary tract surgery. Consider use of negative pressure dressings
	Minimize operating room traffic
	Redose antibiotics on time when appropriate

AUGMENTING HOST CONTAINMENT OF CONTAMINATING BACTERIA

PREOPERATIVE	INTRAOPERATIVE AND POSTOPERATIVE
Resolve malnutrition	Minimize dead space, devitalized tissue, and hematomas
Discontinue tobacco use 30 days before surgery	Perform intraoperative antiseptic lavage
Optimize diabetes control	For procedures not requiring hypothermia, maintain normothermia
Optimize dental/oral hygiene	Avoid perioperative hyperglycemia
	Maintain adequate nutrition and hydration

Adapted from Seidlman JL, Mantyh CR, Anderson DJ. Surgical Site Infection Prevention. *JAMA*. 2023; 329(3):244-252.

of local susceptibility profiles and known patterns of surgical wound infection key to designing surgical prophylaxis regimens that are locally relevant.

Penicillin Allergy

Approximately 10–15% of hospitalized patients report a penicillin allergy, but the label is inappropriate 90% of the time because it is inaccurate or has waned with time. This is consequential as it leads to use of second-line antibiotics that, despite often being more costly, are less efficacious and more hazardous. In the context of surgery, use of alternative antibiotics for surgical prophylaxis has been demonstrated to be associated with a higher SSI risk.[6] The most common reason for avoidance of non-beta-lactam antibiotics is a penicillin allergy label. As immediate hypersensitivity reactions to cephalosporins are determined by the R1 and R2 sidechains, not the beta-lactam ring, 97% of patients with skin-testing proven type 1 hypersensitivity reactions to penicillin will tolerate cephalosporins. The 2022 drug allergy practice parameter update authored by subject matter experts from and jointly authorized by the American Academy of Allergy, Asthma, and Immunology (AAAAI) and the American College of Allergy, Asthma, and Immunology (ACAAI) recommends routine use of a dissimilar cephalosporin in a patient

Algorithm for Surgical Site Infection Prophylaxis

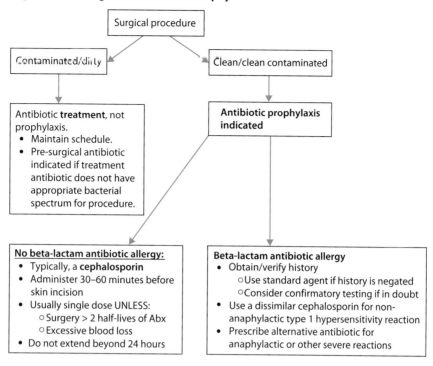

FIGURE 7-1. Algorithm for surgical site infection prophylaxis.

TABLE 7-4. Surgical Wound Classification		
WOUND CLASS	DESCRIPTION	SSI RISK
Class I	Uninfected, primarily closed	1.3–2.9%
Clean	No entry into the respiratory, gastrointestinal, urinary, or genital tract	
Class II Clean-contaminated	With entry into the respiratory, gastrointestinal, urinary, or genital tract under controlled conditions and without unusual contamination. Includes operations involving the oropharynx, biliary tract, appendix, and vagina provided there is no evidence of infection or major break in technique	2.4–7.7%
Class III	Open, fresh accidental wounds	
Contaminated	Operations with major breaks in sterile technique in which acute, nonpurulent inflammation is encountered	6.4–15.2%
Class IV	Old traumatic wound with retained devitalized tissue	
Dirty-infected	Wounds that involve pre-existing clinical infection or perforated viscera	7.1–40.0%

Adapted from Mangram AJ, Horan TC, Pearson ML, et al. Guideline for prevention of surgical site infection, 1999. Hospital infection control practices advisory committee. *Infect Control Hosp Epidemiol.* 1999; 20:250-278.

TABLE 7-5. Organisms That Cause Surgical Site Infections

SITE	ORGANISM
Abdominal	*Escherichia coli, Enterococcus faecalis, Staphylococcus aureus*
Breast	*S. aureus, Pseudomonas aeruginosa*
Cardiac	*S. aureus,* coagulase-negative Staphylococci
Kidney	*S. aureus, E. coli*
Neck	*S. aureus,* coagulase-negative Staphylococci
Neurological	*S. aureus,* coagulase-negative Staphylococci
Ob/Gyn	*S. aureus, E. coli*
Orthopedic	*S. aureus,* coagulase-negative Staphylococci
Prostate	*S. aureus, E. coli*
Transplant	Coagulase-negative Staphylococci, *Enterococcus faecium, E. coli*
Vascular	*S. aureus*

with a non-anaphylactic penicillin allergy reaction.[7] Penicillin allergies should be clarified by history to identify anaphylactic reactions and severe non-type 1 hypersensitivity reactions as either would contraindicate use of cephalosporins unless they have undergone a successful challenge in the past.[8] Penicillin skin testing can provide a definitive verdict for some patients. If the necessary resources are available, this can be safely carried out in a preoperative clinic.[9] Inaccurate labels should be removed or corrected as appropriate, and updated information should be conveyed to a member of the surgical team.

Timing of Antibiotic Prophylaxis

One of the key aspects of successful perioperative antimicrobial prophylaxis is ensuring blood and tissue antibiotic concentrations are maintained above the minimum inhibitory concentration (MIC) of expected pathogens while the surgical wound is open. The factors necessary to accomplish this include appropriate dosing for weight, timing that takes into consideration infusion time and specific pharmacokinetics, and duration of surgery. Cephalosporins and other beta-lactam agents have a short infusion time and achieve target tissue levels rapidly; thus, these should be administered within 60 minutes of incision. Antibiotics with a longer infusion time such as vancomycin should be given within 120 minutes of incision. All antibiotics should be redosed if surgery extends longer than two half-lives of the antibiotic used and if blood loss is excessive (>1,500 mL). Antibiotics are not necessary after wound closure as no benefit has been found and there is potential harm from increased risk of *Clostridioides difficile* infection and contributing to antimicrobial resistance. Clinical practice guidelines for antimicrobial prophylaxis in surgery have been published jointly by the American Society of Healthcare Pharmacists (ASHP), IDSA, Surgical Infection Society (SIS), and SHEA.[10]

IMPORTANT PREOPERATIVE NONANTIBIOTIC MEASURES FOR PREVENTION OF SURGICAL SITE INFECTIONS

Nutritional Status Optimization

Multiple studies have shown obesity to be an independent risk factor with incremental impact on the risk of SSIs in all age groups and across several surgery types, especially neurosurgical, cardiac, colorectal, obstetric, gynecologic, orthopedic, and transplant procedures.[11,12] This is attributed to greater technical difficulty, longer procedure time, greater surgical blood loss, and poorer wound healing in comparison to nonobese patients. While the ideal BMI for avoidance of SSIs is not clearly defined in literature, weight loss to the normal BMI range prior to major surgery should be considered where possible.

Malnutrition is the central component of frailty and is an established risk factor for postoperative morbidity and mortality due to reduced physiological reserve. Protein-calorie and micronutrient deficiencies adversely alter the gut microbiome and depress host immunity, making patients more susceptible to infection. This is magnified postoperatively as surgery induces an inflammatory response and catabolic state with negative nitrogen balance. Underweight patients may benefit from enhanced nutrition starting prior to planned surgery.[4,5]

Glycemic Control

Diabetes contributes to SSIs by way of accompanying neuropathy and vasculopathy that delay wound healing. Poorly controlled disease carries a higher risk for SSIs, and while the definition of optimal control is not strictly defined, several studies have suggested that glycosylated hemoglobin (A1c) levels above 7% or 8% may correlate with a higher SSI rate.[13]

More important is postoperative glycemic control in both diabetic and nondiabetic patients as established by the landmark study in patients undergoing cardiothoracic surgery that showed hyperglycemia defined as serum glucose >200 mg/dL 48 hours after surgery was associated with a 102% increase in SSIs.[14] Similar outcomes have been replicated in studies of patients undergoing noncardiac surgery.[15] It is therefore imperative to identify diabetes and risk for hyperglycemia before surgery and proactively develop a strategy for perioperative glucose management.

Smoking Cessation

Smoking during the perioperative period is associated with delayed wound healing, SSIs, nosocomial pneumonia, and neurological complications.[16] The preoperative visit offers an opportunity to utilize a teachable moment to influence a patient toward smoking cessation. Offering supportive resources such as nicotine replacement therapy and supportive services can further motivate the patient to quit tobacco use.

Skin Antisepsis

The goal of antiseptic skin preparation before surgery is to reduce wound contamination by reducing local bioburden at the incision site. There is high-quality evidence for using an alcohol-based antiseptic agent for intraoperative skin preparation. Chlorhexidine shows superior performance over povidone-iodine.

Preoperative bathing or showering using an antiseptic the night before or morning of surgery is an accepted practice, but the benefits are less well established. Multiple studies and serial meta-analyses have failed to show a benefit over using regular soap. The CDC recommends that patients take a full body shower or bath with soap or an antiseptic agent the night before the operative day.[3] The preoperative clinician should take time to explain the rationale for and reinforce the importance of skin preparation during the patient's visit. Where antiseptic bathing is the accepted practice, the preoperative clinic can be a convenient location for distribution of the selected product.

Staphylococcus aureus Decolonization. Colonization with *S. aureus* has been associated with an increased risk for *S. aureus* SSIs specifically and all SSIs in general. Preoperative nasal decolonization as a single intervention has shown mixed impact on SSI rates,[17] but when used in combination with preoperative chlorhexidine bathing and preoperative antibiotic selection directed by nasal *S. aureus* screening results, it has led to significant SSI reduction, best demonstrated in patients undergoing cardiothoracic and joint arthroplasty surgery.[18] The value of universal nasal *S. aureus* decolonization, best agents, and regimens are areas in need of more precise definition. The preoperative visit provides an opportunity to screen for nasal residence of *S. aureus* and provide decolonization.

SUMMARY

SSIs remain the most common and most costly nosocomial infections. Risk factors can be categorized into those intrinsic and extrinsic to the patient, with varying levels of modifiability. The goal of preventive measures is to eliminate all preventable infections. This is accomplished by interventions to diminish inoculation of bacteria into the surgical wound and to promote host containment and elimination of contaminating bacteria. The preoperative visit should include evaluation and mitigation for individual patient risk for SSI.

Clinical pearls

- Numerous factors place a patient at increased risk for surgical wound infections. Preoperative evaluation provides an opportunity to identify and modify individual risk factors where possible with the goal of avoiding preventable infections.

- Due to appropriate antibacterial spectrum and safety, cephalosporins are first-line options for surgical prophylaxis. A careful history to clarify the likelihood and severity of a penicillin allergy label during preoperative evaluation can avoid unnecessary use of less effective second-line agents.

- Timely administration of appropriately dosed and timed preoperative antibiotics is effective in reducing the risk of surgical wound infections in clean and clean-contaminated procedures.

REFERENCES

1. Seidlman JL, Mantyh CR, Anderson DJ. Surgical site infection prevention. *JAMA*. 2023;329(3):244-252. PMID: 36648463

2. CDC National and State Healthcare-Associated Infections Progress Report, published November 2023. Available at https://www.cdc.gov/hai/data/portal/progress-report.html.

3. Zimlichman, E, Henderson D, Tamir O, et al. Health care-associated infections. A meta-analysis of costs and financial impact on the US health care system. *JAMA Intern Med*. 2013;173(22): 2039-2046. PMID: 23999949

4. Allegranzri B, Bischoff P, de Jonge S, et al. New WHO recommendations on preoperative measures for surgical site infection prevention: an evidence-based global perspective. *Lancet Infect Dis*. 2016;16:e276-e287. PMID: 27816413

5. Calderwood MS, Anderson DJ, Bratzler DW, et al. Strategies to prevent surgical site infections in acute-care hospitals: 2022 update. *Infect Control Hosp Epidemiol*. 2023;44(5):695-720. PMID: 37137483

6. Blumenthal KG, Ryan EE, Li Y, et al. The impact of a reported penicillin allergy on surgical site infection risk. *Clin Infect Dis*. 2018;66(3):329-336. PMID: 29361015

7. Khan DA, Banerji A, Blumenthal KG, et al. Drug allergy: a 2022 practice parameter update. *J Allergy Clin Immunol*. 2022;150(6):1333-1393. PMID: 36122788

8. Wong BBL, Keith PK, Waserman S. Clinical history as a predictor of penicillin skin test outcome. *Ann Allergy Asthma Immunol*. 2006;97:169-174. PMID: 16937746

9. Park M, Markus P, Matesic D, Li JT. Safety and effectiveness of a preoperative allergy clinic in decreasing vancomycin use in patients with a history of penicillin allergy. *Ann Allergy Asthma Immunol*. 2006;97(5):681-687. PMID: 17165279

10. Bratzler DW, Dellinger EP, Olsen KM, et al. American Society of Health-System Pharmacists (ASHP); Infectious Diseases Society of America (IDSA); Surgical Infection Society (SIS); Society for Healthcare Epidemiology of America (SHEA). Clinical practice guidelines for antimicrobial prophylaxis in surgery. *Surg Infect*. 2013;14(1):73-156. PMID: 23461695

11. Gurunathan U, Ramsey S, Mitric G, et al. Association between obesity and wound infection following colorectal surgery: systematic review and meta-analysis. *J Gastrointest Surg*. 2017;21(10):1700-1712. PMID: 28785932

12. Yuan K, Chen H-L. Obesity and surgical site infections risk in orthopedics: a meta-analysis. *Int J Surg*. 2013;11(5):383-388. PMID: 23470598

13. Gabriel RA, Hylton DJ, Burton BN, et al. The association of preoperative haemoglobin A1c with 30-day postoperative surgical site infection following non-cardiac surgery. *J Perioper Pract*. 2019;30(10):320-325. PMID: 31694470

14. Latham R, Lancaster AD, Covington JF, et al. The association of diabetes and glucose control with surgical site infections among cardiothoracic surgery patients. *Infect Control Hosp Epidemiol*. 2001;22:607-612. PMID: 11776345

15. Showen A, Russell TA, Young S, et al. Hyperglycemia is associated with surgical site infections among general and vascular surgery patients. *Am Surg*. 2017;83(10):1108-1111. PMID: 29391105

16. Grønkjær M, Eliasen M, Skov-Ettrup LS, et al. Preoperative smoking status and postoperative complications: a systematic review and meta-analysis. *Ann Surg*. 2014;259(1):52-71. PMID: 23799418

17. Perl TM, Cullen JJ, Wenzel RP, et al. Intranasal mupirocin to prevent postoperative *Staphylococcus aureus* infections. *N Engl J Med*. 2002;346(24):1871. PMID: 12063371

18. Schweizer ML, Chiang HY, Septimus E, et al. Association of a bundled intervention with surgical site infections among patients undergoing cardiac, hip, or knee surgery. *JAMA*. 2015;313(21):2162-2171. PMID: 26034956

## 8

Prevention of Infective Endocarditis

Steven L. Cohn, MD, MACP, SFHM, FRCP

COMMON CLINICAL QUESTIONS

1. Which cardiac conditions place patients at increased risk of adverse outcomes from infective endocarditis?
2. Which procedures are associated with bacteremia warranting endocarditis prophylaxis in high-risk patients?
3. Which antibiotics are indicated for prophylaxis, and what are the alternatives if the patient is allergic?

INTRODUCTION

Infective endocarditis (IE) is thought to result from formation of nonbacterial thrombotic endocarditis (platelets and fibrin) on the surface of a valve or damaged endothelial surface, bacteremia with adherence to the fibrin-platelet matrix, and proliferation of the bacteria within the vegetation. The annual incidence of IE increased from 2000 to 2011, ranging from 3 to 10 episodes/100,000 population worldwide and 11 to 15/100,000 in the United States and has continued to increase in the past decade with a male predominance. Incidence of native-valve IE has decreased, while IE related to prosthetic valves and cardiac devices has increased. Mortality has also increased and is highest in those over 50 years old.

Since 1955 the American Heart Association (AHA) has issued guidelines with various recommendations for prevention of IE with antimicrobial prophylaxis before specific procedures such as dental, gastrointestinal (GI), and genitourinary (GU) procedures in patients considered to be at risk for its development. The underlying principles were that IE is uncommon but life-threatening, and prevention is preferable to treatment; certain underlying cardiac conditions predispose to IE; bacteremia with organisms known to cause IE occurs in association with specific procedures; antimicrobial prophylaxis prevented experimental IE in animals and was thought to be effective in preventing IE in humans undergoing specific procedures. However, incidence and mortality of IE have not decreased in the past 30 years despite prophylaxis, and the guidelines are based on consensus or expert opinion rather than randomized controlled trials (RCT). With the incidence of IE continuing to increase, there have been questions about whether the change in guidelines that resulted in fewer groups of patients receiving prophylaxis was too restrictive. A 2022 Cochrane systematic review concluded that there remained no clear evidence about whether antibiotic prophylaxis is effective or ineffective against IE in people at risk undergoing an invasive dental procedure.[1] The authors could not determine whether the potential harms and costs of prophylactic antibiotics outweighed any potential benefit. However, two subsequent case crossover analyses and cohort studies in over 9.5 million people in Medicare supplemental and Medicaid databases demonstrated a significant temporal association between invasive dental procedures and subsequent IE in high-risk individuals as well as a significant association between antibiotic prophylaxis and reduced IE incidence after these procedures.[2,3] Previous guidelines were complicated, making it difficult for physicians and patients to remember or interpret, resulting in both overuse and underuse of prophylaxis.

This chapter will review and summarize the 2007 AHA guidelines[4] (including the 2020 ACC/AHA guidelines for the management of patients with valvular heart disease[5]) and highlight some of the recommendations from other societies, including the 2023 European Society of Cardiology (ESC)[6] and National Institute for Health and Clinical Excellence (NICE)[7] [http://www.nice.org.uk/CG064].[8]

PATIENT-RELATED RISK FACTORS/ CARDIAC CONDITIONS

Conditions identified by the previous AHA guidelines as being associated with an increased risk of IE with a higher lifetime risk compared to individuals with no known underlying cardiac conditions included prosthetic cardiac valves, rheumatic heart disease (RHD), previous IE, congenital heart disease (CHD), and mitral valve prolapse (MVP) with mitral regurgitation.

However, the 2007 AHA guidelines restricted prophylaxis to those patients with the highest risk of adverse outcome from IE who would derive the greatest benefit from its prevention assuming prophylaxis is effective. This high-risk group included patients with a prosthetic heart valve or prosthetic material used for cardiac valve repair, previous IE, CHD, and cardiac transplant recipients who develop valvulopathy. Guidelines from other societies differ somewhat in their recommendations and definitions of at-risk patients and cardiac conditions (Table 8-1).

PROCEDURE-RELATED RISK FACTORS

Previous AHA guidelines were based on procedures most likely to induce bacteremia and therefore theoretically increase the risk of causing IE in susceptible patients. These procedures included dental, respiratory tract, and GI and GU procedures. Lacking data to prove a cause-and-effect link between these procedures and subsequent development of IE with those organisms, the 2007 AHA guidelines only recommended prophylaxis for dental procedures involving

manipulation of gingival tissue or the periapical region of teeth or perforation of the oral mucosa, and for procedures on the respiratory tract or infected skin, skin structures, or musculoskeletal tissue, and only in patients with the cardiac conditions noted above. Observational studies reported that compared with patients with IE not undergoing an invasive procedure, several invasive nondental medical procedures were associated with increased risk of IE, including cardiovascular interventions, skin procedures and wound management, transfusion, dialysis, bone marrow puncture, and endoscopic procedures. These studies prompted a recent science advisory from the AHA which suggested a re-evaluation of IE prevention advice.[9] However, the etiology of IE in these cases is usually staphylococci rather than streptococci, and standard prophylaxis with amoxicillin would not be expected to be effective. For procedures on infected tissue, the antibiotic regimen should include an agent active against staphylococci and beta-hemolytic streptococci. Endocarditis prophylaxis is no longer recommended by the AHA/ACC for GI or GU procedures solely to prevent IE; however, if an infection is present or the patient will receive antibiotic therapy to prevent a wound infection, it is reasonable for the antibiotic regimen to include a drug active against enterococci. Society guidelines differ in their recommendations and definitions of high-risk procedures (Table 8-2).

ANTIMICROBIAL THERAPY

If IE prophylaxis is recommended, it should be administered as a single dose 30–60 minutes before the procedure. Antibiotic regimens for IE prophylaxis in patients with cardiac conditions who are undergoing procedures warranting prophylaxis (dental and upper respiratory) are listed in Figure 8-1. These antibiotic regimens are based on the most likely causative organisms—*Streptococcus viridans* for dental procedures and various microorganisms for respiratory tract procedures (if infected, consider *S. viridans*, *Staphylococcus aureus* for cardiac surgery).

If a patient will be receiving antibiotic prophylaxis to prevent wound infection after specific procedures, it is reasonable that the regimen includes an agent that is active against the most likely pathogen for that setting. If a patient is already receiving long-term antibiotics with a drug also recommended for IE prophylaxis, and the patient has a cardiac condition

TABLE 8-1. Cardiac Conditions Associated with the Highest Risk of Adverse Outcome from Endocarditis for which Prophylaxis with Procedures in Table 8-2 Is Recommended

	AHA[4,9] (2007/2021)	ESC[6] (2023)	NICE[7,8*] (2015–2016)
Targeted population **for which antibiotic prophylaxis is recommended with high-risk procedures**	Those at highest risk for an adverse outcome from IE	Those at highest risk of IE undergoing a high-risk procedure	Not recommended "routinely"** for people undergoing dental or other procedures
Cardiac conditions **at highest risk of IE**		**Class of recommendation; Level of evidence**	
Prosthetic cardiac valves, including transcatheter-implanted prostheses and homografts[3]: - transcatheter aortic/pulm valve - transcatheter mitral/tricuspid valve or prosthetic material used for valve repair such as annuloplasty rings and chords	Yes (IIa; C-LD)	Yes (I; C) (I; C) (IIa; C)	No
Previous IE	Yes (IIa; C)	Yes (I; B)	No
Congenital heart disease (CHD) • Unrepaired cyanotic CHD, including palliative shunts and conduits • Repaired congenital heart defect with prosthetic material or device during the first 6 months after the procedure or lifelong if residual defect (shunt or valvular regurgitation) remains	Yes (IIa; C)	Yes (I; C)	No
Cardiac transplant recipients who develop valvulopathy Ventricular-assist devices	Yes (IIa; C)	Yes (IIb; C) (I; C)	No

IE, infective endocarditis; GI, gastrointestinal; GU, genitourinary; AHA, American Heart Association; ESC, European Society of Cardiology; NICE, National Institute for Health and Clinical Excellence.

* Only for GI or GU procedures at "infected" or "potentially infected" sites in patients at risk (essentially all conditions listed).

** Doctors and dentists should offer the most appropriate treatment options, in conjunction with the patient and/or caregiver or guardian. In doing so, they should take into account the recommendations in this guideline and the values and preferences of patients and apply their clinical judgment.

warranting prophylaxis, it is prudent to change the antibiotic to a different class for the procedure. For example, in a patient receiving penicillin prophylaxis for rheumatic fever who is scheduled for an invasive dental procedure, azithromycin or doxycycline should be given for IE prophylaxis. Clindamycin is no longer recommended by the AHA[10] or ESC[6] as an alternative due to its association with adverse events, mainly *Clostridium difficile.* Maintenance of optimal oral health and hygiene (brushing twice daily and professional cleaning one to two times per year) may reduce the incidence of bacteremia from daily activities and is more important than prophylactic antibiotics to reduce IE risk for a dental procedure. Other general measures should include strict skin hygiene, wound disinfection, curative antibiotics when indicated, no

TABLE 8-2. Procedures for Which Endocarditis Prophylaxis Is Recommended in the Highest Risk Patients (in Table 8-1)

PROCEDURE	AHA[4,9] (2007/2021)	ESC[6] (2023)	NICE[5,6*] (2015–2016)
Dental*	**(Class of recommendation; Level of evidence)**		
Dental procedures that involve manipulation of either gingival tissue or the periapical region of the teeth or perforation of the oral mucosa	Yes (IIa; B)/(IIa; C)	Yes (I; B)	No
Routine anesthetic injections through noninfected tissue, dental x-rays, placement/removal/adjustment of prosthodontic or orthodontic appliances/brackets, shedding of deciduous teeth, bleeding from trauma to the lips or oral mucosa	No	No (III; C)	No
Respiratory**			
Invasive respiratory tract procedures involving incision or biopsy of the respiratory mucosa (e.g., tonsillectomy or adenoidectomy)	Yes (IIa; C)	Maybe (IIb; C)	No
Bronchoscopy, laryngoscopy, or intubation	No	Maybe (IIb; C)	No
GI/GU***			
Sclerotherapy/dilatation of esophageal varices, esophageal laser therapy, gastroscopy, colonoscopy, ERCP, hepatic/biliary operations, gallstone lithotripsy, surgery involving intestinal mucosa, cystoscopy, urethral dilatation, TURP, transrectal prostate biopsy, vaginal hysterectomy, cesarean section	No (III; B)	Maybe (IIb; C)	No

GI, gastrointestinal; GU, genitourinary; AHA, American Heart Association; ESC, European Society of Cardiology; NICE, National Institute for Health and Clinical Excellence.

* Not recommended routinely but advises informed consent discussion if high-risk.

** *Recommended* for dental procedures that involve manipulation of either gingival tissue or the periapical region of the teeth or perforation of the oral mucosa (not recommended for routine anesthetic injections through noninfected tissue, dental x-rays, placement/removal/adjustment of prosthodontic or orthodontic appliances/brackets, shedding of deciduous teeth, bleeding from trauma to the lips or oral mucosa).

*** *Recommended* for invasive respiratory tract procedures involving incision or biopsy of the respiratory mucosa (e.g., tonsillectomy/adenoidectomy) (not recommended for bronchoscopy, laryngoscopy, or intubation).

**** Sclerotherapy/dilatation of esophageal varices, esophageal laser therapy, gastroscopy, colonoscopy, ERCP, hepatic/biliary operations, gallstone lithotripsy, surgery involving intestinal mucosa, cystoscopy, urethral dilatation, TURP, transrectal prostate biopsy, vaginal hysterectomy, caesarian section.

self-medication with antibiotics, and strict infection control measures for at-risk procedures.

SUMMARY

Multiple guidelines currently recommend IE prophylaxis for significantly fewer patients than in the past. This is related to the lack of scientific evidence linking procedures and bacteremia to subsequent endocarditis and the lack of efficacy for prophylaxis. The effects of these changes need to continue to be monitored. The incidence of IE has been increasing, both before and after guideline changes, but this has been even more pronounced in the United Kingdom, where the 2008

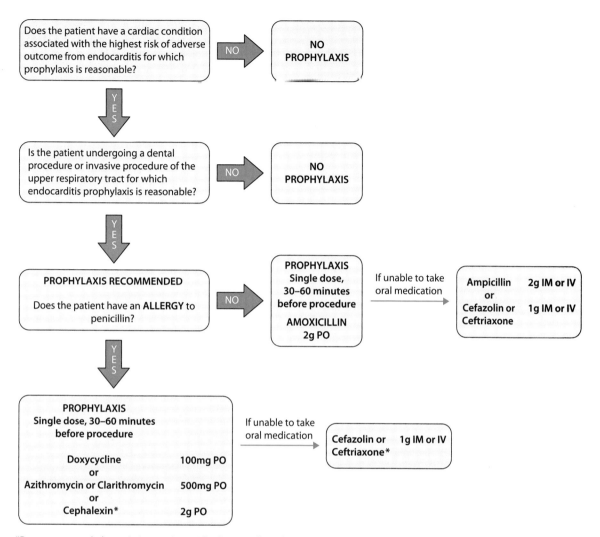

FIGURE 8-1. Algorithm for endocarditis prophylaxis.

guidelines advocated total restriction of prophylaxis.[11] In the United States, antibiotic prophylaxis prescriptions have decreased significantly since the 2007 guidelines, particularly for the moderate-risk group, without a significant increase in IE. There has also been an inappropriate decrease in prescribing for the high-risk group in whom IE continues to increase.[12] In 2021, after reviewing the available evidence, the AHA issued a scientific statement that recommended no changes to the 2007 Viridans Group Streptococci IE prevention guidelines.[10] However, studies showing an association between nondental invasive procedures and subsequent endocarditis prompted a 2023 science advisory from the AHA which suggested a reevaluation of IE prevention advice, particularly for some endoscopic procedures.[9] Because the numbers required for an RCT are unreasonable, additional prospective case-control studies are needed to evaluate current regimens and to provide evidence for future recommendations.

In summary, at the current time, prophylaxis is recommended if the patient has BOTH a cardiac condition least able to tolerate endocarditis AND is undergoing a dental or invasive upper respiratory tract procedure (see Figure 8-1).

Clinical pearls

- Antibiotic prophylaxis should be restricted to those patients with cardiac conditions least able to tolerate IE should they get it. These include prosthetic heart valves, prior endocarditis, CHD, and heart transplant recipients who have developed valvulopathy.

- Procedures most likely to cause bacteremia that may be associated with IE include invasive dental procedures and those invading the respiratory mucosa or any infected tissue.

- The drug of choice is amoxicillin, with clindamycin, azithromycin, doxycycline, or possibly a cephalosporin as alternatives if the patient is allergic to penicillin. Clindamycin is no longer recommended.

- Only give IE prophylaxis to patients who have BOTH a cardiac condition placing them at risk AND are undergoing one of the procedures associated with bacteremia.

REFERENCES

1. Rutherford SJ, Glenny AM, Roberts G, et al. Antibiotic prophylaxis for preventing bacterial endocarditis following dental procedures. *Cochrane Database Syst Rev.* 2022;5(5):CD003813. PMID: 35536541

2. Thornhill MH, Gibson TB, Yoon F, et al. Antibiotic prophylaxis against infective endocarditis before invasive dental procedures. *J Am Coll Cardiol.* 2022;80(11):1029-1041. PMID: 35987887

3. Thornhill MH, Gibson TB, Yoon F, et al. Endocarditis, invasive dental procedures, and antibiotic prophylaxis efficacy in US Medicaid patients. *Oral Dis.* 2024;30(3):1591-1605. PMID: 37103475

4. Wilson W, Taubert KA, Gewitz M, et al. Prevention of infective endocarditis: guidelines from the American Heart Association: a guideline from the American Heart Association Rheumatic Fever, Endocarditis, and Kawasaki Disease Committee, Council on Cardiovascular Disease in the Young, and the Council on Clinical Cardiology, Council on Cardiovascular Surgery and Anesthesia, and the Quality of Care and Outcomes Research Interdisciplinary Working Group. *Circulation.* 2007;116(15):1736-1754. PMID: 17446442

5. Otto CM, Nishimura RA, Bonow RO, et al. 2020 ACC/AHA guideline for the management of patients with valvular heart disease: a report of the American College of Cardiology/American Heart Association Joint Committee on Clinical Practice Guidelines. *Circulation.* 2021;143(5):e72-e227. PMID: 33332150

6. Delgado V, Ajmone Marsan N, de Waha S, et al.; ESC Scientific Document Group. 2023 ESC Guidelines for the management of endocarditis. *Eur Heart J.* 2023;44(39):3948-4042. PMID: 37622656

7. Richey R, Wray D, Stokes T. Prophylaxis against infective endocarditis: summary of NICE guidance. *BMJ.* 2008;336(7647):770-771. PMID: 18390528

8. National Institute for Health and Care Excellence (NICE) Prophylaxis against infective endocarditis 2015 [NICE Clinical Guideline No 64]. Available at http://www.nice.org.uk/guidance/cg64/chapter/Recommendations. Accessed June 20, 2024.

9. Baddour LM, Janszky I, Thornhill MH, et al. American Heart Association Council on Lifelong Congenital Heart Disease and Heart Health in the Young (Young Hearts) and Council on Cardiovascular and Stroke Nursing. Nondental invasive procedures and risk of infective endocarditis: time for a revisit: a science advisory from the American Heart Association. *Circulation.* 2023;148(19):1529-1541. PMID: 37795631

10. Wilson WR, Gewitz M, Lockhart PB, et al. American Heart Association Young Hearts Rheumatic Fever, Endocarditis and Kawasaki Disease Committee of the Council on Lifelong Congenital Heart Disease and Heart Health in the Young; Council on Cardiovascular and Stroke Nursing; and the Council on Quality of Care and Outcomes Research. Prevention of viridans group streptococcal infective endocarditis: a scientific statement from the American Heart Association. *Circulation.* 2021;143(20):e963-e978. PMID: 33853363

11. Cahill TJ, Harrison JL, Jewell P, et al. Antibiotic prophylaxis for infective endocarditis: a systematic review and meta-analysis. *Heart.* 2017;103(12):937-944. PMID: 28213367

12. Thornhill MH, Gibson TB, Cutler E, et al. Antibiotic prophylaxis and incidence of endocarditis before and after the 2007 AHA recommendations. *J Am Coll Cardiol.* 2018;72(20):2443-2454. PMID: 30409564

PREOPERATIVE EVALUATION AND PERIOPERATIVE MANAGEMENT: CO-EXISTING DISEASES AND SPECIAL POPULATIONS

## 9

Cardiac Risk Calculators

Steven L. Cohn, MD, MACP, SFHM, FRCP

COMMON CLINICAL QUESTIONS

1. Which risk calculators are recommended by the ACC/AHA guidelines?
2. How are risk calculators incorporated into the ACC/AHA algorithm?
3. How should you use these calculators to avoid the pitfalls of misinterpreting risk?

INTRODUCTION

Since Goldman's original cardiac risk index in 1977,[1] multiple cardiac risk indices and calculators have been published to facilitate risk stratification for perioperative cardiac complications. The three most widely used and recommended by the 2014 ACC/AHA guidelines[2] are the Lee Revised Cardiac Risk Index (RCRI),[3] and the calculators derived from the National Surgical Quality Improvement Program (NSQIP) database—Gupta MI or Cardiac Arrest (MICA) calculator[4] and the ACS Surgical Risk Calculator (ACS-SRC)[5] (Table 9-1). Although the 2024 ACC/AHA guidelines state that using a validated risk-prediction tool can be useful to estimate risk of perioperative MACE, they did not recommend one calculator over another.[6] However, before using any calculator, it is important to understand the setting in which it was derived, the population studied, types of surgery included, definitions of risk factors, and outcomes studied including the timeframe; otherwise, there is potential for

misuse and incorrect risk stratification. These calculators should be used in the ACC/AHA algorithm to determine if the patient is at low (<1%) or elevated (≥1%) chance of having a major adverse cardiac event (MACE) (see details in Chapter 11).

ACC/AHA RECOMMENDED RISK CALCULATORS

Revised Cardiac Risk Index (RCRI)[3]

https://qxmd.com/calculate/calculator_195/revised-cardiac-risk-index-lee-criteria

Lee and colleagues prospectively evaluated 4,315 patients aged 50 years and older undergoing elective noncardiac, non-neurologic surgery with an *expected hospital length of stay of at least 2 days*. They developed a cardiac risk index composed of six variables, each given equal weighting: high-risk type of surgery (intrathoracic, intraabdominal, suprainguinal vascular), ischemic heart disease (not revascularized), history of congestive heart failure, history of cerebrovascular disease, insulin therapy for diabetes, and serum creatinine >2.0 mg/dL. The frequency of major cardiac complications (MI, pulmonary edema, ventricular fibrillation or primary cardiac arrest, or complete heart block) during hospitalization increased with the number of risk factors present in both the derivation and validation patient cohorts (0.4–1.3% with 0–1 factors, 4–7% with 2 factors, and 9–11% with 3 or more factors). (Note that the higher complication rates

TABLE 9-1. Characteristics of Three Major Risk Calculators

	RCRI (LEE)	MICA (GUPTA)	ACS SRC (BILIMORIA)
Methodology	Prospective (1989–1994)	Historical (NSQIP) (2007–2008)	Historical (NSQIP) (2009–2012)
# of patients (derivation/ validation)	4,315 (2,893/1,422)	468,795 (211,410/257,385)	1,414,006
# of hospitals	1	>200	393
Age	≥50	≥16	≥16
Type of surgery	Nonemergent Noncardiac **LOS ≥ 2 days**	21 categories Excluded trauma and transplant pts	1,557 CPT codes
# risk factors	6 Surg, CAD, HF, CVA, DM, CKD	5 Surg, funct status, ASA, age, CKD	21 Surg, funct status, ASA, age, sex, HF, card event, HTN, DM, COPD, smoker, ARF, HD, dyspnea, emergency, cancer, BMI, sepsis, steroids, ascites, vent-depend
Outcomes	MI, pulm edema, VF/ cardiac arrest/CHB	MI, cardiac arrest	MI, cardiac arrest, multiple noncardiac complications
Time frame	In-hospital	30 days	30 days

LOS, length of stay; CAD, coronary artery disease; HF, heart failure; CVA, cerebrovascular accident (stroke); DM, diabetes mellitus; CKD, chronic kidney disease; MI, myocardial infarction; VF, ventricular fibrillation; CHB, complete heart block; ASA, American Society of Anesthesiologists; HTN, hypertension; COPD, chronic obstructive pulmonary disease; ARF, acute renal failure; HD, hemodialysis; BMI, body mass index.

quoted using MDCalc (3.9% with no risk factors) are based on studies with different patient populations, postoperative monitoring, and outcomes. Because this would classify all patients as elevated risk, we do not recommend using this calculator for the RCRI to estimate risk. (Please see https://www.mdcalc.com/calc/1739/revised-cardiac-risk-index-pre-operative-risk for more details.) Risk was underestimated for patients undergoing abdominal aortic aneurysm. In a single-center prospective cohort study of 9,519 patients, Davis and colleagues[7] found that a simplified five-factor model ("reconstructed RCRI") replacing creatinine >2 mg/dL with a preoperative GFR <30 mL/min and eliminating diabetes treated with insulin resulted in superior prediction of major cardiac complications following elective noncardiac surgery compared with the RCRI. Similar to the RCRI, risk was underestimated for patients undergoing major vascular surgery. The addition of age, as in the

original CRI, also improved risk prediction. However, these models have not been externally validated.

Myocardial Infarction or Cardiac Arrest (MICA) Calculator[4]

https://qxmd.com/calculate/calculator_245/gupta-perioperative-cardiac-risk

Using historical information from 211,410 patients in the NSQIP database, Gupta and colleagues derived a calculator to predict risk of MICA within 30 days of noncardiac surgery, and then validated it using another 257,385 patients. Their risk factors included the type of surgery (21 categories), ASA class, functional dependence, age, and serum creatinine >1.5 mg/dL. A smartphone or computer is required to calculate risk. Using their database of patients and 30-day outcomes, this calculator demonstrated better predictive ability than the RCRI.

American College of Surgeons Surgical Risk Calculator (ACS-SRC)[5]

https://riskcalculator.facs.org/RiskCalculator/index.jsp

Bilimoria and colleagues developed the most comprehensive risk calculator based on information from 1,414,006 patients in the NSQIP database. This calculator used the CPT code for the specific surgical procedure (over 1,500 codes) along with 20 other variables to predict risk of postoperative cardiac complications and death as well as serious complications, any complication, and several others. It provides a color-coded display of risk that is useful to show patients for shared decision making. This also requires the use of a smartphone or computer. Although more cumbersome to use, this calculator is the most comprehensive and is regularly updated with additional data.

NEWER CARDIAC RISK CALCULATORS (TABLE 9-2)

Vascular Quality Initiative (VQI)[8]

https://svs-vqi.shinyapps.io/CRICalculators/

Because the RCRI (and MICA to a lesser extent) underestimated risk in major vascular surgery, the Vascular Study Group of New England (VSGNE) developed a calculator specifically for patients undergoing vascular surgery. This subsequently evolved to the VQI which included a calculator for vascular surgery procedures in general as well as separate risk calculators to predict risk of postoperative MI after specific vascular procedures such as open and endovascular aortic aneurysm repair, carotid endarterectomy, and supra- and infrainguinal bypass surgery. The procedure-specific calculators perform slightly better than the overall vascular surgery calculator, but each one uses different information for risk factors.

Geriatric-sensitive Cardiac Risk Index (GS-CRI)[9]

https://qxmd.com/calculate/calculator_448/geriatric-sensitive-perioperative-cardiac-risk-index-gscri

Although age is incorporated into the NSQIP calculators, it was not an independent risk factor in the RCRI which may underestimate risk in elderly patients. The GS-CRI was developed specifically for use in geriatric patients 65 years of age or older. It replaces history of ischemic heart disease with ASA class and functional capacity and expands upon several of the other RCRI risk factors. In the geriatric setting, it outperformed the RCRI.

Cardiovascular Risk Index (CVRI) or (AUB-HAS-2)[10]

The CVRI was derived prospectively from 3,284 patients at the *American University of Beirut* undergoing noncardiac surgery (but including emergency surgery) and validated on 1,167,414 million patients from the NSQIP database. Risk factors for death, MI, or stroke at 30 days included *H*istory of heart disease, *H*eart disease symptoms of angina or dyspnea, *A*ge ≥75, *A*nemia with Hb <12 mg/dL, vascular *S*urgery, and emergency *S*urgery, renaming the index *AUB-HAS2*.[11] They identified three groups of patients based on the number of risk factors: 0–1 low-risk (0–1.6% complication rate), 2–3 intermediate-risk (2–11%), and >3 high-risk (15–17%). A subsequent analysis by subspecialty type of surgery and by common site-specific surgical procedures confirmed these risk categories and demonstrated better risk estimation than the RCRI. Similar results were found in a substudy of only patients undergoing elective noncardiac surgery. An additional prospective study of 1,918 patients validated the index with an AUC of 0.89.[12]

Updated Cardiac Risk Score (UCRS)[13]

The preOperative assessment of cardiovascular RIsk in patients undergoing nONcardiac surgery (ORION) was an observational prospective cohort study that derived an UCRS from 4,600 patients and validated it on another 2,735 patients. Four variables were significantly associated with the risk of major perioperative cardiovascular events: high-risk surgery, preoperative glomerular filtration rate <30 mL/min, age ≥75 years, and history of heart failure. Based on the UCRS, four risk classes were created (0, 1, 2, or ≥3 risk factors) with a corresponding 30-day risk of a major cardiovascular complication (death due to cardiovascular causes, cardiac arrest, acute myocardial infarction, acute heart failure, type 2 second-degree atrioventricular block or complete atrioventricular block requiring cardiac pacing, and stroke) of 0.8%, 2.5%, 8.7%, and 27.2%, respectively. The ROC curves were marginally better than the RCRI. This risk calculator has not been externally validated and is rarely used.

TABLE 9-2. Characteristics of Newer Risk Calculators

NAME	VQI	GS-CRI	AUB-HAS-2 (CVRI)	UCRS	CARDIAC & STROKE RISK
AUTHOR PUBLICATION DATE	BERTAGE 2016	ALZREK 2017	DAKIK 2019–2020	SCORCU 2019	WOO 2021
Methodology	Historical (VQI registry) (2012–2016)	Historical (NSQIP) (2012–2013)	Prospective derivation Retrospect validation Prospective validation (2016–2017; 2008–2012; 2018–2019)	Prospective (2013–2015)	Retrospective (NSQIP) (2007–2010)
# of patients (derivation/validation)	88,791 (61,236/27,555)	383,819 (210,914/172,905)	1,170,728 (3284/1,167,414); (1918)	7,335 (4600/2735)	1,165,750 (809,880/355,870)
# of hospitals	>350	>200	1/>200	1	393
Age	–	≥65	>40	≥40	>16
Type of surgery	Nonemergent vascular CEA, INFRA, SUPRA, EVAR, OAAA	Elective NCS	Consecutive NCS (incl emergency)	Consecutive Elective/urgent (excl unstable cardiac)	NCS (incl emergency)
# risk factors	Surg, HF, DM, CKD, CAD, age, stress test, +others	7-Surg, HF, DM, CKD, CVA; ASA, functions	6-Surg (vasc/emerg), age ≥ 75, heart dis, angina/SOB, Hb < 12	4-Surg (high-risk), HF, CKD, age ≥ 75	9-surg, emerg, age, CVA, CAD, ASA, Hct ≤ 27, Na+, cr > 1.8
Outcomes	MI/MINS	MI, cardiac arrest	Death, MI, CVA	CV death, MI, CVA, HF, HB/card arrest	CVA, MI, cardiac arrest, all-cause mortality
Time frame	In-hospital	30 days	30 days	30 days	30 days

Woo Perioperative Risk[14]

https://qxmd.com/calculate/calculator_823/woo-perioperative-risk

Using data from the 2007–2010 NSQIP data base, a model to predict stroke, major cardiac events (MI/cardiac arrest), and mortality was derived from 809,880 patients using age, history of coronary artery disease, history of stroke, emergency surgery, preoperative serum sodium ($\leq$130 mEq/L, >146 mEq/L), creatinine >1.8 mg/dL, hematocrit $\leq$27%, American Society of Anesthesiologists physical status class, and type of surgery, and validated using data from another 355,870 patients. The risk prediction model had high predictive accuracy with area under the receiver operating characteristic curve for stroke (training cohort = 0.869, validation cohort = 0.876), major cardiovascular events (training cohort = 0.871, validation cohort = 0.868), and 30-day mortality (training cohort = 0.922, validation cohort = 0.925). However, this model has not been externally validated.

OTHER SURGICAL RISK CALCULATORS (TABLE 9-3)

There are other surgical risk calculators to predict postoperative morbidity and mortality although not specifically cardiac complications. As many of these include intraoperative data such as blood loss and hypotension, they are not useful preoperatively to predict postoperative risk. Some of these include Surgical Risk Score (SRS), Surgical Outcome Risk Tool (SORT), Surgical Apgar Score (SAS), Physiological and Operative Severity Score for the enUmeration of Mortality and morbidity (POSSUM), Portsmouth (P-POSSUM), and oesophageal (O-POSSUM). The Surgical Risk Preoperative Assessment System (SURPAS) uses only 8 variables derived from the NSQIP database and predicted overall morbidity more accurately than the ACS-SRC. It was incorporated into the EMR at the University of Colorado School of Medicine and is currently being evaluated.[15,16]

Using artificial intelligence (AI), specifically machine learning, with institution-specific EMR data, models have been created to better predict postoperative morbidity and mortality. Pythia, developed at Duke, is a calculator requiring input of nine data fields to produce a risk assessment for 14 groupings of postoperative outcomes, and it identifies high-risk patients where further attention can be focused on additional preoperative evaluation, interventions, and postoperative monitoring.[17] Similarly, the University of Pittsburgh Medical Center (UPMC) developed a machine-learning model to identify patients at high risk for postoperative adverse events.[18] Both models outperformed the ACS NSQIP calculator.

COMPARISON OF THE PREOPERATIVE CARDIAC RISK ASSESSMENT TOOLS

Given the variety of cardiac risk assessment methods currently in existence, it is difficult for the clinician to select a given method over any of the others. Several studies have compared the various calculators and risk indices; however, because these tools used different definitions of risk factors (Table 9-4) as well as different complications and timeframes (Table 9-5), results are variable, and true head-to-head comparisons cannot be performed. It is important for the user to understand how each calculator was derived and what complications they predicted (Tables 9-1 and 9-2).

Using comprehensive medical records from a database of 663 patients from our preoperative clinic, we found that all three major risk calculators performed well in the setting in which they were originally studied but were less accurate when applied in a different manner. All three calculators were useful in defining low-risk patients in whom further cardiac testing was unnecessary.[19] Another study using a larger sample of 10,000 patient records from the NSQIP database found wide variability in the predicted risk of cardiac complications using different risk-prediction tools. The MICA and ACS-SRC, both of which were derived from the NSQIP database, correlated well but both had poor agreement with the RCRI. They noted that including more than one prediction tool in clinical guidelines could lead to differences in decision making for some patients.[20] A third analysis studied 11 risk indices involving 2,910,297 patients and noted that they fell into two groups: those with higher accuracy for predicting a narrow range of cardiac outcomes and those with lower accuracy for predicting a broader range of cardiac outcomes. They suggested that using one index from each group may be the most clinically useful approach.[21]

SUMMARY

Tables 9-4 and 9-5 compare the most frequently used tools, illustrating similarities and differences in risk factors and outcomes. Generally, you should select a

TABLE 9-3. Surgical Risk Calculators to Predict Mortality +/− Morbidity

SURGICAL OUTCOME RISK TOOL (SORT)
http://www.sortsurgery.com
• 7 preop variables
  - Specific procedure, severity, urgency, ASA, thoracic/GI/vasc surg, cancer, clinician's risk assessment
  - Predicts 30-day mortality

SURGICAL APGAR SCORE (SAS) https://www.mdcalc.com/calc/1826/surgical-apgar-score-sas-postoperative-risk • 3 variables, 10 points total—lowest HR, lowest MAP, intraop blood loss   - Predicts mortality, surgical complications, systemic complications if > 4 points

SURGICAL RISK SCORE (SRS)—classifies risk based on combination of the CEPOD, ASA, and BUPA
https://www.evidencio.com/models/show/1013#:~:text=Login-,The%20Surgical%20Risk%20Scale%20
    (SRS)%3A%20Mortality%20in%20general%20surgical,across%20the%20entire%20risk%20spectrum
• Confidential Enquiry into Perioperative Deaths (CEPOD)—urgency of surgery
• British United Provident Association (BUPA) scores—minor to major/complex
• American Society of Anesthesiologists (ASA)
  - Predicts mortality in general surgery

POSSUM—*Physiological and Operative Severity Score for the enUmeration of Mortality and Morbidity*
https://www.mdcalc.com/calc/3927/possum-operative-morbidity-mortality-risk
• 12 preop variables
  - Age, cardiac signs, pulm signs, syst BP, HR, coma score, Hb, WBC, Na, K, BUN, ECG
• 6 postop variables
  - Malignancy, urgency, blood loss, operative magnitude, peritoneal contamination, operations w/i 30-d
P-POSSUM (Portsmouth POSSUM)
O-POSSUM for oesophageal cancer surgery
V-POSSUM (vascular surgery)
CR-POSSUM (colorectal surgery)

POSPUM (Preoperative Score to Predict Postoperative Mortality) • 17 preop predictors for in-hospital mortality   - Age, ischemic heart disease, arrhythmia/heart block, HF/cardiomyopathy, PVD, dementia, CVA, hemiplegia, COPD, chronic respiratory failure, alcohol abuse, cancer, diabetes, transplanted organ, dialysis, chronic renal failure, type of surgery
SURPAS (Surgical Risk Preoperative Assessment System) • 8 preop predictors for morbidity and mortality (8 postoperative complications)   - ASA, age, functional status, emergency surgery, inpatient/outpatient operation, systemic sepsis, primary surgeon specialty, work RVUs

method you feel comfortable with that is easily implemented, is appropriate for the patient and setting being evaluated, and represents a reminder of the essential features of history that must be elicited preoperatively. The RCRI has been the most widely used calculator, probably related to its simplicity, but the ACS-SRC is the most comprehensive. Be aware that estimates for cardiac complications in the original RCRI study are lower than those in more recent studies using hsTnT and a 30-day timeframe. Data from VISION reported

1.6%, 4%, 7.9%, and 12.9% complication rates for MI, nonfatal cardiac arrest, and cardiac death with 0, 1, 2, or 3 risk factors, respectively.[22] Also, none of the risk calculators were designed to predict perioperative myocardial ischemia (PMI) or myocardial injury after noncardiac surgery (MINS) which occur far more frequently than MI. The newer calculators are promising but need to be tested further to determine their role. Machine-learning models should be the most accurate but need to be developed using institution-specific

TABLE 9-4. Comparison of Risk Factors in Cardiac Risk Calculators

RISK FACTOR		RCRI	MICA	ACS-SRC	VQI	GS-CRI	AUB-HAS2	UCRS	WOO
Surgery	High risk	X						X	
	Vascular				X				
	Multiple procedures		X	X		X	X		X
	Urgent/emergent						X	X	X
IHD	History of CAD	X		X	X	X	X		X
	Symptoms (angina/dyspnea)				X		X		
	Stress test				X				
Diabetes	On insulin	X							
	Any DM			X	X	X			
Renal	Creat >1.5		X			X			
	Creat >1.8				X				X
	Creat >2	X							
	GFR <30							X	
	ARF			X					
	Dialysis			X	X				
HF	History	X			X	X	X	X	
	Hx in past 30 days			X					
	Signs/symptoms				X		X		
Cerebrovasc disease	Stroke/TIA	X				X			X
ASA class			X	X		X			X
Functional status			X	X		X			
Age			X	X	X		X	X	X
Anemia							X		X
Sodium									X

IHD, ischemic heart disease; HF, heart failure; ASA, American Society of Anesthesiology; TIA, transient ischemic attack; CAD, coronary artery disease; DM, diabetes mellitus; create, creatinine; GFR, glomerular filtration rate; ARF, acute renal failure; Hx, history.

TABLE 9-5. Comparison of Outcomes of Cardiac Risk Calculators

OUTCOMES	RCRI	MICA	ACS-SRC	VQI	GS-CRI	AUB-HAS2	UCRS	WOO
Timeframe:								
In-hospital	X			X				
30 days		X	X		X	X	X	X
MI	X	X	X	X	X	X	X	X
MINS				X				
Heart block	X						X	
Cardiac arrest	X	X					X	X
Death			X					X
CV death							X	
Stroke			X			X	X	X
HF/pulm edema	X					X	X	
Noncardiac complications			X					

MI, myocardial infarction; MINS, myocardial injury after noncardiac surgery; CV, cardiovascular; HF, heart failure.

EMR data. Most importantly, these calculators are only tools to assist you in risk stratification and should not be used as a number or percentage in isolation without clinical judgment.

Clinical pearls

- It is important to understand how each risk calculator was derived (inclusion/exclusion criteria), the patient population studied, the setting, procedures included, definitions of risk factors, outcomes studied, and the timeframe. Because of these differences, true valid comparisons cannot really be performed to determine which risk calculator is best.
- The RCRI has been the most widely used calculator, probably related to its simplicity, but the ACS-SRC is the most comprehensive.
- Do not use the RCRI for ambulatory surgery and low-risk procedures with a length of stay less than 2 days or it will overestimate risk. It also underestimates risk in major vascular surgery.
- The NSQIP database lacks certain information, and calculators based on it may fail to include NSTEMIs if troponin was less than three times the upper limit of normal.
- Some of the newer risk calculators look promising, but they need to be tested in other settings to determine their role in future guidelines. Machine-learning calculators based on institution-specific EMR data are the wave of the future.
- Risk calculators are merely tools to assist in decision making. The ultimate decision has to be made by the physician using good judgment.

REFERENCES

1. Goldman L, Caldera DL, Nussbaum SR, et al. Multifactorial index of cardiac risk in noncardiac surgical procedures. *N Engl J Med*. 1977;297(16):845-850. PMID: 904659
2. Fleisher LA, Fleischmann KE, Auerbach AD, et al. 2014 ACC/AHA guideline on perioperative cardiovascular evaluation and management of patients undergoing noncardiac surgery: a report of the American College of Cardiology/American Heart Association Task Force

on practice guidelines. *J Am Coll Cardiol*. 2014;64(22): e77-e137. PMID: 25091544

3. Lee TH, Marcantonio ER, Mangione CM, et al. Derivation and prospective validation of a simple index for prediction of cardiac risk of major noncardiac surgery. *Circulation*. 1999;100(10):1043-1049. PMID: 10477528

4. Gupta PK, Gupta H, Sundaram A, et al. Development and validation of a risk calculator for prediction of cardiac risk after surgery. *Circulation*. 2011;124(4):381-387. PMID: 21730309

5. Bilimoria KY, Liu Y, Paruch JL, et al. Development and evaluation of the universal ACS NSQIP surgical risk calculator: a decision aid and informed consent tool for patients and surgeons. *J Am Coll Surg*. 2013;217(5):833-842. PMID: 24055383

6. Writing Committee Members; Thompson A, Fleischmann KE, Smilowitz NR, et al. 2024 AHA/ACC/ACS/ASNC/HRS/SCA/SCCT/SCMR/SVM guideline for perioperative cardiovascular management for noncardiac surgery: a report of the American College of Cardiology/American Heart Association Joint Committee on Clinical Practice Guidelines. *J Am Coll Cardiol*. 2024;84(19):1869-1969. doi:10.1016/j.jacc.2024.06.013. PMID: 39320289

7. Davis C, Tait G, Carroll J, et al. The Revised Cardiac Risk Index in the new millennium: a single-centre prospective cohort re-evaluation of the original variables in 9,519 consecutive elective surgical patients. *Can J Anaesth*. 2013;60(9):855-863. PMID: 23813289

8. Bertges DJ, Neal D, Schanzer A, et al. Vascular quality initiative. The vascular quality initiative cardiac risk index for prediction of myocardial infarction after vascular surgery. *J Vasc Surg*. 2016;64(5):1411-1421. PMID: 27449347

9. Alrezk R, Jackson N, Al Rezk M, et al. Derivation and validation of a geriatric-sensitive perioperative cardiac risk index. *J Am Heart Assoc*. 2017;6(11):e006648. PMID: 29146612

10. Dakik HA, Chehab O, Eldirani M, et al. A new index for pre-operative cardiovascular evaluation. *J Am Coll Cardiol*. 2019;73(24):3067-3078. PMID: 31221255

11. Dakik HA, Sbaity E, Msheik A, et al. AUB-HAS2 cardiovascular risk index: performance in surgical subpopulations and comparison to the revised cardiac risk index. *J Am Heart Assoc*. 2020;9(10):e016228. PMID: 32390481

12. Dakik HA, Eldirani M, Kaspar C, et al. Prospective validation of the AUB-HAS2 cardiovascular risk index. *Eur Heart J Qual Care Clin Outcomes*. 2022 Jan 5;8(1):96-97. PMID: 33017006. PMID: 32025039

13. Scorcu G, Pilleri A, Contu P, et al. Preoperative assessment of cardiovascular risk in patients undergoing noncardiac surgery: the Orion study. *Monaldi Arch Chest Dis*. 2020;90(1). doi:10.4081/monaldi.2020.1169. PMID: 32025039

14. Woo SH, Marhefka GD, Cowan SW, Ackermann L. Development and validation of a prediction model for stroke, cardiac, and mortality risk after non-cardiac surgery. *J Am Heart Assoc*. 2021;10(4):e018013. PMID: 33522252

15. Meguid RA, Bronsert MR, Juarez-Colunga E, et al. Surgical Risk Preoperative Assessment System (SURPAS): III. Accurate preoperative prediction of 8 adverse outcomes using 8 predictor variables. *Ann Surg*. 2016 Jul;264(1):23-31. PMID: 26928465

16. Khaneki S, Bronsert MR, Henderson WG, et al. Comparison of accuracy of prediction of postoperative mortality and morbidity between a new, parsimonious risk calculator (SURPAS) and the ACS Surgical Risk Calculator. *Am J Surg*. 2020 Jun;219(6):1065-1072. PMID: 31376949

17. Corey KM, Kashyap S, Lorenzi E, et al. Development and validation of machine learning models to identify high-risk surgical patients using automatically curated electronic health record data (Pythia): a retrospective, single-site study. *PLoS Med*. 2018;15(11):e1002701. PMID: 30481172

18. Mahajan A, Esper S, Oo TH, et al. Development and validation of a machine learning model to identify patients before surgery at high risk for postoperative adverse events. *JAMA Netw Open*. 2023;6(7):e2322285. PMID: 37418262

19. Cohn SL, Fernandez Ros N. Comparison of 4 cardiac risk calculators in predicting postoperative cardiac complications after noncardiac operations. *Am J Cardiol*. 2018;121(1):125-130. PMID: 29126584

20. Glance LG, Faden E, Dutton RP, et al. Impact of the choice of risk model for identifying low-risk patients using the 2014 American College of Cardiology/American Heart Association perioperative guidelines. *Anesthesiology*. 2018;129(5):889-900. PMID: 30001221

21. Wright DE, Knuesel SJ, Nagurur A, et al. Examining risk: a systematic review of perioperative cardiac risk prediction indices. *Mayo Clin Proc*. 2019;94(11): 2277-2290. PMID: 31202481

22. Roshanov PS, Sessler DI, Chow CK, et al. Predicting myocardial injury and other cardiac complications after elective noncardiac surgery with the revised cardiac risk index: the VISION study. *Can J Cardiol*. 2021;37(8):1215-1224. PMID: 33766613

10

Cardiac Biomarkers

Emmanuelle Duceppe, MD, PhD

COMMON CLINICAL QUESTIONS

1. What is the utility of preoperative biomarkers for cardiac risk evaluation?
2. Which biomarkers are recommended?
3. Is there additional prognostic benefit over clinical risk scores alone?

INTRODUCTION

Perioperative cardiac complications are common and associated with increased morbidity and mortality, which makes the evaluation of cardiac risk a central component of the preoperative assessment of patients at higher risk. Several tools are available for cardiac risk stratification, including risk scores and cardiac imaging, but have limited risk discrimination. Biomarkers offer an interesting additional option to improve cardiac risk prediction. They can be measured at the same time as routine preoperative blood-work, without requiring additional preoperative visits, and provide incremental risk prediction. This chapter reviews biomarkers that can be used for the cardiac evaluation of patients undergoing noncardiac surgery.

PREOPERATIVE BIOMARKERS

Recent decades have seen an increasing number of studies showing the utility of biomarkers for preoperative cardiac risk prediction in noncardiac surgery.[1]

While the most studied biomarkers are brain natriuretic peptides (BNPs) followed by cardiac troponins, other biomarkers show promising results for cardiac risk stratification. Some are also available as point-of-care, which is a helpful option to have in preoperative clinics. More importantly, however, is that some of these biomarkers have been shown to improve risk prediction beyond clinical evaluation alone using cardiac risk scores.

BRAIN NATRIURETIC PEPTIDES

It was first reported more than 40 years ago that the myocardium produces biologically active peptides and that the heart exerts an endocrine function. BNPs, which are predominantly produced by cardiomyocytes, include the active component BNP and the inactive peptide N-terminal pro-BNP (NT-proBNP). Both represent the same hormonal activity, although their laboratory range differs. Initially described in heart failure, it has since been demonstrated that BNPs are released in response to various pathophysiological mechanisms such as inflammatory, ischemic, hemodynamic, mechanical, and humoral stimuli.[2] Several conditions are associated with elevated BNP/NT-proBNP, many of which are relevant in the perioperative setting (Table 10-1).

In contrast to the 2014 ACC/AHA guidelines, the updated 2024 ACC/AHA guidelines on perioperative cardiovascular management state it is reasonable to measure BNP/NT-proBNP in patients aged ≥65 years,

TABLE 10-1. Conditions Associated with Elevated BNP/NT-proBNP

Cardiac conditions
  Left ventricular hypertrophy
  Diastolic dysfunction
  Acute or chronic heart failure
  Cardiomyopathy
  Ischemic heart disease
  Atrial fibrillation
  Significant valvular heart disease
  Inflammatory cardiac disease
  Carcinoid heart disease

Extra-cardiac conditions
  Poorly controlled hypertension
  Primary and secondary pulmonary hypertension
  Cirrhosis
  Severe chronic renal disease/dialysis
  Endocrine disorder (e.g., Cushing's syndrome, hyperthyroidism, hyperaldosteronism)

patients with known cardiovascular disease, or patients aged 45–64 years with symptoms suggestive of cardiovascular disease undergoing higher-risk noncardiac surgery.[3] Similarly, the perioperative guidelines from the Canadian Cardiovascular Society (CCS) recommend measuring preoperative BNP/NT-proBNP in patients aged ≥65 years, aged 45–64 years with significant cardiovascular disease, or with a Revised Cardiac Risk Index (RCRI) score ≥1 (i.e., ischemic heart disease, cerebrovascular disease, heart failure, diabetes treated with insulin, chronic kidney disease with serum creatinine >2.0 mg/dL (177 μmol/L), and high-risk surgery).[4] The 2022 European Society of Cardiology (ESC) guidelines also consider preoperative BNP/NT-proBNP measurement in patients with established cardiovascular disease, aged ≥65 years old, patients with cardiovascular risk factors (i.e., hypertension, smoking, dyslipidemia, diabetes, family history of cardiovascular disease) undergoing intermediate to high-risk noncardiac surgery, or aged 45–64 years old undergoing high-risk noncardiac surgery.[5] The ESC also recommends measuring BNP/NT-proBNP in patients with unexplained shortness of breath of peripheral edema. The CCS guidelines recommend using a threshold of ≥92 ng/L for BNP and ≥300 ng/L for NT-proBNP, although more recent evidence suggests using a threshold of ≥200 ng/L.[6] The

CCS guidelines also recommend postoperative troponin surveillance in patients with elevated preoperative BNP/NT-proBNP.

BNP/NT-proBNP in Addition to Cardiac Risk Scores

BNP/NT-proBNP can be used preoperatively to inform the patient and their treating team on the risk of perioperative cardiac complications.

NT-proBNP can improve risk prediction of postoperative cardiac events when used in addition to the RCRI.[1] A large study in patients undergoing noncardiac surgery found that preoperative NT-proBNP thresholds of <100 ng/L, 100 to <200 ng/L, 200 to <1,500 ng/L, and ≥1,500 ng/L were associated with the risk at 30 days of all-cause mortality or myocardial infarction of 1.7%, 3.0%, 7.9%, and 15.8%, respectively.[6] These thresholds can be used alone to predict perioperative cardiac risk, or in combination with the RCRI (Table 10-2). An online calculator combining RCRI and NT-proBNP is also available on QxMed (https://qxmd.com/calculate). In this study, the addition of NT-proBNP to the RCRI improved risk prediction in one in four patients. Adding NT-proBNP to the NSQIP MICA score has also been shown to improve risk prediction of in-hospital and 30-day major adverse cardiac events (MACE), although no calculator is available.[7]

BNP can also predict the risk of postoperative cardiac events and mortality alone and in combination with the RCRI.[1] A single threshold of ≥92 ng/L for BNP has been suggested, but no calculator is available to add BNP results to the RCRI. Alternative BNP threshold values of 0 to 100, >100 to 250, and >250 ng/L can be used, with associated risk estimates of 30-day myocardial infarction or mortality of 5.1%, 11.6%, and 26.3%, respectively.[8] No data are available for the combination of preoperative BNP and NSQIP-based risk scores.

BNP/NT-proBNP and Functional Capacity

The evaluation of functional capacity has been recommended to risk stratify patients before undergoing noncardiac surgery, but recent studies have raised questions as to whether it can improve prediction of perioperative cardiovascular outcomes. Formal functional capacity testing by measuring peak oxygen

TABLE 10-2. Incidence of MI or Death According to NT-proBNP Thresholds and RCRI

RCRI	NT-proBNP			
	<100 ng/L	100 to <200 ng/l	200 to <1,500 ng/L	≥1,500 NG/L
0	1.0% (95% CI 0.8–1.4)	1.9% (95% CI 1.2–2.9)	4.7% (95% CI 3.6–6.0)	7.5% (95% CI 4.1–13.2)
1	2.6% (95% CI 1.9–3.5)	3.6% (95% CI 2.4–5.4)	8.9% (95% CI 7.2–10.9)	13.4% (95% CI 9.3–19.1)
2	5.6% (95% CI 3.4–9.0)	7.2% (95% CI 4.2–12.1)	10.1% (95% CI 7.5–13.5)	15.4% (95% CI 10.4–22.2)
≥3	4.1% (95% CI 1.1–13.7)	5.1% (95% CI 1.4–16.9)	22.1% (95% CI 15.9–29.7)	28.0% (95% CI 21.1–36.2)

CI, confidence intervals; NT-proBNP, N-terminal pro-brain natriuretic peptide; RCRI, Revised Cardiac Risk Index.

The Revised Cardiac Risk Index score includes the following risk factors, each worth one point: history of ischemic heart disease, history of cerebrovascular disease, history of congestive heart failure, preoperative insulin use, preoperative creatinine >2 mg/dL (176.8 µmol/L), and high-risk surgery (i.e., intraperitoneal, intrathoracic, and suprainguinal vascular surgery).

consumption has not been found to predict postoperative cardiac events,[9] and subjective assessment of functional capacity (e.g., asking patients if they can climb two flight of stairs) has shown conflicting results in large studies.[9,10] Assessing functional capacity using the Duke Activity Status Index (DASI) questionnaire is preferable to predict cardiac outcomes at 30 days, and adding NT-proBNP can further improve risk prediction.[7,11] Notably, in a large study, adding NT-proBNP to NSQIP-MICA resulted in greater risk discrimination than when functional capacity was added to the risk score.[7]

BNP/NT-proBNP and Cardiac Testing

Guidelines do not recommend routine cardiac imaging in asymptomatic patients.[3,4] Preoperative echocardiogram findings have been shown to mildly improve prediction of cardiac events in patients with risk factors, but preoperative NT-proBNP was significantly superior.[12] BNP/NT-proBNP can, however, be useful in guiding which patients may be considered for further preoperative cardiac testing. For example, an echocardiogram could be considered to a patient with new shortness of breath and elevated BNP/NT-proBNP. On the contrary, in many conditions detailed in Table 10-1, BNP/NT-proBNP has a good negative predictive value. In a patient with low

BNP/NT-proBNP, shortness of breath is unlikely to be caused by undiagnosed heart failure, severe left-sided valvular disease, or other severe cardiac conditions. In determining if a patient with elevated BNP/NT-proBNP should undergo further cardiac testing (e.g., echocardiogram, cardiac stress test), the patient's risk factors, symptoms, risk and urgency of surgery, and magnitude of BNP/NT-proBNP elevation should be taken into consideration.

CARDIAC TROPONIN

Measuring preoperative cardiac troponin (cTn) was not recommended by previous guidelines, it can be considered in patients with risk factors. The 2022 ESC guidelines recommend measuring hs-cTn before intermediate- and high-risk surgery in patients with known cardiovascular disease, cardiovascular risk factors (including age >65 years), or symptoms suggestive of cardiovascular disease.[4] The 2024 ACC/AHA guidelines state that in these patients, it may be reasonable to measure cTn before surgery to supplement evaluation of perioperative risk.[3] Preoperative cTn can be used for baseline comparison in patients where postoperative cTn measurement is ordered, to distinguish between chronic elevation and dynamic cTn changes consistent with myocardial injury. Patients with preoperative cTn elevation are at higher risk of

30-day and 1-year mortality, and those who also have a postoperative myocardial injury have worse prognosis than patients with normal preoperative cTn or postoperative myocardial injury alone.[13]

It remains uncertain which cTn cutoff should be used to define preoperative elevation because each cTn manufacturer and type of cTn has a different laboratory range and the 99th percentile may be too sensitive, in particular with high-sensitivity assays. In a study of noncardiac surgery patients who were ≥65 years of age or 45–64 years with a history of coronary artery disease, peripheral artery disease, or stroke, half of the patients had a preoperative high-sensitivity cTn value above the 99th percentile.[13] Nonetheless, measuring preoperative cTn has been shown to improve risk prediction of perioperative cardiac events when added to the RCRI, and may be considered in at-risk patients.[1]

OTHER BIOMARKERS

C-reactive Protein (CRP)

Systemic inflammation is known to play a role in the formation and destabilization of atherosclerosis.[14] CRP is a well-established marker of systemic inflammation and a few studies aimed to determine if preoperative CRP could predict postoperative cardiovascular events.[1] However, when added to the RCRI, CRP yielded only modest improvement in risk prediction.[1] The evidence is too limited at this time to recommend measuring preoperative CRP for prediction of cardiac events in noncardiac surgery.

Growth Differentiation Factor-15 (GDF-15)

GDF-15 is a cytokine that is expressed in response to tissue injury and inflammation and has been associated with increased mortality in various cardiovascular diseases. In both cardiac and noncardiac surgery, it was shown to significantly improve risk prediction of perioperative cardiac events, in addition to cardiac risk scores and NT-proBNP.[15] Although promising, it remains a novel biomarker that is not yet available in most clinical laboratory.

SUMMARY

Preoperative biomarkers for cardiac risk stratification before noncardiac surgeries are an interesting alternative to conventional cardiac testing that should be considered in at-risk patients. BNP/NT-proBNP are the most studied biomarkers in this setting, and thresholds have been proposed that can be used in clinical practice, including when added to cardiac risk scores. Preoperative cTn can also be considered for comparison with postoperative cTn elevation, and potentially for risk prediction, although cTn cutoffs remain uncertain. How to manage patients with elevated preoperative cardiac biomarkers should be individualized to the patient's clinical presentation, risk factors, and risk of surgery. A proposed algorithm is illustrated in Figure 10-1.

Clinical pearls

- The use of preoperative BNP/NT-proBNP may be helpful in determining which patients could benefit from further preoperative cardiac testing and postoperative surveillance for cardiac events.

- Preoperative NT-proBNP can be added to the RCRI score to provide better risk estimates of perioperative cardiac events.

- BNP ≥92 ng/L and NT-proBNP ≥200 ng/L can be used as cutoffs to define elevated perioperative risk.

- Preoperative cTns may be helpful for comparison with postoperative results, to distinguish between chronic elevation and myocardial injury. It may also be useful for cardiac risk prediction, although the cutoffs to define elevation remain uncertain.

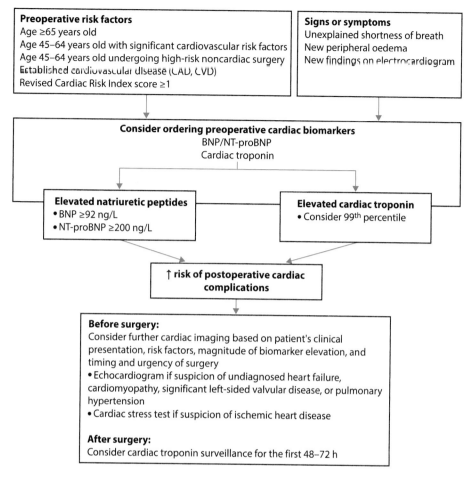

FIGURE 10-1. Proposed decision-making algorithm for cardiac biomarkers.

REFERENCES

1. Vernooij LM, van Klei WA, Moons KG, et al. The comparative and added prognostic value of biomarkers to the Revised Cardiac Risk Index for preoperative prediction of major adverse cardiac events and all-cause mortality in patients who undergo noncardiac surgery. *Cochrane Database Syst Rev.* 2021;12:Cd013139. PMID: 34931303

2. Clerico A, Giannoni A, Vittorini S, Passino C. Thirty years of the heart as an endocrine organ: physiological role and clinical utility of cardiac natriuretic hormones. *Am J Physiol Heart Circ Physiol.* 2011;301:H12-H20. PMID: 21551272

3. Thompson A, Fleischmann KE, Smilowitz NR, et al. 2024 AHA/ACC/ACS/ASNC/HRS/SCA/SCCT/ SCMR/SVM guideline for perioperative cardiovascular management for noncardiac surgery: a report of the American College of Cardiology/American Heart Association Joint Committee on Clinical Practice Guidelines. *J Am Coll Cardiol.* 2024;84(19):1869-1969. doi: 10.1016/j.jacc.2024.06.013. PMID: 39320289

4. Duceppe E, Parlow J, MacDonald P, et al. Canadian Cardiovascular Society guidelines on perioperative cardiac risk assessment and management for patients who undergo noncardiac surgery. *Can J Cardiol.* 2017;33: 17-32. PMID: 27865641

5. Halvorsen S, Mehilli J, Cassese S, et al. 2022 ESC guidelines on cardiovascular assessment and management of patients undergoing non-cardiac surgery. *Eur Heart J.* 2022;43:3826-3924. PMID: 36017553

6. Duceppe E, Patel A, Chan MTV, et al. Preoperative N-terminal Pro-B-type natriuretic peptide and cardiovascular events after noncardiac surgery: a cohort study. *Ann Intern Med.* 2020;172:96-104. PMID: 32539503

7. Lurati Buse G, Larmann J, Gillmann HJ, et al. NT-proBNP or self-reported functional capacity in estimating risk of cardiovascular events after noncardiac surgery. *JAMA Netw Open.* 2023;6:e2342527. PMID: 37938844

8. Rodseth RN, Biccard BM, Le Manach Y, et al. The prognostic value of pre-operative and post-operative B-type natriuretic peptides in patients undergoing noncardiac surgery: B-type natriuretic peptide and N-terminal fragment of pro-B-type natriuretic peptide: a systematic review and individual patient data meta-analysis. *J Am Coll Cardiol.* 2014;63:170-180. PMID: 24076282

9. Wijeysundera DN, Pearse RM, Shulman MA, et al. Assessment of functional capacity before major noncardiac surgery: an international, prospective cohort study. *Lancet* 2018;391:2631-2640. PMID: 30070222

10. Lurati Buse GAL, Puelacher C, Gualandro DM, et al. Association between self-reported functional capacity and major adverse cardiac events in patients at elevated risk undergoing noncardiac surgery: a prospective diagnostic cohort study. *Br J Anaesth* 2021;126:102-110. PMID: 33081973

11. Wijeysundera DN, Beattie WS, Hillis GS, et al. Integration of the Duke Activity Status Index into preoperative risk evaluation: a multicentre prospective cohort study. *Br J Anaesth.* 2020;124:261-270. PMID: 31864719

12. Park SJ, Choi JH, Cho SJ, et al. Comparison of transthoracic echocardiography with N-terminal pro-brain natriuretic peptide as a tool for risk stratification of patients undergoing major noncardiac surgery. *Korean Circ J.* 2011;41:505-511. PMID: 2202232

13. Puelacher C, Lurati Buse G, Seeberger D, et al. Perioperative myocardial injury after noncardiac surgery: incidence, mortality, and characterization. *Circulation.* 2018;137:1221-1232. PMID: 29203498

14. Matter MA, Paneni F, Libby P, et al. Inflammation in acute myocardial infarction: the good, the bad and the ugly. *Eur Heart J.* 2023;45:89-103. PMID: 37587550

15. Duceppe E, Borges FK, Conen D, et al. Association of preoperative growth differentiation factor-15 concentrations and postoperative cardiovascular events after major noncardiac surgery. *Anesthesiology.* 2023;138:508-522. PMID: 37039711

## 11

Ischemic Heart Disease

Steven L. Cohn, MD, MACP, SFHM, FRCP

COMMON CLINICAL QUESTIONS

1. What is the 2024 ACC/AHA guideline step-wise approach to preoperative cardiac risk evaluation?
2. How do functional capacity and biomarkers assist in risk estimation and decision making related to stress testing?
3. Is there a role for preoperative coronary revascularization?
4. How should antiplatelet therapy after percutaneous coronary intervention (PCI) be managed before noncardiac surgery?

INTRODUCTION

Over 300 million surgical procedures are performed worldwide each year, and it is estimated that over 4 million people die within 30 days of surgery, making it the third greatest contributor to mortality. Cardiac complications are one of the leading causes of postoperative morbidity and mortality, accounting for more than one-third of these deaths. This chapter will review preoperative evaluation and perioperative management of the patient with ischemic heart disease undergoing noncardiac surgery and is based on the 2024 ACC/AHA guideline for perioperative cardiac management.[1]

PATIENT-RELATED RISK FACTORS

History and Physical Exam

The most important element in preoperative cardiac risk assessment is a comprehensive history encompassing all relevant components of the cardiovascular system. These include symptoms of cardiovascular disease (CVD), prior cardiac disease, evaluation and interventions, risk factors, functional status, associated comorbid diseases, and medications (Table 11-1). The physical exam is important to corroborate history or elicit/assess risk factors focusing on vital signs and cardiopulmonary exam.

SURGERY-RELATED RISK FACTORS

Type of Surgery

Factors to consider that influence surgical risk include the site and type of incision, open or laparoscopic, hemodynamic compromise, estimated blood loss, duration of procedure, and type of anesthesia. The highest-risk procedures are aortic and major vascular surgery and prolonged procedures with significant blood loss or fluid shifts. Table 11-2 lists the risks of various surgical procedures.

Urgency of Surgery

The 2024 ACC guidelines changed some of their definitions regarding urgency of surgery, shortening

TABLE 11-1. Key Components in Cardiac Risk Assessment

PATIENT-RELATED HISTORY	SPECIFICS	SURGERY-RELATED
Prior cardiac disease	Previous MI (<2, 2–6, 6–12, >12 months) Angina (stable?/NYHA Class) HF (syst/diast/symptoms/EF) Arrhythmias/pacemaker/AICD Valvular disease (AS/MS, severity, symptoms) Syncope Congenital heart disease Pulmonary hypertension	High risk: major vascular surgery (AAA, infrainguinal bypass), major operations with significant blood loss or fluid shifts Intermediate risk: intraperitoneal, intrathoracic (nonmajor), major orthopedic, CEA, endovascular surgery
Prior cardiac intervention	CABG PCI (BA, BMS, DES) What? When? Recurrent symptoms?	Emergency procedure
Prior cardiac evaluation	ECG, exercise/pharmacologic, ECHO/nuclear/CCTA, ICA	Type of anesthesia? (GA vs. neuraxial)
Risk factors for CAD	Age, HTN, DM, dyslipidemia, smoking	
Associated comorbid diseases	CVA, PAD, CKD, COPD, OSA	
Current clinical status (symptoms)	Chest pain, dyspnea Functional status (independent?) Exercise capacity (>4 METs?)	
Cardiovascular medications	Antiplatelet, beta-blocker, ACEI/ARB, nitrate, other antianginal, antihypertensive, statin, anticoagulant	
Physical Exam	BP (hyper-hypotensive), HR (tachy/reg/irregular), RR (tachypnea), JVD, murmur, S3, rales, edema	
Cardiac Tests	ECG, stress test, CCTA, ICA, BNP/troponin	

MI, myocardial infarction; NYHA, NY Heart Association; HF, heart failure; EF, ejection fraction; AICD, automatic implantable cardiac defibrillator; AS, aortic stenosis; MS, mitral stenosis; AAA, abdominal aortic aneurysm; CEA, carotid endarterectomy; CABG, coronary artery bypass graft; PCI, percutaneous coronary intervention; BA, balloon angioplasty; BMS, bare metal stent; DES, drug-eluting stent; ECG, electrocardiogram; ECHO, echocardiogram; CA, coronary computerized tomography angiography; ICA, invasive coronary angiography; GA, general anesthesia; HTN, hypertension; DM, diabetes mellitus; CVA, cerebrovascular accident; PAD, peripheral arterial disease; CKD, chronic kidney disease; COPD, chronic obstructive pulmonary disease; METs, metabolic equivalents; ACEI, angiotensin-converting enzyme inhibitor; ARB, angiotensin receptor blocker; BP, blood pressure; HR, heart rate; RR, respiratory rate; JVD, jugular venous distention; BNP, brain natriuretic peptide; OSA, obstructive sleep apnea.

the definition of emergency from <6 to <2 hours and increasing that for time-sensitive surgery from 6 weeks to up to 3 months.

Surgery is considered an emergency when there is an immediate threat to life or limb as in a ruptured aortic aneurysm. Emergency surgery increases the risk for cardiac complications two- to fourfold due to increased physiological and emotional stress, a lack of time, typically <2 hours, to perform a detailed cardiac evaluation and optimize management, and potentially fewer personnel and resources at off-hours. Urgent surgery, usually required within 24 hours for

TABLE 11-2. Estimated Risks* Associated with Various Surgical Procedures

LOW RISK (<1%)	INTERMEDIATE RISK (1–5%)	HIGH RISK (>5%)
Superficial	Head and neck surgery	Aortic and major vascular surgery
Dental (extractions, endodontal)	Carotid endarterectomy	Peripheral vascular surgery
Eye (cataract)	Peripheral arterial angioplasty	Major abdominal surgery with significant blood loss or fluid shifts (pancreatic, liver resection, bile duct, esophagectomy, perforated bowel, radical cystectomy)
Breast (biopsy, mastectomy)	Endovascular aortic aneurysm repair	Major thoracic surgery (pneumonectomy)
Minor urologic (cystoscopy, TURBT, TURP)	Major urologic surgery (open prostatectomy)	Lung or liver transplant
Minor gynecologic (tubal ligation)	Major gynecologic surgery (hysterectomy/oophorectomy)	
Minor orthopedic (arthroscopy, meniscectomy)	Orthopedic surgery (hip, knee, spine)	
Endoscopic (EGD, colonoscopy, bronchoscopy)	Intraperitoneal (cholecystectomy, splenectomy)	
Inguinal herniorrhaphy	Nonmajor thoracic surgery Renal transplant	

TURBT/TURP, transurethral resection of bladder tumor/prostate; EGD, esophagogastroduodenoscopy.
*Estimated risk of 30-day cardiovascular death or myocardial infarction based only on surgical procedure.

a condition like a hip fracture, allows minimal time for limited preoperative evaluation and risk reduction strategies. Time-sensitive surgery, typically for malignancy, can often be delayed for up to 3 months and allows for preoperative evaluation and management without affecting outcome. Elective surgery, for example, a total joint replacement, can be delayed as long as necessary to complete a full evaluation and management plan.

Type of Anesthesia

There is a perception that neuraxial (spinal or epidural) anesthesia is safer than general anesthesia, but it remains controversial. However, the decision as to the type of anesthesia is still best left to the anesthesiologist. For minor procedures performed with local anesthesia, the expected risk of coronary ischemia is minimal (see Chapter 3).

PREOPERATIVE EVALUATION

The ACC guideline defines two categories of risk based on clinical/patient risk factors and surgical risk factors—low risk, which is <1% risk of major adverse cardiovascular events (MACE), and elevated risk with ≥1% risk of MACE. Earlier guidelines had low, intermediate, and high-risk categories (<1, 1–5, >5%), but the current categories were designed to have a low-risk group where everyone would agree that no further workup is necessary. Many clinicians, however, will approach patients with a slightly higher risk (i.e., 2%) in a similar fashion to low-risk patients.

Cardiac Risk Indices/Calculators

Since Goldman's original cardiac risk index in 1977, multiple cardiac risk indices and calculators have been published to facilitate risk stratification for perioperative cardiac complications. Those recommended by the 2014 ACC guidelines include the Lee Revised Cardiac Risk Index (RCRI), Gupta Myocardial Infarction or Cardiac Arrest (MICA) calculator, and the Bilimoria American College of Surgeons Surgical Risk Calculator (ACS-SRC). However, the current versions of the ACC and ESC guidelines do not recommend a specific calculator. These calculators and several newer tools are discussed in Chapter 9.

Diagnostic Tests

In addition to recommendations from the ACC perioperative guidelines,[1] the ACC/AHA along with other societies published "Appropriate Use Criteria for Multimodality Imaging in Cardiovascular Evaluation of Patients Undergoing Nonemergent, Noncardiac Surgery" which gives ratings for various imaging modalities in different clinical scenarios.[2]

Resting Tests. *Electrocardiogram:* The ECG remains a standard, inexpensive preoperative screening tool for patients with or at risk for coronary artery disease (CAD). It allows an immediate assessment of cardiac rate and rhythm and identification of new arrhythmias or conduction defects. The presence of pathological Q-waves may alert the clinician to previously undetected CAD or new infarction, and new ST segment changes associated with ongoing ischemia may be identified. Preoperative ECGs should be ordered selectively and not for low-risk patients undergoing low-risk surgery or based solely on age (see Chapter 2).

Echocardiogram: No evidence supports routine resting transthoracic echocardiography (TTE) to evaluate CAD in the preoperative setting. However, this test may provide essential information for patients with known or suspected significant valvular heart disease or left ventricular dysfunction (see Chapters 12 and 13).

Dynamic/Functional Noninvasive Tests

In general, stress tests should only be done if they would have been indicated regardless of the need for surgery or if the results are likely to change management in patients at elevated risk with poor exercise capacity. Cardiac biomarkers may be of help in making this decision.

Exercise Testing. Although exercise stress testing is not routinely recommended, information about recently performed stress tests may be useful, particularly if functional imaging was performed concurrently. A patient with a negative stress test of good quality has a low risk of significant perioperative ischemia. However, for patients with limited exercise capacity, such as those undergoing major joint replacement or peripheral vascular bypass, treadmill exercise testing is likely to be a futile endeavor, and for patients with adequate exercise capacity, the test is not indicated.

Pharmacologic Stress Testing. *Dipyridamole or adenosine stress testing* with nuclear imaging (technetium or thallium) may be indicated for selected elevated-risk patients with limited exercise capacity if the results will change management. Although the positive predictive value (PPV) of such testing is limited (PPV 15–25%), a negative test confers a low likelihood of cardiac complications (negative predictive value [NPV] > 95%). Additionally, the degree of abnormal stress perfusion predicts the likelihood of subsequent cardiac events. Fixed defects or small reperfusion abnormalities confer lower perioperative cardiac risk. The presence of ventricular dilatation or a significant drop in ejection fraction (EF) with stress suggests more significant underlying ischemia. Because dipyridamole and adenosine may cause bronchospasm, they are relatively contraindicated in patients with obstructive lung disease particularly if they are wheezing.

Dobutamine stress echocardiogram (DSE) is another noninvasive testing option. This is more physiological, as dobutamine increases heart rate and blood pressure more than dipyridamole or adenosine and can provide a double product (maximum heart rate times systolic blood pressure) or ischemic threshold that is reproducible for an individual patient. The number and degree of cardiac wall motion abnormalities detected with this method are associated with short- and long-term outcomes. The PPVs and NPVs of DSE are similar to those of nuclear imaging techniques, although DSE may have fewer false positives. Contraindications to DSE include uncontrolled hypertension (systolic > 180 mmHg) and suspected critical aortic stenosis.

Anatomic Tests. *Cardiac CT angiography (CCTA):* Although data are limited for noncardiac surgery, CCTA is a noninvasive method of evaluating coronary anatomy. It can demonstrate multivessel disease, rule out left main disease, and diagnose nonobstructive coronary disease. It tends to correlate reasonably well with ischemia on stress testing and has comparable rule-out capabilities (i.e., absence of multivessel disease even in the setting of predicted elevated risk by clinical indices has a high NPV). However, it has been reported that CCTA misclassifies some low-risk patients as high-risk, potentially subjecting them to unnecessary coronary angiography.

Invasive coronary angiography (ICA) is the invasive gold standard for evaluating coronary anatomy. Potential indications include having a significantly abnormal noninvasive test or symptomatic patients with Class III–IV or unstable angina. The decision to perform ICA should be made independent of the planned noncardiac operation.

Biomarkers (See Chapter 10)

BNP/NT-proBNP. The 2024 ACC guidelines[1] now state that it is reasonable to obtain preoperative BNP/NT-proBNP for patients who have known CVD, are 65 years of age or older, or have symptoms suggestive of CAD. The 2022 ESC guidelines[3] suggest consideration of these biomarkers in similar high-risk patients. The CCS guidelines[4] recommend them in the same setting plus for patients with an RCRI score ≥ 1. If elevated, there is a correlation with increased risk, and in conjunction with the RCRI, they may improve risk prediction. Cut-off values for elevated risk in the CCS guidelines are ≥ 92 pg/mL for BNP and ≥ 300 pg/mL for NT-proBNP, although a more recent study suggested that ≥ 200 pg/mL might be a better cut-off for NT-proBNP.[5]

Troponin. Preoperative troponin is not recommended by the CCS guidelines.[4] However, the ACC[1] states that preoperative troponin may be reasonable in patients with known CVD, symptoms suggestive of CVD, or age ≥ 65. The ESC[3] recommends obtaining troponin preoperatively and postoperatively in these patients undergoing intermediate- or high-risk surgery. If elevated, it is associated with increased risk. It may also be helpful as a baseline for comparison with postoperative troponin.

SOCIETY GUIDELINES (TABLE 11-3)

American College of Cardiology (ACC)[1]

https://www.jacc.org/doi/epdf/10.1016/j.jacc.2024.06.013

The 2024 ACC/AHA guideline provides a stepwise approach to preoperative cardiac risk assessment using urgency of surgery, clinical and surgery-specific risk factors, exercise capacity, biomarkers, and multidisciplinary team decision making.

1. Patients with no known CV disease, risk factors, or symptoms can proceed to surgery. Otherwise, continue to the next step.
2. Patients requiring *emergency surgery* will proceed to surgery without further testing and with limited medical optimization as time permits.
3. Patients with a *recent acute coronary syndrome* represent the highest-risk group and should not undergo elective surgery without further evaluation and therapy as per guideline recommendations. Similarly, elective surgery should be delayed for patients with *unstable arrhythmias or decompensated HF* to manage their cardiac condition.
4. Although not in the ACC algorithm, patients with *ischemic symptoms or history of CAD* should be questioned whether symptoms are new, worse, or stable; whether they had ACS, percutaneous coronary intervention (PCI), or coronary artery bypass graft (CABG) in the past year; and whether they have stable CAD with any *coronary evaluation/testing* in the past year and what the results were. Patients who were revascularized or had low-risk test results do not require further testing in the absence of new symptoms.
5. For all other patients, *estimate risk* based on clinical predictors and surgery-specific risk using one of the recommended *risk calculators*. If low risk (<1% risk of major adverse cardiac events—MACE), they should proceed to surgery without further testing. However, new to the 2024 ACC algorithm is a list of *risk modifiers* not in most risk calculators (severe valvular disease, pulmonary hypertension, recent stroke, prior PCI/CABG, congenital heart disease, Cardiac Implantable Electrical Device [CIED], frailty) that need to be evaluated and treated regardless of any calculated risk. These are discussed in other chapters.

TABLE 11-3. Comparison of the Three Major Society Guidelines—Testing

	ACC	ESC	CCS
Risk assessment tools	RCRI, MICA, ACS-SRC; (AUB-HAS2, SORT, GS-CRI)	RCRI, MICA, ACS-SRC; (AUB-HAS2, SORT)	RCRI (conditional recommend; low quality evidence)
Preop biomarkers	BNP/NT-proBNP (IIa/B) or troponin (IIb/B) if CVD, age ≥ 65, or ≥ 45 years with symptoms suggestive of CVD for elev risk NCS	Troponin (I/B) or BNP/NT-proBNP (IIa/B) if CVD, CV risk factors (incl age ≥ 65), or symptoms suggestive of CVD in interm-high-risk NCS	BNP/NT-proBNP if ≥65, 18–64 + CAD, or RCRI ≥ 1 (strong recommendation; mod quality evidence)
Use of exercise/ functional capacity	DASI ≥ 34 (IIa/B) (± > 2 flights of stairs)	DASI (IIa/B) >2 flights of stairs (IIa/B)	No recommendation
Echocardiogram (resting)	For new dyspnea, heart failure (Ib) or worsening symptoms with known HF (IIa/C), suspected mod-severe AS or MR (I/C)	If poor functioning capacity and/or high NT-proBNP/BNP, or if murmurs are detected before high-risk NCS (I/B); suspected new CVD or unexplained signs or symptoms before high-risk NCS (IIa/B); with poor funct capacity, abnormal ECG, high NT-proBNP/BNP, or ≥1 clinical risk factor before intermediate-risk NCS (IIb/B)	No (strong recommendation; low-quality evidence)
Stress testing (DSE/MPI)	If elevated clinical risk, elevated risk NCS, & poor/unknown exercise capacity (IIb/B)	If high clinical risk, high-risk NCS, & poor/unknown functional capacity; (I/B) high-risk NCS in asympt pts with poor funct capacity, & previous PCI or CABG; (IIa/C) interm-risk NCS when ischaemia is of concern in pts with clin risk factors & poor funct capacity (IIb/B)	No (strong recommendation; low/moderate quality evidence)
CCTA	If elevated clinical risk, elevated risk NCS, & poor/unknown exercise capacity (IIb/B)	To rule out CAD in pts with suspected CCS or biomarker-neg NSTE-ACS with low-to-interm clinical likelihood of CAD; in pts unsuitable for noninvasive funct testing undergoing interm-, & high-risk NCS (IIa/C)	No (strong recommendation; low-quality evidence)

ACC, American College of Cardiology; ESC, European College of Cardiology; CCS, Canadian Cardiovascular Society; RCRI, Revised Cardiac Risk Index; MICA, myocardial infarction or cardiac arrest; ACS-SRC, American College of Surgeons Surgical Risk Calculator; BNP/NT-proBNP, brain natriuretic peptide; CAD, coronary artery disease; CCTA, coronary computerized tomography angiography; CPET, cardiopulmonary exercise testing; METs, metabolic equivalents.

6. For patients classified as *elevated risk (≥1%)*, determine their functional capacity. The cut-off for adequate exercise capacity has classically been *4 METs (metabolic equivalents)*, and if ≥4 METs, the patient can proceed to surgery without further testing. Typically, a clinician would ask the patient if he/she could walk 2 to 4 blocks at a brisk pace or climb a flight of stairs without symptoms. Two large studies of elevated-risk patients, BASEL-PMI[6] and MET-REPAIR,[7] did show an association of postoperative cardiac complications with the self-reported inability to climb *two flights of stairs*, but the incremental value over risk indices was marginal. The *Measurement of Exercise Tolerance before Surgery* (METS) trial demonstrated that a clinician's subjective assessment was unreliable, and that use of the *Duke Activity Status Index (DASI)* (Table 11-4) was more accurate in predicting postoperative death or myocardial infarction (MI) at 30 days.[8] Of note, the majority of patients in this study were not at elevated risk, and the number of postoperative events was somewhat limited.

A DASI score > 34 was associated with a decreased risk of cardiac complications, although it corresponded to approximately 5 METs on cardiopulmonary exercise testing (CPET).[9] Note that scores using DASI calculators derived from nonsurgical patients will result in higher values of METs than those from surgical patients in the study (in this case a score of 34 results in 7 METs with the calculator rather than 5 METs on CPET). As many patients will be unable to achieve a DASI score of 34, a score of 25, which corresponded to approximately 4 METs in the study, may be a more reasonable cut-off although associated with a slightly higher risk of complications.

7. For patients whose *exercise capacity is <4 METs* or unable to be assessed, a decision must be made as to *whether further cardiac testing will change management*. Options may include potential

TABLE 11-4. Duke Activity Status Index (Max. Score 58.2)

ACTIVITY	WEIGHT
Can you ...	
1. take care of yourself, that is, eating, dressing, bathing, or using the toilet?	2.75
2. walk indoors, such as around your house?	1.75
3. walk a block or two on level ground?	2.75
4. climb a flight of stairs or walk up a hill?	5.50
5. run a short distance?	8.00
6. do light work around the house like dusting or washing dishes?	2.70
7. do moderate work around the house like vacuuming, sweeping floors, or carrying in groceries?	3.50
8. do heavy work around the house like scrubbing floors or lifting or moving heavy furniture?	8.00
9. do yardwork like raking leaves, weeding, or pushing a power mower?	4.50
10. have sexual relations?	5.25
11. participate in moderate recreational activities like golf, bowling, dancing, doubles tennis, or throwing a baseball or football?	6.00
12. participate in strenuous sports like swimming, singles, tennis, football, basketball, or skiing?	7.50

Source: Reproduced with permission from Hlatky MA, Boineau RE, Higginbotham MB, et al. A brief self-administered questionnaire to determine functional capacity. *The American Journal of Cardiology*. 1989;64(10):651-654.

revascularization, performing a less invasive procedure, nonsurgical treatment such as radiation or chemotherapy for cancer, or not having elective surgery at all. Consider whether surgery is *time-sensitive* and may not allow for further testing or interventions. *If the results will not change management and surgery is the only option, further cardiac testing should not be done.* If uncertain, the use of *cardiac biomarkers (BNP/NT-proBNP, troponin)* may be helpful in making this decision. If below the cut-off, which suggests low risk, no further testing would be indicated.

8. *If test results will change management, pharmacologic stress testing, CCTA, and/or invasive coronary angiography (ICA) can be performed.* If normal or low-risk results, the patient can proceed to surgery. If markedly abnormal, further cardiac intervention or nonsurgical options can be considered.

9. If deemed to be high risk, consider *postoperative troponin surveillance.*

10. All patients with CV disease or risk factors should be *treated as per GDMT.*

European Society of Cardiology (ESC)[3]

https://academic.oup.com/eurheartj/article/43/39/3826/6675076?login=false

The ESC approach is similar to the ACC and uses the urgency of surgery, presence of active or unstable cardiac conditions, risk of the surgical procedure, functional capacity, biomarkers, and consideration of noninvasive testing for those with poor functional capacity, multiple cardiac risk factors, and planned intermediate- to high-risk surgery if it aids counseling and decision making or changes management. Their approach is a bit more liberal than the ACC recommendations in terms of recommending additional cardiac tests, particularly echocardiography.

Canadian Cardiovascular Society (CCS)[4]

https://www.onlinecjc.ca/article/S0828-282X(16)30980-1/fulltext

The CCS approach differs significantly from the ACC and ESC by recommending use of the RCRI specifically, no role for stress testing, obtaining preoperative BNP/NT-proBNP in patients with age ≥ 65, RCRI score ≥ 1, or 45–64 with significant cardiac risk factors, and if elevated (or for patients undergoing urgent/emergent surgery), postoperative troponins, and comanagement.

Figure 11-1 illustrates a proposed algorithm based on the ACC guidelines incorporating various modifiers, measures of functional capacity, and biomarkers.

PERIOPERATIVE MANAGEMENT

Interventions to Reduce Risk

For high-risk patients with ischemic heart disease, options to lower that risk include coronary revascularization (CABG, PCI), medical therapy, invasive monitoring, changing to a lesser surgical procedure, or canceling surgery. Whether revascularization decreases surgical risk, how long the protection lasts, the optimal time to perform noncardiac surgery after these procedures, and which patients are likely to benefit are controversial, and there are few randomized controlled trials to evaluate these choices.

Preoperative Strategies

Coronary Revascularization. Regarding *CABG and PCI*, **studies of prophylactic revascularization are limited and to date have not been able to demonstrate a beneficial effect compared with medical therapy alone.**

Although not a study of prophylactic CABG prior to noncardiac surgery, a registry of patients with angina from the Coronary Artery Surgery Study (CASS) who were randomized to CABG versus those treated medically and who subsequently underwent major noncardiac surgery at a later date had a lower risk of death (1.7% vs. 3.3%) and nonfatal MI (0.8% vs. 2.7%).[10] There was no benefit for low-risk surgery, and this "protective" effect of CABG appeared to last for 4–6 years.

Data from the *Coronary Artery Revascularization Prophylaxis (CARP)* trial[11] failed to demonstrate either a short-term benefit (no reduction in perioperative MI or death, although underpowered) or improved long-term survival (22–23% mortality at 2.7 years in both groups) after CABG or PCI in patients with stable cardiac symptoms scheduled for elective vascular surgery. However, both groups received intensive perioperative medical therapy, and patients with >50% stenosis of the left main coronary artery, severe aortic stenosis, or left ventricular ejection fraction (LVEF) < 20% were excluded. The risk of morbidity and mortality associated with prophylactic revascularization in this study was 1.7% mortality, 5.8% perioperative MI, and 2.5%

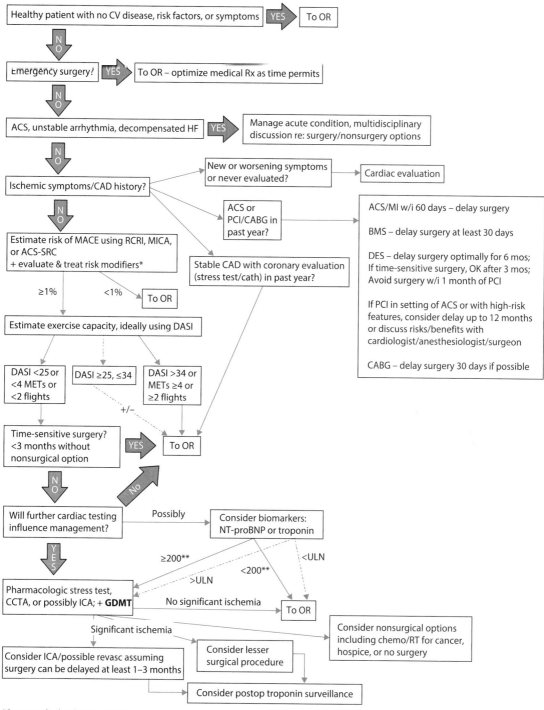

FIGURE 11-1. Proposed algorithm for preoperative cardiac evaluation.
Adapted from Thompson A, Fleischmann KE, Smilowitz NR, et al. *J Am Coll Cardiol*. 2024;84(19):1869-1969.

reoperation. Although there were no perioperative strokes, this complication may occur in up to 2%.

DECREASE V[12] was a pilot study of 200 patients with multiple cardiac risk factors and significant abnormalities on DSE previously who were shown not to benefit from beta-blockers. Results failed to demonstrate a decrease in MI or death at 30 days or 1 year in those patients undergoing noncardiac surgery who were randomized to prophylactic revascularization on top of medical therapy alone. (Although not showing positive results, this study from the Poldermans group was questioned for scientific integrity.)

Regarding the timing of subsequent noncardiac surgery, several studies have demonstrated an increased surgical risk if the noncardiac surgery was performed within 30 days of CABG.

Because PCI has a lower risk for adverse events than CABG, in theory it might be better, but there are no studies to confirm a benefit of prophylactic PCI. On the other hand, there are multiple studies demonstrating an increased risk associated with noncardiac surgery if performed soon after PCI, primarily related to stent thrombosis and associated STEMI and death. Timing of noncardiac surgery after PCI depends on the urgency of surgery and type of intervention performed, although some data suggest there may be no difference in risk between a bare metal stent (BMS) or drug-eluting stent (DES). **The preferred management of patients on dual antiplatelet therapy (DAPT) is to delay elective noncardiac surgery until completion of the full course of therapy if possible—6 months after elective PCI or 12 months after ACS or high-risk/complex PCI. ACC/AHA guidelines[1] recommend delaying elective surgery for at least 14 days after PTCA (balloon angioplasty), 30 days (possibly up to 90 days) after placement of a BMS, and optimally 6 months after a DES in order to complete the course of DAPT with aspirin and a P2Y12 inhibitor. However, if surgery is required sooner, it may be considered after 3 months (1 month as per ESC guidelines) if the risk of delaying surgery is thought to be greater than the risk of stent thrombosis, and aspirin should be continued whenever possible. Elective surgery in the first month after stent placement is not recommended. Risk of stent thrombosis is increased in high-risk settings including patient factors (age, diabetes mellitus [DM], low EF, severe renal disease), as well as procedural and anatomical factors (setting of ACS, LAD/LM stenting,** **multiple stents/multiple vessels, bifurcation, long, narrow, and multiple lesions).** These recommendations may change as shorter durations of DAPT are now being used more frequently in the nonsurgical setting.

Medical Therapy (Table 11-5)

Antiplatelet Drugs. *Aspirin:* Aspirin should be continued in patients with coronary stents, recent cardiovascular events (MI or stroke), and for carotid endarterectomy. The POISE-2 trial found no benefit to starting or continuing aspirin perioperatively in other patients, and it was associated with an increased risk of bleeding overall but not in the aspirin continuation subgroup.[13]

P2Y12 inhibitors: Typically, these drugs are stopped 5–7 days before surgery unless they are part of DAPT for recent stents (within 3 months). If they are monotherapy for stents, they can be continued, or aspirin can be substituted.

Beta-blockers. Two randomized controlled trials, by Mangano using atenolol and by Poldermans using bisoprolol, demonstrated beneficial effects of prophylactic beta-blockers before noncardiac surgery. Both studies titrated the beta-blocker dose to maintain heart rate between 55 and 65 beats per minute. Despite having only 312 patients in these two trials and methodologic criticisms, agencies and society guidelines recommended prophylactic beta-blockers.

Three subsequent RCTs (POBBLE, DiPOM, and MaVS) with approximately 1,500 patients failed to show any benefit of metoprolol in various cardiovascular outcomes. These studies started metoprolol on the day of or day before surgery and did not titrate the dose to control heart rate.

POISE,[14] the largest perioperative beta-blocker trial, randomized 8,351 patients to metoprolol succinate extended release or placebo. Patients received the first dose (metoprolol ER 100 mg or placebo) 2–6 hours before surgery, a second dose (100 mg) within 6 hours after the end of surgery, and then a maintenance dose of 200 mg daily started 12 hours after the postoperative dose. The drug was withheld for heart rate < 45 beats per minute or systolic BP < 100 mmHg and then restarted at half the dose 12 hours later if BP and pulse improved.

Primary outcome, a composite of cardiac death, nonfatal MI, and cardiac arrest, was significantly better

TABLE 11-5. Perioperative Cardiac Medication Management

MEDICATION	RECOMMENDATIONS
Aspirin	• Continue if for PCI/CABG (I/B) or if <1 year for ACS/MI/CVA • Do not start prophylactically except for CEA • If necessary to discontinue, stop 4–5 days before surgery
P2Y12 inhibitors	• Continue if 1st month after PCI or ACS • Optimally continue for ≥6 months after PCI (12 for ACS) but at least 3 months if surgery is time-sensitive • If necessary to discontinue, stop clopidogrel 5–7 days before, prasugrel 7 days before, and ticagrelor 3–5 days before surgery
Beta-blockers	• Continue if already taking it (I/B) • If new indication, beta-blockers may be initiated far enough before surgery (optimally >7 days) to permit assessments of tolerability and drug titration if needed (IIb/B)—not within 24 hours of surgery (III/B)
Statins	• Continue if already taking it (I/B) • Consider starting prophylactically if there are other independent indications for statins (I/B)
ACEIs/ARBs	• May withhold on AM of surgery if taken for HTN and BP is controlled (IIb/B) but restart by 48 hours postop if hemodynamically stable • If on chronic RAASi for HFrEF, perioperative continuation is reasonable (IIa/C)
Alpha agonists	• Continue if already taking it • Do not start prophylactically (III/B)
Calcium blockers	• Continue
Nitrates	• Continue (if for anginal control)

PCI, percutaneous coronary intervention; CABG, coronary artery bypass graft; ACS, acute coronary syndrome; MI, myocardial infarction; CVA, cerebrovascular accident; CEA, carotid endarterectomy; RCRI, Revised Cardiac Risk Index; ACEI, angiotensin-converting enzyme inhibitor; ARB, angiotensin receptor blocker; HF, heart failure; BP, blood pressure; RAASi, renin-angiotensin-aldosterone system inhibitor.

in the metoprolol-treated group due to a statistically significant reduction in nonfatal MIs from 5.1% to 3.6%. However, this benefit came at the expense of a statistically significant increase in secondary outcome events—nonfatal stroke (0.5–1%) and total mortality (2.3–3.1%) in the treatment group, in part due to significantly more episodes of hypotension and bradycardia.

This study was criticized because of the high dose of metoprolol that was started shortly before surgery in beta-blocker naïve patients, many of whom underwent emergency surgery or had sepsis.

DECREASE IV evaluated intermediate-risk patients who were given bisoprolol, fluvastatin, both, or neither. Bisoprolol was started approximately 1 month before surgery and titrated to a heart rate between 50 and 70 beats per minute. Cardiac death and nonfatal MI were significantly reduced from 6% to 2.1% in the group receiving bisoprolol versus the control group.

Multiple meta-analyses have been published with varying results depending on which studies were included. (Also note that the DECREASE trials from the Poldermans group have been questioned regarding scientific integrity.) A Cochrane systematic review demonstrated that perioperative beta-blockers were associated with lower rates of ischemia and MI but higher rates of hypotension and bradycardia. The 2019 Cochrane review stated that there was no increase in postoperative stroke and the effect on mortality was uncertain,[15] whereas the previous review stated both were increased with beta-blockers.

Patients currently taking beta-blockers should continue them perioperatively. If *prophylactic* beta-blockers are to be used, they should probably be started *at least 7 days before surgery* and titrated to achieve a heart rate of 55–65. The more cardioselective beta-blockers (bisoprolol and atenolol) may be preferable to metoprolol.

Alpha Agonists. Although several small studies reported potentially beneficial effects with clonidine, the POISE-2 trial using clonidine, aspirin, both, or neither in over 10,000 patients found no benefit with prophylactic clonidine, and instead it was associated with more hypotension, bradycardia, and nonfatal cardiac arrests.[16] A Cochrane systematic review of various alpha agonists also found adverse effects and no benefit. However, clonidine should be continued in patients already taking it to prevent withdrawal effects.

ACEIs/ARBs. Perioperative management of these agents is controversial. Since they have been associated with increased risk of intraoperative hypotension, they are often withheld on the morning of surgery unless the patient has HF or uncontrolled hypertension. However, recent studies (POISE-3, SPACE, STOP or NOT) have not shown harm in continuing these drugs preoperatively despite the risk of hypotension. If discontinued preoperatively, they should be restarted within 48 hours after surgery, assuming the patient is hemodynamically stable. Failure to restart these drugs within 14 days has been associated with adverse outcomes (see Chapter 4).

Calcium Blockers. Limited data found no evidence of any beneficial effect of calcium channel blockers in noncardiac surgery, but they are typically continued perioperatively.

Nitrates. A Cochrane systematic review found nitroglycerin or isosorbide dinitrate was not associated with a beneficial effect on mortality or cardiac complications in patients undergoing noncardiac surgery, but more patients experienced hypotension, tachycardia, and headache. However, a patient requiring nitrates for control of angina should continue them perioperatively.

Statins. Limited RCTs as well as observational studies and meta-analyses suggest that statin therapy is associated with a decrease in perioperative MI and possibly lower mortality. This is thought to be most likely related to its pleiotropic and anti-inflammatory properties rather than lowering cholesterol. Unanswered questions regarding perioperative statin use are whether this is a class effect, what dose should be used, how long in advance to start it prophylactically for it to be effective, whether loading or reloading doses are beneficial, and which patients are most likely to benefit from them. **Statins should be continued in patients already taking them. Additionally, in view of the potential benefit with little to no risk, an intermediate to high dose of a more potent statin (atorvastatin or rosuvastatin) should be started as early as possible preoperatively for patients undergoing vascular surgery as well as for those with any indications (e.g., peripheral arterial disease [PAD], DM, hyperlipidemia) for statins who are undergoing intermediate- to high-risk procedures.**

Intraoperative Monitoring

Intraoperative monitoring falls under the purview of the anesthesiologist. The consultant should communicate all pertinent information related to the patient's cardiac status, including the results of any recent cardiac investigations, to the anesthesiologist in advance (see Chapter 3).

Standard intraoperative monitoring includes heart rate and rhythm, blood pressure (noninvasive or arterial line), respiratory rate, pulse oximetry, and temperature. Additional modalities may include transesophageal echocardiography (TEE), pulmonary artery catheters, or ST segment monitors. Early identification of potential problems and prompt intervention are key to reducing adverse outcomes. The ACC recommends maintaining an intraoperative mean arterial pressure (MAP) $\geq$ 60 to 65 mmHg or SBP $\geq$ 90 mmHg to reduce the risk of myocardial injury. Maintenance of normothermia is also recommended.

Postoperative Management

Blood Pressure. Hypotension, particularly when unrecognized, is associated with postoperative cardiac complications. Treatment of hypotension (MAP < 60–65 mmHg or SBP < 90 mmHg) in the postoperative period is recommended to limit the risk of cardiovascular, cerebrovascular, renal events, and mortality. In addition to monitoring high-risk patients in step-down or telemetry units, real-time hemodynamic monitoring is being investigated in other settings including post-discharge. Evaluation and management of postoperative hypotension and hypertension are discussed in Chapter 36.

Pain Management. The surgical team and anesthesiologist are generally responsible for pain management postoperatively. Poorly controlled pain increases rates of cardiac ischemia due to increased sympathetic tone (tachycardia, hypertension). The consultant should alert the surgical team to assess the patient's pain control if this appears to be inadequate (see Chapter 45).

Continuation of Medical Therapy. Continue antiischemic medications throughout the perioperative period. This is especially true for beta-blockers or centrally acting alpha agonists, as there is a known rebound phenomenon associated with abrupt discontinuation of these drugs. Continue other cardiac medications postoperatively unless specifically contraindicated (e.g., hypotension, septic shock, acute renal failure). See Chapter 4 for a detailed discussion of perioperative medication management.

Surveillance with Biomarkers. Postoperative troponins (and ECGs) are recommended by the CCS guidelines for patients with a baseline risk > 5% for cardiovascular death or nonfatal MI at 30 days after surgery (i.e., patients with an elevated NT-proBNP/BNP measurement before surgery or, if there is no NT-proBNP/BNP measurement before surgery, in those who have an RCRI score ≥ 1, age 45–64 years with significant cardiovascular disease, or age 65 years or older). In the previous ESC and ACC guidelines, surveillance was only recommended for patients with signs or symptoms suggestive of ischemia. One reason for this discrepancy is that postoperative myocardial injury (MINS) has multiple etiologies that may need to be approached differently, and there is no clear, evidence-based treatment for MINS other than for Type I MI (see Chapter 37). However, the 2022 ESC guidelines recommend postoperative troponin surveillance, and the 2024 ACC guidelines say it is reasonable for at-risk patients (similar to the CCS criteria) undergoing intermediate- to high-risk surgery. Future studies may better identify the patient and surgical risk factors for which troponin screening may be beneficial.

Medical Comanagement. Shared-care management between surgeons and medical specialists was recommended for high-risk patients by the CCS guidelines. These models can coordinate care and provide more readily available help for evaluation and management of postoperative cardiac complications.

SUMMARY

Preoperative assessment of the patient with CAD should include a focused history and physical exam based upon established guidelines. A minority of patients may require noninvasive cardiac investigation and/or angiography, which should only be done if the results will change management. Employ risk reduction strategies including beta-blockers and statins for high-risk patients as per guideline recommendations. Using this approach for medical optimization, the consultant can hopefully improve the likelihood that a patient with CAD will have a better outcome after noncardiac surgery.

Clinical pearls

- History and physical exam are most important in preoperative evaluation. Cardiac risk calculators are helpful in defining low- and elevated-risk patient groups, but they are only tools to assist in risk assessment and decision making and have limitations.

- Subjective clinician assessment of a patient's exercise was found to be unreliable and should be replaced by a standardized questionnaire such as the DASI.

- Do not perform stress testing if the results will not change management.

- The use of cardiac biomarkers (BNP/NT-proBNP and troponin) may be helpful in deciding whether to pursue further cardiac testing.

- Because prophylactic coronary revascularization has not been shown to be beneficial, the indication for CABG and PCI in the preoperative period is the same as for the nonsurgical patient, and it should not be performed solely to get the patient through noncardiac surgery.

- ACC/AHA guidelines recommend delaying elective surgery for at least 14 days after PTCA (balloon angioplasty), 30 days (possibly up to 90 days) after placement of a BMS, and optimally 6 months after a DES to complete the course of DAPT with aspirin and a P2Y12 inhibitor. However, if surgery is required sooner, it may be considered after 3 months (1 month as per ESC guidelines) if the risk of delaying surgery is thought to be greater than the risk of stent thrombosis, and aspirin should be continued whenever possible. Elective surgery in the first month after stent placement is not recommended.

- Perioperative beta-blockers were associated with lower rates of ischemia and MI but higher rates of hypotension and bradycardia. There may be an increase in postoperative stroke (primarily in POISE) and the effect on mortality is uncertain.

- If *prophylactic* beta-blockers are to be used, they should probably be started at least 7 days before surgery and titrated to achieve a heart rate of 55–65. The more cardioselective beta-blockers (bisoprolol and atenolol) may be preferable to metoprolol.

- In view of the potential benefit with little to no risk, an intermediate to high dose of a more potent statin (atorvastatin or rosuvastatin) should be started as early as possible preoperatively for patients with indications for them who are undergoing intermediate- to high-risk procedures, particularly vascular surgery. Statins should be continued in patients already taking them.

REFERENCES

1. Writing Committee Members; Thompson A, Fleischmann KE, Smilowitz NR, et al. 2024 AHA/ACC/ACS/ASNC/HRS/SCA/SCCT/SCMR/SVM guideline for perioperative cardiovascular management for noncardiac surgery: a report of the American College of Cardiology/American Heart Association Joint Committee on Clinical Practice Guidelines. *J Am Coll Cardiol*. 2024;84(19):1869-1969. doi: 10.1016/j.jacc.2024.06.013. PMID: 39320289

2. Writing Group Members; Doherty JU, Daugherty SL, Kort S, et al. ACC/AHA/ASE/ASNC/HFSA/HRS/SCAI/SCCT/SCMR/STS 2024 appropriate use criteria for multimodality imaging in cardiovascular evaluation of patients undergoing nonemergent, noncardiac surgery. *J Am Coll Cardiol*. 2024;84(15):1455-1491. PMID: 39207318

3. Halvorsen S, Mehilli J, Cassese S, et al.; ESC Scientific Document Group. 2022 ESC guidelines on cardiovascular assessment and management of patients undergoing non-cardiac surgery. *Eur Heart J*. 2022;43(39):3826-3924. PMID: 36017553

4. Duceppe E, Parlow J, MacDonald P, et al. Canadian Cardiovascular Society guidelines on perioperative cardiac risk assessment and management for patients who undergo noncardiac surgery. *Can J Cardiol*. 2017;33(1):17-32. PMID: 27865641

5. Duceppe E, Patel A, Chan MTV, et al. Preoperative N-terminal pro-B-type natriuretic peptide and cardiovascular events after noncardiac surgery: a cohort study. *Ann Intern Med*. 2020;172(2):96-104. PMID: 31869834

6. Lurati Buse GA, Puelacher C, Menosi Gualandro D, et al. Association between self-reported functional capacity and major adverse cardiac events in patients at elevated risk undergoing noncardiac surgery: a prospective diagnostic cohort study. *Br J Anaesth*. 2021;126(1):102-110. PMID: 33081973

7. Roth S, M'Pembele R, Nienhaus J, et al; MET: Reevaluation for Perioperative Cardiac Risk Investigators. Association between self-reported functional capacity and general postoperative complications: analysis of predefined outcomes of the MET-REPAIR international cohort study. *Br J Anaesth*. 2024;132(4):811-814. PMID: 38326210

8. Wijeysundera DN, Pearse RM, Shulman MA, et al. Assessment of functional capacity before major noncardiac surgery: an international, prospective cohort study. *Lancet*. 2018;391(10140):2631-2640. PMID: 30070222

9. Wijeysundera DN, Beattie WS, Hillis GS, et al. Integration of the Duke activity status index into preoperative risk evaluation: a multicentre prospective cohort study. *Br J Anaesth*. 2020;124(3):261-270. PMID: 31864719

10. Eagle KA, Rihal CS, Mickel MC, et al. Cardiac risk of noncardiac surgery: influence of coronary disease and type of surgery in 3368 operations. CASS Investigators and University of Michigan Heart Care Program. Coronary artery surgery study. *Circulation*. 1997;96(6):1882-1887. PMID: 9323076

11. McFalls EO, Ward HB, Moritz TE, et al. Coronary-artery revascularization before elective major vascular surgery. *N Engl J Med*. 2004;351(27):2795-2804. PMID: 15625331

12. Poldermans D, Schouten O, Vidakovic R; DECREASE Study Group. A clinical randomized trial to evaluate the safety of a noninvasive approach in high-risk patients undergoing major vascular surgery: the DECREASE-V pilot study. *J Am Coll Cardiol*. 2007;49(17):1763-1769. PMID: 17466225

13. Devereaux PJ, Mrkobrada M, Sessler DI, et al. Aspirin in patients undergoing noncardiac surgery. *N Engl J Med*. 2014;370(16):1494-1503. PMID: 24679062

14. POISE Study Group, Devereaux PJ, Yang H, et al. Effects of extended-release metoprolol succinate in patients undergoing non-cardiac surgery (POISE trial): a randomised controlled trial. *Lancet*. 2008;371(9627):1839-1847. PMID: 18479744

15. Blessberger H, Lewis SR, Pritchard MW, et al. Perioperative beta-blockers for preventing surgery-related mortality and morbidity in adults undergoing non-cardiac surgery. *Cochrane Database Syst Rev*. 2019;9:CD013438. PMID: 31556094

16. Devereaux PJ, Sessler DI, Leslie K, et al. Clonidine in patients undergoing noncardiac surgery. *N Engl J Med*. 2014;370(16):1504-1513. PMID: 24679061

## 12

Heart Failure

Gregary D. Marhefka, MD, FACP, FACC and Howard H. Weitz, MD, MACP, FACC, FRCP

COMMON CLINICAL QUESTIONS

1. Which patients with heart failure are at the highest risk for postoperative cardiac complications?
2. When should noncardiac surgery be postponed in patients with heart failure?
3. How should medications for heart failure be managed perioperatively?

RISK FACTORS (SEE TABLE 12-1)

Heart Failure and Risk of Mortality

As early as 1977 the Goldman Risk Index identified the presence of heart failure physical exam signs (jugular venous distension or S3 gallop) as one of nine variables associated with an increased risk of cardiac complications in noncardiac surgery.[1] The Goldman Risk Index was revised in 1999 to facilitate ease of use and increased accuracy. This Revised Cardiac Risk Index (RCRI), still in popular use today, considers a "history of congestive heart failure" as one of the six predictors of perioperative nonfatal myocardial infarction, pulmonary edema, ventricular fibrillation, nonfatal cardiac arrest, and complete heart block.[2] Despite advances in the treatment of heart failure since 1999, preexisting heart failure before noncardiac surgery continues to be a marker of increased perioperative risk that is often underestimated.

- In a large Canadian cohort of 38,047 patients undergoing noncardiac surgery, the unadjusted 30-day postoperative mortality was significantly higher in patients with preexisting nonischemic and ischemic heart failure than in those with preexisting atrial fibrillation and coronary artery disease.[3] The higher risk was observed even in minor risk procedures.

- In a study of 1,172,632 patients undergoing noncardiac surgery, 7,544 (0.64%) had preexisting heart failure. The group with heart failure was more likely to require cardiopulmonary resuscitation and ventilator support for more than 48 hours, and experienced higher rates of 30-day mortality, readmission to the hospital, and myocardial infarction.[4]

- In a large retrospective cohort of 609,735 Veteran's Affairs patients, 47,997 (7.87%) had preexisting heart failure. The 90-day postoperative mortality was significantly higher in those with heart failure compared to those without. Furthermore, the lower the ejection fraction, the higher the mortality.[5] Despite the association of heart failure with postoperative mortality, after multivariable regression analysis, heart failure itself was not the clinical cause of mortality, but rather served as a marker for a multitude of comorbidities that heart failure patients typically have. Patients with heart failure were older and had more coexisting conditions.

- A retrospective study of 296,057 heart failure patients from the Nationwide Readmissions Database found that patients with HFrEF had a higher inhospital mortality rate and more 30-day readmissions than patients with HFpEF.[6]

TABLE 12-1. Heart Failure and Perioperative Risk

RISK FACTORS	HF SYMPTOMS	STAGE	LV FUNCTION	EJECTION FRACTION (EF)	
• Stage (D>C>B) • LV function (reduced>preserved) • EF (<30–40%) • Symptomatic>asymptomatic • Med Rx: Suboptimal Rx > optimally Rx'd • Acute or recently Dx HF • RV dysfunction • Associated valvular disease • Elevated BNP/NT-proBNP • Age • Other comorbidities • High-risk surgery (vascular/ortho) • Urgent/emergency surgery	Asymptomatic	B (pre-HF)	Preserved (diastolic dysfunction)	>50%	Increasing Risk
			Reduced (systolic dysfunction)	<50%	
	Prior symptoms but currently asymptomatic	C (HF)	Preserved (HFpEF)	>50%	
			Mildly reduced (HFmrEF)	41–49%	
			Reduced (HFrEF)	<40%	
	Currently symptomatic	C or D (advanced HF)	Preserved (HFpEF)	>50%	
			Mildly reduced (HFmrEF)	41–49%	
			Reduced (HFrEF)	30–40%	
			Severely reduced	<30%	

- Utilizing the Healthcare Cost and Utilization Project National Inpatient Sample, an analysis of 21,560,996 adults undergoing noncardiac surgery from 2012 and 2014 found that 1,063,405 (4.9%) had a concomitant diagnosis of heart failure (of which 4.7% were acute, 11.3% were acute on chronic, 27.8% were chronic, and 56.2% were unspecified).[7] Inhospital perioperative mortality was significantly more common in heart failure patients (4.8% vs. 0.78%). Acute heart failure and acute on chronic heart failure had the highest mortality rates, 8% and 7.8%, respectively. Heart failure patients were older and more likely male with more cardiovascular disease comorbidities.

- In a secondary analysis of a prospective, international study of cardiac complications following noncardiac surgery in both Switzerland and Brazil, 9,164 patients (based on age > 65 years old or ≥ 45 years old plus coronary, peripheral or cerebral vascular disease) underwent 11,262 surgeries were analyzed.[8] The incidence of postoperative heart failure was 2.5% (mostly within

2 days of surgery), including 51% in patients without known heart failure. In patients with known chronic heart failure, 10% developed postoperative acute heart failure, whereas in those without preexisting heart failure, 1.5% developed acute heart failure. Independent predictors of acute heart failure were preexisting heart failure, diabetes, urgent or emergent surgery, atrial fibrillation, troponin elevation above 99th percentile, chronic obstructive pulmonary disease, anemia, peripheral artery disease, coronary artery disease, and older age. Acute heart failure postoperatively was associated with higher all-cause mortality at 1 year, 44% versus 11%, with early separation of the curves, as well as higher 1-year readmission rates for acute heart failure, 15% versus 2%.

The acuity and treatment status of heart failure is also important. Active signs of heart failure confer the highest risk. Association of heart failure with valvular heart disease such as severe aortic stenosis or severe mitral regurgitation also correlates with worse outcomes.

PREOPERATIVE EVALUATION

Indications to Delay or Cancel Surgery (Acute HFrEF or HFpEF) (See Figure 12-1)

Based on standard history, review of systems, and physical exam, heart failure can often be suspected and identified. Eliciting a history of peripheral edema and weight gain, diminished exercise tolerance, dyspnea with exertion, orthopnea, and paroxysmal nocturnal dyspnea can suggest clinical heart failure. Asking if a patient no longer sleeps in a bed, but is sleeping in a chair or recliner, and assessing for bendopnea (dyspnea within 30 seconds of bending forward while seated) can sometimes uncover a new suspicion for heart failure in an undiagnosed patient, or signal an acute exacerbation in a patient with chronic heart failure. Careful assessment for physical exam findings of conversational dyspnea, jugular venous distension, S3 gallop, murmurs of aortic stenosis or mitral regurgitation, peripheral edema, and chest x-ray findings of pulmonary vascular

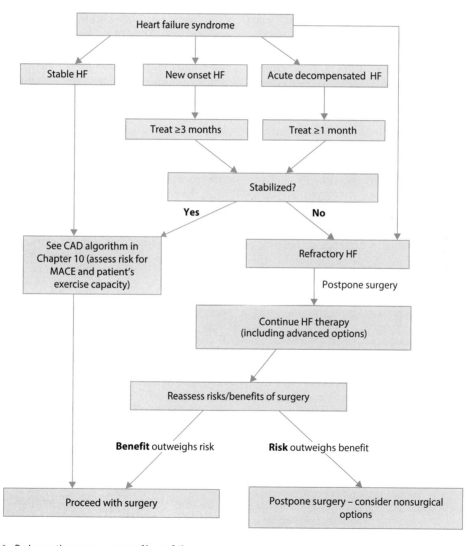

FIGURE 12-1. Perioperative management of heart failure.
Adapted from Meyer TE. Perioperative management of heart failure in patients undergoing noncardiac surgery.

redistribution or pulmonary edema can help confirm the presence of acute heart failure. These patients are at significant risk for perioperative complications, and acute heart failure should be treated with guideline-directed medical therapy (GDMT) before elective noncardiac surgery. Furthermore, these findings should prompt cancellation or delay of elective noncardiac surgery when possible.

For the patient with acute heart failure with reduced ejection fraction (HFrEF), the goal is diuresis and titration of medications modulating the renin-angiotensin-aldosterone system, including angiotensin receptor neprilysin inhibitors, as well as sodium glucose cotransporter-2 (SGLT2) inhibition, when indicated. Once acute heart failure is improved or resolved, then introducing, reintroducing, or slowly retitrating maximally tolerated doses of proven chronic heart failure benefiting beta-blockade is the next step. Patients with acute heart failure with preserved ejection fraction (HFpEF) do not appear to have as high a risk for perioperative cardiovascular events, but they are still at increased risk compared to patients without heart failure. Optimization and stabilization of blood pressure and judicious diuretics to eliminate volume overload are important. SGLT2 inhibitors are indicated to reduce cardiovascular death and heart failure hospitalizations in patients with symptomatic chronic HFpEF, unrelated to presence or absence of diabetes mellitus type 2.[9] If not being used to treat hypertension, beta-blockers, angiotensin-converting enzyme inhibitors, angiotensin receptor blockers, angiotensin receptor neprilysin inhibitors, and aldosterone inhibitors have not been found to be effective in the treatment of HFpEF. Lastly, the ideal duration of clinical stability once acute heart or chronic failure has been treated prior to proceeding to noncardiac surgery has never been elucidated.

Preoperative Management of Heart Failure Guideline GDMT (RAAS Inhibitors, Beta-Blockers, Mineralocorticoid Inhibitors, SGLT2 Inhibitors)

Continued use of chronic preoperative renin-angiotensin-aldosterone system (RAAS) inhibitors (angiotensin-converting enzyme inhibitors, angiotensin receptor blockers) may be associated with intraoperative or postoperative hypotension which may result in acute kidney injury and contribute to myocardial injury in noncardiac surgery. It is controversial as to whether these agents should be discontinued prior to surgery. Our approach for the patient who is receiving these medications for hypertension is to discontinue them the day before surgery and to resume them when the patient is stable following the surgical procedure. For the patient who is taking these medications as key agents in the treatment of chronic HFrEF, we determine whether they should be discontinued prior to surgery on a case-by-case basis (Table 12-2).[10-12]

TABLE 12-2. National Guidelines Recommendations for Management of Perioperative Angiotensin Converting Enzymes Inhibitors, Angiotensin Receptor Blockers, and Aldosterone Inhibitors[10-12]

NATIONAL GUIDELINE	RECOMMENDATION REGARDING ACEI/ARB
2022 ESC/ESA Guidelines	In patients without HF, withholding RAAS inhibitors on the day of noncardiac surgery should be considered to prevent perioperative hypotension. These medications should be restarted as soon as possible in order to prevent unintended long-term omission. In patients with stable HF, perioperative continuation of RAAS inhibitors may be considered.
2017 CCS Guideline	Withhold ACEI/ARB 24 hours before noncardiac surgery and restart ACEI/ARB on day 2 after surgery, if the patient is hemodynamically stable.
2024 ACC/AHA Guideline	In patients on chronic ACEI/ARBs for HFrEF, continuation is reasonable perioperatively. In patients undergoing elevated-risk noncardiac surgery who are on chronic ACEIs/ARBs for hypertension whose BP is controlled, omission 24 hours before surgery may be beneficial to limit intraoperative hypotension. If ACEIs or ARBs are held before surgery, it is reasonable to restart as soon as clinically feasible postoperatively.

In patients on chronic beta-blockers, these agents should be continued perioperatively when possible to avoid withdrawal. Because beta-blockers can result in perioperative bradycardia or hypotension, these patients should be observed carefully in the perioperative period. In patients never previously treated with a beta-blocker or in whom beta-blockers were discontinued for a significant period of time, these medications should not be started in close proximity to surgery. For the patient receiving mineralocorticoid blockers, for example, spironolactone or eplerenone, we typically continue these agents up to the time of surgery and resume them when oral intake resumes. If surgery is complicated by acute kidney injury, we withhold these agents. SGLT2 inhibitors should be held at least 3 days prior to elective noncardiac surgery to avoid the risk of diabetic ketoacidosis, which may be precipitated by these agents when used in the fasting state (see Chapter 4).

Role of Heart Failure Biomarkers (BNP and NT-proBNP) in Preoperative Risk Stratification (See Chapter 10)

History and physical exam alone can have some limitations in terms of diagnosing heart failure and assessing cardiovascular risk prior to noncardiac surgery. A systematic review and meta-analysis of 3,281 patients demonstrated that an elevated preoperative BNP was an independent predictor of 30-day postoperative cardiac death, nonfatal myocardial infarction, and atrial fibrillation.[13] A prospective cohort study of 10,402 patients 45 years or older undergoing noncardiac surgery studied preoperative NT-proBNP and postoperative troponin T measurements for up to 3 days following surgery. The higher the preoperative NT-proBNP, the higher the risk of vascular death and myocardial injury after noncardiac surgery (MINS).[14] The authors propose that a preoperative NT-proBNP > 200 pg/mL could guide clinicians to order postoperative troponins. The Canadian Cardiovascular Society Guidelines on Perioperative Cardiac Risk Assessment and Management for Patients Undergoing Noncardiac Surgery recommend measuring BNP or NT-BNP (using cut-offs to order postoperative troponins of 92 pg/mL and 300 pg/mL, respectively) before noncardiac surgery in those ≥ 65 years old or those aged 45–65 with known cardiovascular disease, or an RCRI score ≥ 1.[12] If heart failure is suspected, the strength

of measuring preoperative BNP or NT-proBNP is its high negative predictive value for excluding heart failure and predicting lower risk related to noncardiac surgery. It is important to note that many of the patients with an elevated BNP or NT-proBNP did not have clinical heart failure. Patients, families when appropriate, and surgeons should be counseled on the clinical significance of an elevated preoperative BNP or NT-BNP and its association with worse outcomes, recognizing that ideal optimization or risk reduction in such patients is unknown. If noncardiac surgery is totally elective and of marginal clinical value, then perhaps considering cancellation of the surgery would be the most practical recommendation when appropriate. The European Society of Cardiology recommends that in patients with known or suspected heart failure scheduled for high-risk noncardiac surgery unless already performed, left ventricular function should be assessed before surgery with measurement of NT-proBNP/BNP and echocardiogram.[15]

PERIOPERATIVE MANAGEMENT

Role for Echocardiography

Transthoracic echocardiography is useful in known or suspected heart failure, not only to assess ejection fraction because of its correlation with perioperative prognosis as indicated previously in Table 12-1, but also to assess valvular abnormalities that can often be associated with heart failure, as well as to assess diastolic indices. Diastolic dysfunction has been associated with events, length of stay, and increased incidence of postoperative heart failure. However, routine echocardiography is not imperative in the absence of suspected or known heart failure and has never been proven to be of clinical benefit in the perioperative period. As per the recommendations of the European Society of Cardiology, it is our practice for patients with known or suspected heart failure with new or worsening symptoms who are to undergo high-risk surgery to perform a transthoracic echocardiogram before surgery to evaluate ventricular function if it has not been recently performed.[10]

The Patient with a Ventricular Assist Device (VAD)

VAD as therapy to bridge to heart transplant or as destination therapy is playing an increasing role in the care of the patient with advanced heart failure. Noncardiac surgery for patients with these devices should be performed in a center that has the experience and infrastructure to manage these devices.

Management of Acute Heart Failure in the Perioperative Period

Current perioperative and heart failure guidelines do not address the acute management of heart failure in the perioperative period. Approaching acute heart failure identified in the postoperative period is similar to the approach in nonoperative settings. Evaluation should center on physical examination, ECG, chest x-ray, BNP or NT-proBNP assessment, troponin assessment, and selective echocardiography. In the perioperative setting, high volume fluid resuscitation often occurs, which, after mobilization in the body, can result in acute pulmonary edema requiring diuresis. The same is true for postoperative acute HFrEF or HFpEF. Attention to volume status with control of hypertension and arrhythmias should be employed to reduce a similar risk of acute pulmonary edema. Pulmonary artery catheters in the perioperative period have never been proven to be of benefit, but in select cases in experienced centers may be of utility in extreme cases of heart failure combined with suspected cardiogenic shock to guide management.

One type of heart failure warranting further discussion is hypertrophic cardiomyopathy (HCM). An inherited form of cardiomyopathy with varied phenotypic expression, up to 70% can have associated left ventricular outflow tract (LVOT) obstruction. This can often go unrecognized and prove to be highly problematic in the postoperative period. Its presence should be suspected with a dynamic or changing harsh systolic murmur over the precordium that increases with Valsalva (LVOT obstruction) and sometimes a dynamic or changing holosystolic murmur at the apex (mitral regurgitation from systolic anterior motion of the anterior mitral valve leaflet from LVOT obstruction) that may have been less or nonexistent preoperatively. Conditions that can exacerbate LVOT obstruction, with or without associated mitral regurgitation, are often encountered in the postoperative period, such as tachycardia and increased sympathetic tone, hypovolemia, and arrhythmias. These unrecognized conditions, combined with inappropriate utilization of

medications for hypotension that can increase inotropy, can further exacerbate LVOT obstruction and lead to worsening clinical deterioration and hemodynamic collapse. One small study of 30-day outcomes in 92 patients with HCM compared to 184 patients without HCM undergoing intermediate or high-risk noncardiac surgery showed an increased event rate of heart failure and atrial fibrillation during the hospitalization and increased readmission for heart failure.[15] A higher provocable LVOT gradient and a longer duration of intraoperative hypotension were also associated with higher incidence of events. In a retrospective publication of perioperative outcomes of HCM patients between 2016 and 2019 from the National Readmission Database of the Agency for Healthcare Research and Quality through the Healthcare Cost and Utilization Project, there were 16,098 hospitalizations in patients with HCM with obstruction and 21,895,699 hospitalizations in patients without HCM with obstruction.[16] Both groups were about 60% female, but the HCM with obstruction group had more preexisting HF (43% vs. 13%), valvular disease (31% vs. 5%), peripheral vascular disease (20% vs. 6%), diabetes (10% vs. 9%), hypertension (48% vs. 18%), prior myocardial infarction (MI) (8.5% vs. 4.3%), and CAD (44% vs. 17%). There were more deaths during the index surgical hospitalization in the HCM with obstruction group (6.86% vs. 3%), acute MI (8.57% vs. 2.6%), more acute HF (16.8% vs. 4.3%), cardiogenic shock (4.9% vs. 0.9%), and more cardiac arrests (2.3% vs. 0.9%). There were also more readmissions in the HCM with obstruction group (2.9% vs. 2.1%); however, there were no difference in mortality after readmission (1% vs. 1.5%), or major adverse cardiac and cerebrovascular events (5.7% vs. 5.1%), but there were more exacerbations of HF during readmission (12.7% vs. 3.3%). Therefore, in patients with HCM with LVOT obstruction, we recommend avoiding hypovolemia, tachycardia, and any medications that can increase inotropy. Recognizing that hypotension could be due to LVOT obstruction is paramount, and auscultation of the harsh precordial systolic murmur can be the first indication, with confirmation by point-of-care ultrasound or formal echocardiography with color flow and spectral Doppler. Continued use of beta-blockers in the perioperative period can be essential, even in the face of hypotension at times. For induction of anesthesia, etomidate is associated with less hypotension. For true vasoplegia-related hypotension, use judicious volume loading, along with phenylephrine and/or vasopressin +/− angiotensin II as the pharmacologic agents of choice, as they have no inotropic properties.

Clinical pearls

- Preexisting heart failure is often underestimated and portends a higher risk of postoperative mortality than preexisting coronary artery disease or atrial fibrillation.
- Acute HFrEF or HFpEF should prompt delay of noncardiac surgery and appropriate treatment and stabilization.
- Postoperative HF is associated with higher 1-year mortality and hospital readmission rates.
- Controversy remains regarding optimal preoperative management of angiotensin-converting enzyme inhibitors and angiotensin receptor blockers. Holding these medicines when prescribed for hypertension is reasonable, while trying to continue these medicines when prescribed for heart failure seems appropriate, on a case-by-case basis. Beta-blockers should be continued if chronically taken, but never started in proximity to surgery if not chronically taking. SGLT2 inhibitors should be stopped 3 days before surgery.
- The biomarkers BNP and NT-proBNP are highly predictive of postoperative events and mortality.
- Heart failure in the perioperative period should be managed similarly to noncardiac surgery-related heart failure, with attention to volume, hypertension, and arrhythmia control, which can exacerbate the condition.
- In HCM with obstruction, avoiding hypovolemia, tachycardia, and inotropes is essential.

REFERENCES

1. Goldman L, Caldera DL, Nussbaum SR, et al. Multifactorial index of cardiac risk in noncardiac surgical procedures. *N Engl J Med.* 1977;297(16):845-850. PMID: 904659
2. Lee TH, Marcantonio ER, Mangione CM, et al. Derivation and prospective validation of a simple index for prediction of cardiac risk of major noncardiac surgery. *Circulation.* 1999;100(10):1043-1049. PMID: 10477528
3. van Diepen S, Bakal JA, McAlister FA, et al. Mortality and readmission of patients with heart failure, atrial fibrillation, or coronary artery disease undergoing noncardiac surgery: an analysis of 38 047 patients. *Circulation.* 2011;124(3):289-296. PMID: 21709059
4. Turrentine FE, Sohn MW, Jones RS. Congestive heart failure and noncardiac operations: risk of serious morbidity, readmission, reoperation, and mortality. *J Am Coll Surg.* 2016;222(6):1220-1229. PMID: 27106641
5. Lerman BJ, Popat RA, Assimes TL, et al. Association of left ventricular ejection fraction and symptoms with mortality after elective noncardiac surgery among patients with heart failure. *JAMA.* 2019;321(6):572-579. PMID: 30747965
6. Huang YY, Chen L, Wright JD. Comparison of perioperative outcomes in heart failure patients with reduced versus preserved ejection fraction after noncardiac surgery. *Ann Surg.* 2022;275(4):807-815. PMID: 32541225
7. Smilowitz NR, Banco D, Katz SD, et al. Association between heart failure and perioperative outcomes in patients undergoing non-cardiac surgery. *Eur Heart J – Qual Care Clin Outcomes.* 2021;7:68-75. PMID: 31873731
8. Gualandro DM, Puelacher C, Chew MS, et al. Acute heart failure after non-cardiac surgery: incidence, phenotypes, determinants and outcomes. *Eur J Heart Fail.* 2023;25:347-357. PMID: 36644890
9. Heidenreich PA, Bozkurt B, Aguilr D, et al. 2022 AHA/ACC/HFSA guideline for the management of heart failure. *J Am Coll Cardiol.* 2022;79:e263-e421. PMID: 35379503
10. Halvorsen S, Mehilli J, Cassese S, et al. 2022 ESC guidelines on cardiovascular assessment and management of patients undergoing noncardiac surgery. *Eur Heart J.* 2022;43(39):3826-3924. PMID: 36017553
11. Thompson A, Fleischmann KE, Smilowitz NR, et al. 2024 AHA/ACC/ACS/ASNC/HRS/SCA/SCCT/SCMR/SVM guideline for perioperative cardiovascular management for noncardiac surgery: a report of the American College of Cardiology/American Heart Association Joint Committee on Clinical Practice Guidelines. *J Am Coll Cardiol.* 2024;84(19):1869-1969. doi:10.1016/j.jacc.2024.06.013. PMID: 39320289.
12. Duceppe E, Parlow J, MacDonald P, et al. Canadian Cardiovascular Society Guidelines on perioperative cardiac risk assessment and management for patients who undergo noncardiac surgery. *Can J Cardiol.* 2017;33(1):17-32. PMID: 27865641

13. Karthikeyan G, Moncur RA, Levine O, et al. Is a pre-operative brain natriuretic peptide or N-terminal pro-B-type natriuretic peptide measurement an independent predictor of adverse cardiovascular outcomes within 30 days of noncardiac surgery? A systematic review and meta-analysis of observational studies. *J Am Coll Cardiol.* 2009;54(17):1599-1606. PMID: 19833258

14. Duceppe E, Patel A, Chan MTV, et al. Preoperative N-terminal pro–B-type natriuretic peptide and cardiovascular events after noncardiac surgery: a cohort study. *Ann Intern Med.* 2020;172(2):96-104. PMID: 31869834

15. Dhillon A, Khanna A, Randhawa MS, et al. Perioperative outcomes of patients with hypertrophic cardiomyopathy undergoing noncardiac surgery. *Heart.* 2016;102(20):1627-1632. PMID: 27288277

16. Barssoum K, Abumoawad A, Chowdhury M, et al. Perioperative outcomes of hypertrophic cardiomyopathy: an insight from the National Readmission Database. *Int J Cardiol.* 2024;398:131601. PMID: 37979792

## 13

Valvular Heart Disease

Gregary D. Marhefka, MD, FACP, FACC and Howard H. Weitz, MD, MACP, FACC, FRCP

COMMON CLINICAL QUESTIONS

1. Which patients with aortic stenosis are at highest risk for postoperative cardiac complications?
2. How soon after TAVR can a patient undergo noncardiac surgery?
3. What are the indications for echocardiography?

RISK FACTORS

Up to 2.9% of adults without known valvular heart disease have moderate to severe valve pathology on screening studies, and some of these patients will be faced with undergoing noncardiac surgery.[1] Older patients are more likely to undergo noncardiac surgery and are also more likely to have significant valvular heart disease. In a cohort study of patients over 65 years old undergoing screening echocardiography, newly detected moderate or severe valve disease was uncovered in 6.4%.[2] Advanced age and significant coronary artery disease are associated with calcific and degenerative aortic stenosis. Apart from being older, other risk factors for significant valvular heart disease are listed in Table 13-1.

For many patients, identification of severe valvular heart disease is first made during the preoperative evaluation before noncardiac surgery. For the patient who is planned for elective noncardiac surgery who is found to have severe valvular heart disease, we typically delay the noncardiac surgery to evaluate the valve disease.

VALVULAR HEART DISEASE AND RISK FOR PERIOPERATIVE COMPLICATIONS

Aortic Stenosis

Severe aortic stenosis is defined as an echocardiographic-derived aortic valve area ≤ 1 cm^2 or indexed to body surface area ≤ 0.6 cm^2/m^2, and typically an aortic valve velocity ≥ 4 m/s and mean gradient ≥ 40 mmHg. In general, symptomatic severe aortic stenosis portends a higher perioperative risk than asymptomatic disease, with up to 10% to 30% risk of cardiovascular complications.[3,4] The landmark 1977 Goldman Cardiac Risk Index included physical exam-identified important aortic stenosis as one of the nine variables prospectively predictive of worse postoperative outcomes. In about half of the cases, aortic stenosis severity was determined by cardiac auscultation alone.[5] However, in the 1999 Revised Cardiac Risk Index (RCRI), critical aortic stenosis was relatively underrepresented and found in only 5 of the 2,893 derivation cohort patients (0.2%) and did not correlate with postoperative complications.[6] Our contemporary view of the role of aortic stenosis as a risk factor in noncardiac surgery comes from two single-institution tertiary care center reviews, a small prospective observational study, and a large meta-analysis. In a review of 256 patients with severe aortic stenosis who were estimated to be at intermediate or high risk and underwent noncardiac surgery

TABLE 13-1. Risk Factors for Significant Valvular Heart Disease

Murmur more significant than flow murmur
>65 years old
Heart failure
Atrial fibrillation
Hypertension
Coronary artery disease
Diabetes mellitus
End-stage renal disease
Pulmonary hypertension
Smoking
History of other congenital heart and vascular abnormalities
History of rheumatic fever
History of infective endocarditis
History of chest radiation

at the Mayo Clinic, aortic stenosis was found to be a risk factor for postoperative heart failure but was not a risk for perioperative mortality.[7] In a review of the Cleveland Clinic experience, moderate or severe aortic stenosis was associated with a small increased risk of perioperative mortality and a risk for perioperative myocardial infarction.[3] In a small prospective observational study, 61 patients undergoing noncardiac surgery with echocardiogram-identified severe aortic stenosis were compared to 86 patients with moderate aortic stenosis. Severe aortic stenosis had four times higher 30-day mortality (16% vs. 4%, $p = 0.007$). In addition, symptomatic aortic stenosis portended a higher risk for major adverse cardiovascular events including acute myocardial infarction, acute heart failure, arrhythmia, and cardiac arrest (36% vs. 16%, $p = 0.011$).[8] However, in a meta-analysis of mostly retrospective studies including 29,327 patients undergoing noncardiac surgery, there was no increased mortality, myocardial infarction, heart failure, or stroke observed, but there was an increase in length of stay,

prolonged intubation, reintubation, and intensive care unit admission.[9] Furthermore, in this meta-analysis, there was no difference in outcomes in symptomatic versus asymptomatic disease. Heterogeneity in reporting of severity of aortic stenosis, symptoms, and specific anesthesia management utilized made interpretation of this meta-analysis limited.

Therefore, in the current era, we believe that severe aortic stenosis is a risk factor for postoperative myocardial infarction, congestive heart failure, and, to a lesser degree, death. The risk of major adverse cardiac events in the perioperative period in the patient with severe aortic stenosis is increased in the presence of symptomatic aortic stenosis, high-risk noncardiac surgery, coexisting severe mitral regurgitation, preexisting significant coronary artery disease, and emergency surgery.

Increasingly, patients with preexisting transcatheter aortic valve replacements (TAVR) are encountered prior to noncardiac surgery. In a study from the University of Bern, Switzerland, of 300 patients undergoing noncardiac surgery after TAVR, 63 of 2,238 patients (21%) had surgery within 30 days of TAVR. Timing (≤30 days), urgency, and surgical risk category were not associated with an increase in the composite of death, stroke, myocardial infarction, and major, life-threatening bleeding within 30 days of noncardiac surgery. ACC guideline states it is reasonable to noncardiac surgery early (<30 days) after successful TAVR if clinically indicated.[10] However, increased risk was associated with moderate or severe prosthesis-patient mismatch (adjusted hazard ratio 2.33 [1.37–3.95], $p = 0.002$) and moderate or severe paravalvular regurgitation adjusted hazard ratio 3.61 (1.25–10.41, $p = 0.02$).[11] Prosthesis-patient mismatch occurs when a prosthetic valve's area is relatively small for the patient's body surface area, restricting cardiac output (moderate defined as prosthetic valve area 0.65–0.85 cm^2/m^2, severe < 0.65 cm^2/m^2), which occurs in 25% and 12% of patients, respectively.[12]

Mitral Regurgitation

Severe mitral regurgitation is also associated with worse outcomes in patients undergoing noncardiac surgery. In a study of 298 patients with severe mitral regurgitation compared to 1,172 control patients undergoing noncardiac surgery (84% intermediate or high risk), the incidence of 30-day mortality, myocardial infarction, heart failure, and stroke was more common (22.2% vs. 16.4%, $p = 0.02$), driven mostly by myocardial infarction and heart failure.[13] Patients with ischemic mitral regurgitation (34% of the study population), and those with an ejection fraction < 35% (20% of the study population), had worse outcomes. This may be explained by the impact of severe mitral regurgitation on the interpretation of left ventricular ejection fraction. In severe mitral regurgitation, left ventricular function should be "supra-normal" or hyperdynamic, to accommodate both the blood ejected normally across the aortic valve to the systemic circulation, as well as the regurgitant blood pathologically across the mitral valve into the left atrium. Therefore, a left ventricular ejection fraction that is "normal" in the presence of severe mitral regurgitation is, in effect, indicative of left ventricular systolic dysfunction. Furthermore, a left ventricular ejection fraction < 35% signals very severe left ventricular dysfunction.

Aortic Regurgitation

Though less has been published on patients undergoing noncardiac surgery with significant aortic regurgitation, one study noted worse outcomes. A retrospective study of 167 patients with moderate to severe aortic regurgitation, mean age of 75 years, compared outcomes to 167 control patients undergoing noncardiac surgery (72.5% intermediate or high risk). In the patients with moderate to severe aortic regurgitation, there were more cardiopulmonary complications (16.2% vs. 5.4%, $p = 0.003$; primarily driven by tracheal intubation > 24 hours and pulmonary edema) and in-hospital deaths (9% vs. 1.8%, $p = 0.008$).[14] Ejection fraction < 55% and creatinine > 2 mg/dL were associated with higher risk. In critically ill postoperative patients with severe aortic regurgitation, deciding on a mean arterial pressure or systolic blood pressure goal can prove challenging given the wide pulse pressure > 50 mmHg typically observed.

Mitral Stenosis

Mitral stenosis is classically rheumatic in etiology but can be due to degenerative calcific mitral valve disease, often seen in the elderly. Severe mitral stenosis is defined as an echocardiographic-derived mitral valve area ≤ 1.5 cm^2. Patients with severe mitral stenosis are at increased risk for noncardiac surgery,[10] particularly when symptomatic and/or associated with atrial fibrillation or pulmonary hypertension. Valvular atrial fibrillation is that associated with rheumatic mitral stenosis and has a significantly higher risk for embolic events than non-valvular atrial fibrillation.

Hypertrophic Cardiomyopathy

Though not strictly valvular in nature, hypertrophic cardiomyopathy (HCM) with obstruction can be considered under the rubric of valvular heart disease in noncardiac surgery because of its characteristic hemodynamic pathophysiology. Left ventricular outflow tract obstruction is the pathognomonic finding present in up to 70% of patients. In two contemporary observational studies totaling 149 patients with HCM undergoing noncardiac surgery at experienced centers, postoperative complications were low, when close attention was given to choice of induction agent (more frequently etomidate, which has less effect on hemodynamics than others), volume status (avoiding hypovolemia which can predispose to left ventricular outflow tract obstruction), and choice of vasopressor (avoiding agents with inotropic effects which could likewise increase left ventricular outflow tract obstruction).[15,16] Patients with HCM, particularly with higher preexisting New York Heart Association stage III and IV heart failure, had higher postoperative rates of acute heart failure compared to patients without HCM. In addition, left ventricular outflow obstruction can be induced or worsened by hypovolemia, tachycardia, and inotropes. To further compound the process, when left ventricular outflow tract obstruction is present, there can be resultant systolic anterior motion of the mitral valve and significant mitral regurgitation which can result in acute pulmonary edema and heart failure. HCM with obstruction is also reviewed in Chapter 12.

PREOPERATIVE EVALUATION

Indications for Echocardiography

Echocardiography is indicated in known or suspected significant valvular heart disease by history and physical exam. If there is no change in clinical course, an echocardiogram within the last year is usually sufficient.[4] Innocent murmurs are classically described as short, early systolic murmurs along the left sternal border of no more than grade 1 or 2 intensity and require no further evaluation. The following conditions would warrant further investigation with an echocardiogram: (1) A harsh, crescendo decrescendo murmur at the base (second right intercostal space radiating to the carotids) or across the precordium, particularly when associated with a diminished or absent S2 sound, is classic for aortic stenosis. (2) A holosystolic murmur is typically found in mitral or tricuspid regurgitation and also in ventricular septal defect. (3) A mid-systolic click and murmur is found in mitral valve prolapse. (4) Any diastolic murmur is considered pathologic and could indicate aortic regurgitation or mitral stenosis. Aortic regurgitation can be diagnosed when a diastolic murmur is heard along the left sternal border at end-expiration while leaning forward, and particularly when associated with a wide pulse pressure > 50 mmHg. Mitral stenosis is characterized by an early diastolic opening snap and low-pitched diastolic murmur at the apex, particularly accentuated in the left lateral decubitus position after ten leg flutter kicks.

Routine preoperative echocardiography in patients with prosthetic valve replacements or repairs is rarely necessary in the absence of known or suspected valve dysfunction. In patients with TAVR, evaluating for the presence of moderate to severe prosthesis-patient mismatch, or moderate to severe paravalvular regurgitation is important. There are certain appropriate use criteria for echocardiography after prosthetic valve replacements or repairs that are reasonable to consider. If noncardiac surgery is planned within 3 months of recent prosthetic valve replacement or repair, echocardiography should be performed if not already done to establish a new baseline.[17] Likewise, routine echocardiography may be appropriate more than 3 years after bioprosthetic or mechanical valve replacement or valve repair regardless of symptoms or suspected valve dysfunction before noncardiac surgery.

Indications for Further Evaluation and Intervention Prior to Noncardiac Surgery

The known presence or finding of severe valvular heart disease is one of the conditions necessitating evaluation, stabilization, and at times, intervention

before noncardiac surgery according to the guidelines from the European Society of Cardiology (ESC)/European Society of Anaesthesiology (ESA) and the American College of Cardiology (ACC)/American Heart Association (AHA).[10,18] Severe, symptomatic valvular heart disease warrants evaluation for valvular intervention independent of impending noncardiac surgery. Severe, asymptomatic aortic stenosis or aortic regurgitation with an ejection fraction < 50% and severe, asymptomatic mitral regurgitation with an ejection fraction < 60% also warrant assessment for valve surgery independent of noncardiac surgery. In severe aortic stenosis, if aortic valve replacement is contraindicated or deemed too high risk, balloon aortic valvuloplasty or TAVR may be considered (see algorithm in Figure 13-1). It must be noted though that TAVR is not done on an emergency basis and requires comprehensive preprocedure evaluation. Similarly balloon aortic valvuloplasty offers only a temporary and partial reduction in the degree of aortic stenosis and is not an innocuous procedure, associated with an up to 15% risk of major complication.[19]

In patients who are not candidates for corrective mitral or aortic valve surgery, noncardiac surgery should be performed only if absolutely necessary, recognizing the increased risk. If there is any question as to patients being asymptomatic, stress testing can be performed in certain situations to elicit symptoms and assess hemodynamic response. Patients with mitral stenosis are much less commonly encountered but represent a unique pathophysiologic situation. Since tachycardia results in reduced diastolic filling time, patients with severe mitral stenosis can rapidly develop pulmonary edema in the setting of tachyarrhythmias, with the most common being atrial fibrillation with rapid ventricular response. These patients typically do not tolerate atrial fibrillation, even at lower rates ordinarily tolerated by patients without mitral stenosis. In addition, rheumatic mitral stenosis-associated atrial fibrillation, or valvular atrial fibrillation, has a significantly higher risk of left atrial thrombus formation and embolization compared to non-valvular atrial fibrillation, and perioperative attention to anticoagulation becomes important. Just as in aortic stenosis, mitral regurgitation, and aortic regurgitation, intervening on mitral stenosis should follow the standard of care, independent of impending noncardiac surgery. Percutaneous mitral balloon valvuloplasty

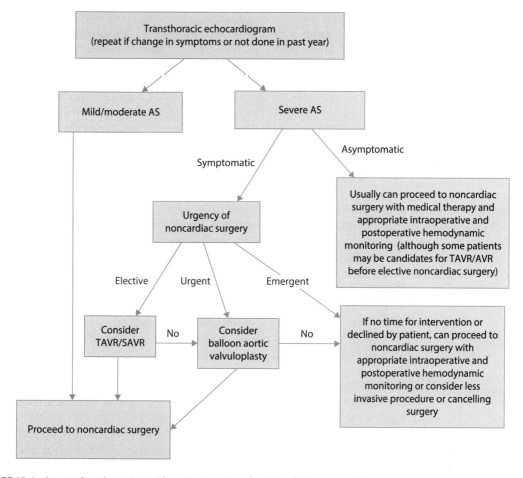

FIGURE 13-1. Approach to the patient with aortic stenosis undergoing elective noncardiac surgery.

or mitral valve replacement should be considered in symptomatic patients with a mitral valve area ≤ 1.5 cm^2. In asymptomatic moderate or severe aortic stenosis with preserved left ventricular function, there is no reason to delay elective noncardiac surgery.[4] However, in asymptomatic severe aortic stenosis, it is reasonable to exclude concomitant severe coronary artery disease (e.g., coronary computed tomography angiogram or cardiac catheterization). Likewise, in asymptomatic moderate or severe mitral regurgitation with preserved left ventricular function in the absence of severe pulmonary hypertension, there is no reason to delay elective noncardiac surgery. Patients with asymptomatic moderate or severe aortic regurgitation and those with asymptomatic moderate or severe rheumatic mitral stenosis without severe pulmonary hypertension do not need to delay elective noncardiac surgery.

PERIOPERATIVE MANAGEMENT

In general, patients with significant valvular heart disease should avoid excessive volume expansion to avoid acute pulmonary edema. Early recognition of patients who develop pulmonary edema in the perioperative period is important for timely administration of intravenous diuretic therapy. Patients with severe aortic stenosis, hypotension, and tachycardia should be avoided and corrected quickly. Coronary hypoperfusion with resultant ischemia and arrhythmias could rapidly ensue, with resultant myocardial injury, heart failure, and death. Guidelines recommend close perioperative hemodynamic monitoring and treatment when applicable, sometimes in an intensive care unit setting. Patients with severe mitral or aortic regurgitation and heart failure should be maximally stabilized with appropriate pharmacologic management in the perioperative period. In particular, patients with severe aortic regurgitation should avoid bradycardia since this increases diastolic regurgitation time. On the contrary, in patients with severe mitral stenosis, maintenance of a lower heart rate to increase diastolic filling time and reduce the gradient across the mitral valve helps reduce the propensity to develop acute pulmonary edema. Atrial fibrillation even without a rapid ventricular response can be detrimental and rate and/or rhythm control becomes critically important in severe mitral stenosis in the perioperative period. Judicious fluid management is also imperative. In addition, attention to early anticoagulation in moderate or severe rheumatic mitral stenosis as soon as safe perioperatively is essential given the increased risk of left atrial thrombus formation and embolization compared to non-valvular atrial fibrillation (Table 13-2).

Endocarditis prophylaxis is recommended prior to dental procedures and surgery that involves manipulation of gingival tissue or potential perforation of oral mucosa in patients with prior endocarditis, with prosthetic valve replacements or repairs including by transcatheter techniques, with unrepaired cyanotic congenital heart disease, with repaired congenital heart disease with residual shunts or valvular regurgitation at or adjacent to prosthetic material, and in those with heart transplant and valvular regurgitation from a structurally abnormal valve.[4] Antibiotic prophylaxis is not recommended for nondental procedures in the absence of active infection. Infective endocarditis prophylaxis is addressed in Chapter 8.

Perioperative Management of Patients with Mechanical Valve Prostheses

We recommend following the ACC/AHA valve guideline recommendation to not bridge patients with a bileaflet tilting disc mechanical aortic valve unless they also have atrial fibrillation, previous thromboembolism, left ventricular dysfunction, or a hypercoagulable state. For bileaflet tilting disc mechanical aortic valve patients with these risk factors, or older generation mechanical aortic valve or mechanical mitral valve replacement patients (mechanical tricuspid valves are rarely used since this position has the highest risk of thrombosis), bridging is typically recommended when the INR is subtherapeutic, balancing the risk of bleeding on an individual basis. Current guidelines also address emergency, major noncardiac surgery in patients with mechanical valves: administration of four-factor prothrombin complex concentrate is reasonable.[4] Perioperative management of anticoagulation is discussed in Chapter 5.

TABLE 13-2. Perioperative Management of Valvular Heart Disease

VALVULAR HEART DISEASE	PERIOPERATIVE MANAGEMENT
All valvular disease	Avoid, recognize, and treat hypervolemia
Aortic stenosis	Avoid and treat hypotension and tachycardia
Mitral regurgitation	Maximal pharmacologic stabilization of heart failure and hypertension management
Aortic regurgitation	Maximal pharmacologic stabilization of heart failure and hypertension management; avoid bradycardia
Mitral stenosis	Maintain low heart rate, avoid and treat tachycardia and arrhythmias; early anticoagulation in atrial fibrillation in rheumatic mitral stenosis
Hypertrophic cardiomyopathy*	Avoid hypovolemia, hypotension, tachycardia, and inotropes

*Though not strictly valvular disease, hypertrophic cardiomyopathy can dynamically present like valvular heart disease.

Clinical pearls

- Severe aortic stenosis and mitral and aortic regurgitation are associated with worse perioperative outcomes.
- Though not strictly valve disease, HCM, particularly with dynamic left ventricular outflow tract obstruction, can increase the risk of perioperative cardiovascular events and warrants special attention.

- Decision making on corrective valve surgery should follow standard valve guidelines independent of impending noncardiac surgery.
- Avoid excessive volume expansion in all valvular heart disease. Avoid and treat hypotension and tachycardia in severe aortic stenosis, bradycardia in severe aortic regurgitation, and tachycardia in severe mitral stenosis.

REFERENCES

1. Chambers JB. Valve disease and noncardiac surgery. *Heart*. 2018;104(22):1878-1887. PMID: 29853487
2. d'Arcy JL, Coffey S, Loudon MA, et al. Large-scale community echocardiographic screening reveals a major burden of undiagnosed valvular heart disease in older people: the OxValVe Population Cohort study. *Eur Heart J*. 2016;37(47):3515-3522. PMID: 27354049
3. Agarwal S, Rajamanickam A, Bajaj NS, et al. Impact of aortic stenosis on postoperative outcomes after noncardiac surgeries. *Circ Cardiovasc Qual Outcomes*. 2013;6(2):193-200. PMID: 23481524
4. Otto CM, Nishimura RA, Bonow RO, et al. 2020 ACC/AHA guideline for the management of patients with valvular heart disease. *Circulation*. 2021;143:e72-e227. PMID: 33332150
5. Goldman L, Caldera DL, Nussbaum SR, et al. Multifactorial index of cardiac risk in noncardiac surgical procedures. *N Engl J Med*. 1977;297(16):845-850. PMID: 904659
6. Lee TH, Marcantonio ER, Mangione CM, et al. Derivation and prospective validation of a simple index for prediction of cardiac risk of major noncardiac surgery. *Circulation*. 1999;100(10):1043-1049. PMID: 10477528
7. Tashiro T, Pislaru SV, Blustin JM, et al. Perioperative risk of major noncardiac surgery in patients with severe aortic stenosis: a reappraisal in contemporary practice. *Eur Heart J*. 2014;35(35):2372-2381. PMID: 24553722
8. MacIntyre PA, Scott MA, Seigne R, et al. An observational study of perioperative risk associated with aortic stenosis in noncardiac surgery. *Anaesth Intensive Care*. 2018;46(2):207-214. PMID: 29519225
9. Kwok CS, Bagur R, Rashid M, et al. Aortic stenosis and noncardiac surgery: a systematic review and meta-analysis. *Int J Cardiol*. 2017;240:145-153. PMID: 29519225
10. Thompson A, Fleischmann KE, Smilowitz NR, et al. 2024 AHA/ACC/ACS/ASNC/HRS/SCA/SCCT/SCMR/SVM guideline for perioperative cardiovascular management for noncardiac surgery: a report of the American College of Cardiology/American Heart Association Joint Committee on Clinical Practice Guidelines. *J Am Coll Cardiol*. 2024;84(19):1869-1969. doi:10.1016/j.jacc.2024.06.013. PMID: 39320289.
11. Okuno T, Demirel C, Tomii D, et al. Risk and timing of noncardiac surgery after transcatheter aortic valve implantation. *JAMA Network Open*. 2022;5(7):e2220689. PMID: 35797045
12. Herrmann HC, Daneshvar AS, Fonarow GC, et al. Prosthesis-patient mismatch in patients undergoing transcatheter aortic valve replacement (from the STS/ACC TVT Registry). *J Am Coll Cardiol*. 2018;72:2701-2711. PMID: 30257798
13. Bajaj NS, Agarwal A, Rajamanickam A, et al. Impact of severe mitral regurgitation on postoperative outcomes after noncardiac surgery. *Am J Med*. 2013;126(6):529-535. PMID: 23587300
14. Lai HC, Lai HC, Lee WL, et al. Impact of chronic advanced aortic regurgitation on the perioperative outcome of noncardiac surgery. *Acta Anaesthesiol Scand*. 2010;54(5):580-588. PMID: 19930243
15. Barbara DW, Hyder JA, Behrend TL, et al. Safety of noncardiac surgery in patients with hypertrophic cardiomyopathy at a tertiary center. *J Cardiothorac Vasc Anesth*. 2016;30(3):659-664. PMID: 26703970
16. Dhillon A, Khanna A, Randhawa MS, et al. Perioperative outcomes of patients with hypertrophic cardiomyopathy undergoing noncardiac surgery. *Heart*. 2016;102:1627-1632. PMID: 27288277
17. Doherty JU, Dehmer GJ, Bailey SR, et al. ACC/AATS/AHA/ASE/ASNC/HRS/SCAI/SCCT/SCMR/STS 2017 appropriate use criteria for multimodality imaging in valvular heart disease. *J Am Soc Echocardiogr*. 2018;31(4):381-404. PMID: 29066081
18. Halvorsen S, Mehilli J, Cassese S, et al. 2022 guidelines on cardiovascular assessment and management of patients undergoing noncardiac surgery. *Eur Heart J*. 2022;43(39):3826-3924. PMID: 36017553
19. Ben-Dor I, Pichard AD, Satler LF, et al. Complications and outcome of balloon aortic valvuloplasty in high risk or inoperable patients. *JACC Card Int*. 2010;3(11):1150-1156. PMID: 21087751

Arrhythmias, Conduction System Disorders, and Cardiovascular Implant Electronic Devices

14

Nidhi Rohatgi, MD, MS, SFHM and Paul J. Wang, MD, FAHA, FACC, FHRS, FESC

COMMON CLINICAL QUESTIONS

1. What are the optimal approaches for evaluation and management of common arrhythmias in the perioperative setting?
2. In the context of an arrhythmia, when should elective surgery be delayed?

INTRODUCTION

Arrhythmias and conduction system disorders are common perioperatively with a reported incidence of 4–20% after noncardiac surgery and 15–60% after cardiac surgery.[1] Prior to noncardiac surgery, a resting 12-lead electrocardiogram (ECG) is recommended for patients with known coronary artery disease, significant structural heart disease, significant arrhythmia, cerebrovascular disease, or peripheral arterial disease, except for patients undergoing low-risk surgery.[2] Comparison with prior ECGs is helpful, and detailed cardiac history should be obtained preoperatively from the patient's cardiologist or primary care physician in addition to the patient and/or caregiver.

There is a paucity of studies addressing the perioperative risk conferred by arrhythmias. Most of the perioperative cardiac risk calculators (e.g., Revised Cardiac Risk Index [RCRI], American College of Surgeons National Surgical Quality Improvement Program [ACS-NSQIP] surgical risk calculator) do not include arrhythmias or conduction system disorders as a predictor of perioperative cardiac complications.

Arrhythmias can be broadly classified as (a) tachyarrhythmias—the underlying mechanism is enhanced automaticity, triggered arrhythmias, or reentry, and (b) bradyarrhythmias—the underlying mechanism is disturbance in impulse formation or disturbance in conduction.

SUPRAVENTRICULAR TACHYARRHYTHMIAS

Supraventricular tachyarrhythmias include a variety of rhythms (Figure 14-1) and are more common than ventricular arrhythmias.[3–6]

Approach to Patients Presenting with Supraventricular Tachyarrhythmias

Clinical presentation may include chest pain, dyspnea on exertion, fatigue, palpitations, presyncope, syncope, or rarely cardiac arrest (in case of Wolff-Parkinson White syndrome or severe cardiomyopathy). ECG is the most important test, especially if recorded during the symptoms. Other options for evaluation include ECG monitoring and event recording, exercise ECG, implantable long-term monitors, and electrophysiological testing. Atrial premature beats (APBs) are usually benign and do not require further workup or delay in surgery. APBs may occur in healthy individuals or those with coronary artery disease, valvular heart disease, or

Preoperative			**Postoperative**

Preoperative (Sinus tachycardia)

1. **Assess for causes** of appropriate sinus tachycardia (e.g., hyperthyroidism, anemia, infection, pain, anxiety)
2. Assess if inappropriate sinus tachycardia (typically women in the third or fourth decade, may present with palpitations, dizziness, fatigue)
3. Preoperative heart rate over 90 may be associated with postoperative myocardial injury after noncardiac surgery

1. 12 lead ECG
2. Holter monitoring occasionally

Work up if surgery can be delayed

Sinus tachycardia

Postoperative (Sinus tachycardia)

1. Obtain 12-lead ECG
2. Determine preoperative heart rate
3. Address cause of sinus tachycardia (e.g., pain, anemia, dehydration, sepsis, pulmonary embolism, urinary retention, ileus, drug/alcohol abuse or withdrawal, agitation, withdrawal from medications such as beta-blockers, rarely myocardial ischemia)

Patients with known history of AF/AFl
1. If resting heart rate 50–100 bpm: Proceed with surgery, continue rate control medications. Minimize perioperative interruption of anticoagulation and risk of bleeding versus risk of stroke should be addressed with surgical team
2. If resting heart rate >100 or <50 bpm: Delay surgery if possible and adjust rate control medications

If new AF/AFl noted during preoperative visit
1. Delay surgery if possible for rate control and work up (if planned for very low-risk procedure and has new AF/AFl, ensure rate is controlled and no hypotension
2. Address any precipitants or underlying causes

Preoperative prophylaxis prior to cardiac surgery
1. Continue home beta-blockers
2. Low-dose beta-blocker can be initiated 2–3 days prior to surgery
3. Amiodarone can be started 5–6 days prior to surgery

1. 12-lead ECG
2. Prior echocardiogram
3. Electrolytes
If new AF/AFl:
1. Electrolytes
2. Thyroid function
3. Echocardiogram
4. Holter monitoring

Delay surgery if new diagnosis of AF/AFl or rate uncontrolled

Atrial fibrillation Atrial flutter

1. See Chapter 38
2. Address precipitating causes and drivers of sympathetic tone (e.g., fluid overload, hypovolemia, anemia, uncontrolled pain)
3. Obtain 12-lead ECG
4. Cardiac monitoring
5. Consider echocardiogram
6. Consider checking thyroid function test
7. Check electrolytes, hematocrit
8. Continue home rate and rhythm control medications
9. Anticoagulation as soon as bleeding risk permits based on CHA2DS2-VASc score
10. Rate or rhythm control medications
11. Electrical cardioversion for unstable AF/AFl
12. Holter monitoring at discharge
13. Cardiology follow up

---

1. **Assess for causes** (e.g., pulmonary disease, digitalis toxicity, prior catheter ablation)
2. Frequent atrial premature beats and focal AT may be a precursor to AF/AFl
3. **If asymptomatic, hemodynamically stable and ventricular rate < 100, proceed with surgery**
4. **Multifocal AT:** Treat underlying pulmonary disease, correct electrolytes, rate control agents if needed are the mainstay. Surgery usually does not have to be delayed unless needed for optimization of pulmonary disease or rate control.
5. **If symptomatic or hemodynamically unstable or ventricular rate > 100, delay surgery** if possible, address any precipitants, work up, consider rate control medications such as beta-blockers or calcium channel blockers
6. Cardiology consultation if delaying surgery

1. 12-lead ECG
2. Echocardiogram
3. Electrolytes
4. Holter monitoring
5. Event monitor

Delay surgery if symptomatic, poor rate control or hemodynamic instability

Atrial tachycardia

1. Address precipitating causes and drivers of sympathetic tone (e.g., fluid overload, hypovolemia, anemia, hypoxia, hypokalemia, uncontrolled pain)
2. Obtain 12-lead ECG
3. Cardiac monitoring
4. Consider echocardiogram
5. Check electrolytes
6. Continue home rate control medications
7. Because focal AT does not depend on AV node for conduction, it does not terminate with AV blockers
8. Adenosine or vagal maneuvers may lead to transient AV block without affecting the atrial rate
9. Beta-blocker and calcium channel blockers may slow the ventricular rate. Incessant AT may cause tachycardia-induced cardiomyopathy
10. Intravenous amiodarone, ibutilide or procainamide can be considered for acute management
11. Holter monitoring at discharge
12. Cardiology consultation

FIGURE 14-1. Management of supraventricular tachyarrhythmias.

Preoperative

Postoperative

1. Usually well tolerated in young patients and no workup may be needed → **Okay to proceed to surgery if asymptomatic**
2. If symptomatic (e.g., chest pain, hypotension, syncope) or in those with sustained tachycardia, delay surgery, work up, initiate rate control medications, and obtain cardiology consultation

1. 12-lead ECG
2. Echocardiogram
3. Electrolytes
4. Holter monitoring
5. Event monitor

AVNRT

Delay surgery if symptomatic or sustained tachycardia

1. Address precipitating causes and drivers of sympathetic tone (e.g., fluid overload, hypovolemia, anemia, uncontrolled pain)
2. Obtain 12-lead ECG
3. Cardiac monitoring
4. Consider echocardiogram
5. Check electrolytes
6. Reassurance and valsalva maneuvers may suffice
7. Adenosine is the treatment of choice for acute management
8. For chronic management: Beta-blockers, calcium channel blockers or catheter ablation are options
9. Holter monitoring at discharge
10. Cardiology follow up

1. **Asymptomatic known pre-excitation without a history of tachycardia or syncope usually does not require treatment → Okay to proceed with surgery after consulting with treating cardiologist;** the patient should have continuous ECG monitoring
2. **If new Wolff-Parkinson-White (WPW) morphology is noted → Delay surgery** for electrophysiological workup, rate control medications or catheter ablation. These patients may be prone to supraventricular arrhythmias with high ventricular rate
   a. WPW with extremely rapid conduction in AF (usually >250 bpm) via the accessory pathway is associated with risk of progression to ventricular fibrillation and cardiac arrest
3. **If the patient has a known history of WPW:**
   a. Discussion between patient's cardiologist and electrophysiologist, anesthesiologist and postoperative medical team should occur to create a plan for minimizing sympathetic and vagal activity and pharmacological therapy in case of tachyarrhythmias
   b. Intra-op: Cautious use of sympathomimetics (e.g., epinephrine, ketamine, ephedrine), vagolytics (e.g., atropine). High spinal blocks and agents that increase vagal tone (e.g., succinylcholine, neostigmine) should be used cautiously to avoid conduction of impulses down the accessory pathway

1. 12-lead ECG
2. Echocardiogram
3. Electrolytes
4. Holter monitoring
5. Event monitor

AVRT

Delay surgery if symptomatic or new WPW

1. Obtain 12-lead ECG
2. Cardiac monitoring
3. Obtain echocardiogram
4. Check electrolytes
5. Reassurance and valsalva maneuvers may suffice
6. Adenosine is the treatment of choice for acute management of narrow complex tachycardia
7. AF/AFl with pre-excitation is usually treated with intravenous amiodarone or procainamide. AV nodal blockers like beta-blockers or digoxin are avoided as they may reduce the refractoriness of the accessory pathway in WPW and progress to ventricular fibrillation
8. Patients with rapid conduction via the accessory pathway will frequently require catheter ablation
9. For chronic management: Flecainide or propafenone with beta-blockers, calcium channel blockers or catheter ablation are options
10. Holter monitoring at discharge
11. Electrophysiology consult

ECG, electrocardiogram; AF/AFl, atrial fibrillation/flutter; AT, atrial tachycardia; AV, atrioventricular; AVNRT, AV nodal re-entrant tachycardia; AVRT, AV re-entrant tachycardia.

FIGURE 14-1. (*Continued*)

cardiomyopathy. Frequent APBs (>100/day) may predict new occurrence of atrial fibrillation. Although data are limited, newly discovered atrial fibrillation may lead to further evaluation and in some cases postponement of surgery.

VENTRICULAR ARRHYTHMIAS

Clinical presentation of ventricular arrhythmias includes palpitations, skipped or extra beats, sustained palpitations, dyspnea, chest pain, dizziness, presyncope, syncope, and cardiac arrest. Patients with ventricular bigeminy or trigeminy can present with effective bradycardia and result in inaccurate estimation of the heart rate. Perioperative approach to patients with ventricular arrhythmias is presented in Figure 14-2.[2,6-8]

BRADYARRHYTHMIAS

Several risk factors have been reported for the development of significant bradyarrhythmias intraoperatively during noncardiac surgery such as age > 60 years, American Society of Anesthesia Class III or IV, preoperative heart rate < 60 bpm, and use of beta-blockers. A few noncardiac procedures may have higher risk of intraoperative bradyarrhythmia such as carotid endarterectomy or carotid artery stenting (could potentially activate the trigeminal cardiac reflex or vagus nerve), neurosurgical procedures that involve manipulation of the spine or dura mater, peritoneal insufflation during abdominal surgeries, and eye surgery.[9] Eye surgeries, traction of the extraocular muscles, direct pressure on the eyeball, severe ocular pain, or increase in intraocular pressure (e.g., by use of inhalational beta-agonists, sulfa drugs) in patients undergoing maxillofacial surgeries involving the eye may drop the heart rate by over 20% due to oculocardiac or trigeminovagal reflex.

General Approach to Patients with Bradyarrhythmia

Most of the patients with bradyarrhythmia are asymptomatic, particularly those with mild bradycardia or during sleep, and bradycardia may be noticed incidentally during routine perioperative monitoring. Presence of bradyarrhythmia during preoperative evaluation should prompt further investigation

depending on the nature and acuity of the arrhythmia and the patient's medical history.[2] The more severe the clinical presentation, the more aggressive is the evaluation and treatment.

Clinical presentation of bradyarrhythmia may range from asymptomatic to exercise intolerance, fatigue, dyspnea on exertion, presyncope, transient dizziness or lightheadedness, confusion states, syncope, and cardiac arrest. ECG is the most important test, especially if recorded during the symptoms. However, longer-term continuous ECG monitoring for 2–4 weeks may be most effective in quantifying arrhythmias and establishing the relationship between symptoms and the heart rhythm. Implantable loop monitors are particularly useful for documenting the rhythm during infrequent symptoms such as syncope that occurs every several months. Perioperative approach to patients with bradyarrhythmias is presented in Figure 14-3.[9]

Sinus Node Dysfunction (SND)

SND can be intrinsic or extrinsic and presents with exercise intolerance, presyncope, and syncope. Extrinsic SND, which may arise perioperatively, is often reversible and should be corrected before pacemaker therapy is considered whenever possible. Extrinsic causes may include acute inferior or posterior myocardial ischemia, medications (e.g., beta-blockers, calcium channel blockers, clonidine, narcotics, lithium, class I/III antiarrhythmics), hyperkalemia, hypokalemia, hypothermia, acidosis, hypoxemia, increased intracranial pressure, surgery involving the carotid artery, endotracheal suctioning causing activation of the vagus nerve, hypothyroidism, or sleep apnea.[1]

Young athletes may have asymptomatic sinus bradycardia with a heart rate under 40 bpm or sinus pause over 5 seconds during rest or sleep when the parasympathetic tone is dominant. SND could also occur due to direct injury to the sinus node during cardiac surgery. SND increases with age and other disorders (e.g., coronary artery disease, some inflammatory and familial disorders) and may be worsened with additional extrinsic factors perioperatively.

Atrioventricular (AV) Block

AV block may be fixed or intermittent, and the clinical manifestations will depend on the ventricular rate

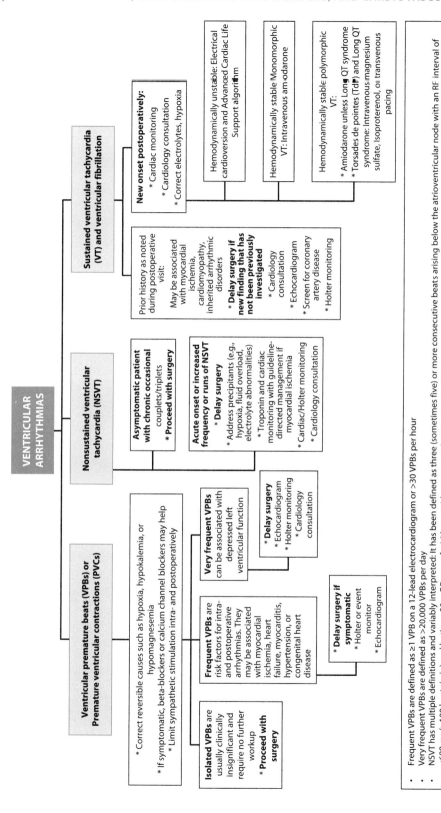

FIGURE 14-2. Perioperative approach to patients with ventricular arrhythmias.

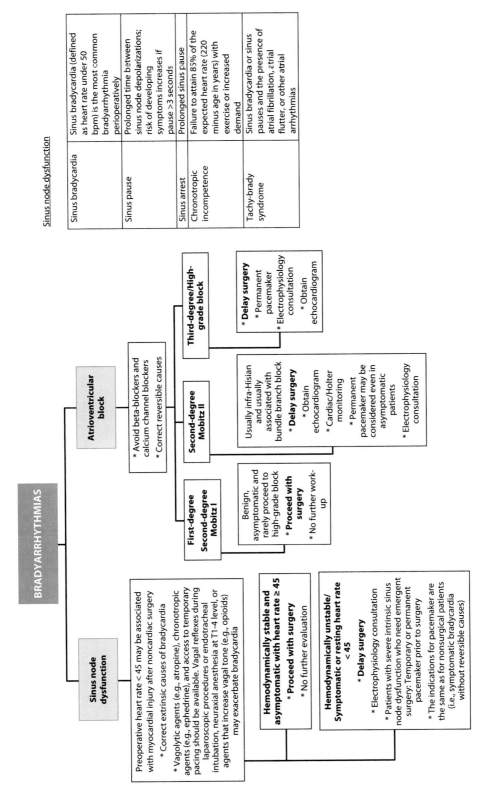

FIGURE 14-3. Perioperative approach to patients with bradyarrhythmias.

and/or duration of ventricular asystole, with variability in the reliability of the escape rhythm. Patients may be asymptomatic, particularly if the escape rhythm is adequate in rate. AV block may be vagally mediated and occur during sleep. The clinical hallmark of vagally mediated AV block is concomitant sinus rate slowing, indicating a vagal effect on the sinus and AV nodes. The clinical consequence of AV block depends on the location and severity of the block, with the most severe forms of AV block being infra-Hisian and those with underlying bundle branch block. AV block in the absence of bundle branch block is overwhelmingly likely at the level of the AV node. AV block should prompt an evaluation of underlying heart disease, including ischemic heart disease, hypertrophic cardiomyopathy, and infiltrative disorders such as sarcoidosis and amyloidosis.

Conduction System Disease

Conduction system disease includes bundle branch and fascicular blocks. Perioperative approach to patients with conduction system disease is presented in Figure 14-4. Bifascicular block refers to complete left bundle branch block (LBBB) or right bundle branch block (RBBB) along with conduction block in one of the fascicles of the left bundle. Patients with isolated RBBB or fascicular blocks are usually asymptomatic and rarely develop high-grade block perioperatively. However, RBBB may be present in patients with pulmonary disease, congenital heart disease, ischemic heart disease, or cardiomyopathy. Progression of bifascicular block to AV block and bradycardia is low, approximately 1% per year, with approximately half of the patients presenting with syncope and the other half with a constellation of symptoms including fatigue, chest pain, or dyspnea.[9] After transcatheter aortic valve replacement (TAVR), new LBBB occurs in 19–55% of the patients and new high-degree AV block occurs in up to 10% of the patients; half of these resolve prior to discharge from the hospital and the remainder may require a permanent pacemaker prior to discharge.[9]

Patients with LBBB have a higher likelihood of underlying structural heart disease or coronary artery disease. If a patient is noted to have LBBB preoperatively, a transthoracic echocardiogram should be obtained electively, but surgery does not need to be postponed in asymptomatic patients in whom there is no concern for underlying heart failure or myocardial ischemia.[9,10] A new bundle branch block should be evaluated preoperatively if the patient is symptomatic, there is suspicion for silent cardiopulmonary disease, or the patient is planned for high-risk surgery.

Most patients with chronic bifascicular block or "trifascicular block" (defined as RBBB with left anterior or left posterior fascicular block and first-degree or higher-grade AV block), a term that is not favored since the PR prolongation may be due to AV nodal disease rather than infra-Hisian disease, do not have an increased risk of progression to AV block and do not warrant pacemakers. Although the perioperative risk is low, transcutaneous and transvenous pacing should be readily available.

Most patients with high grade or complete AV block will need permanent pacemaker implantation unless it is reversible or occurs during periods of increased vagal tone. In most cases, this will need to be performed prior to the planned surgical procedure.

CARDIOVASCULAR IMPLANTABLE ELECTRONIC DEVICES

Patients with cardiovascular implantable electronic devices (CIED) such as an implantable cardioverter defibrillator (ICD) or permanent pacemaker may undergo cardiac and noncardiac surgeries and require special attention perioperatively. Key considerations in the care of patients with CIED in the perioperative setting are shown in Table 14-1.[11] The 2024 ACC/AHA guidelines also offer detailed recommendations for preoperative management of patients with CIEDs undergoing noncardiac surgery.[2]

CIED includes a pulse generator that is typically placed in the chest pocket and is attached to one or more leads for sensing and pacing. Single chamber pacemakers may have a lead in the right atrium or right ventricle and single chamber transvenous ICDs have a lead in the right ventricle. Dual chamber pacemakers or ICDs have a right atrial lead and a right ventricular lead. For ICDs, the right ventricular lead also delivers shock energy. In biventricular pacemakers or ICDs, a third lead is usually placed in the right atrium and then advanced to the cardiac venous system to permit pacing of the left ventricle for resynchronization. A chest x-ray may also help distinguish

Complete Right Bundle Branch Block (RBBB)	• QRS duration ≥ 120 ms • rsr', rsR', rSR' in V1/2 • S wave of longer duration than R wave or >40 ms in I/V6
Incomplete RBBB	• Same morphology as complete RBBB but QRS duration is 110–119 ms
Complete Left Bundle Branch Block (LBBB)	• QRS duration ≥ 120 ms • Broad notched or slurred R wave in I/aVL/V5/V6 • No Q waves in I/V5/V6 • ST and T waves usually opposite direction to QRS
Incomplete LBBB	• Same morphology as complete LBBB but QRS duration is 110–119 ms • Left ventricular hypertrophy pattern • No Q waves in I/V5/V6
Nonspecific intraventricular conduction delay (IVCD)	• QRS duration > 110 ms but criteria for RBBB or LBBB is not met
Left anterior fascicular block	• QRS duration < 120 ms • Left axis deviation (frontal plane axis −45° to −90°)
Left posterior fascicular block	• QRS duration < 120 ms • Right axis deviation (frontal plane axis 90° to 180°)

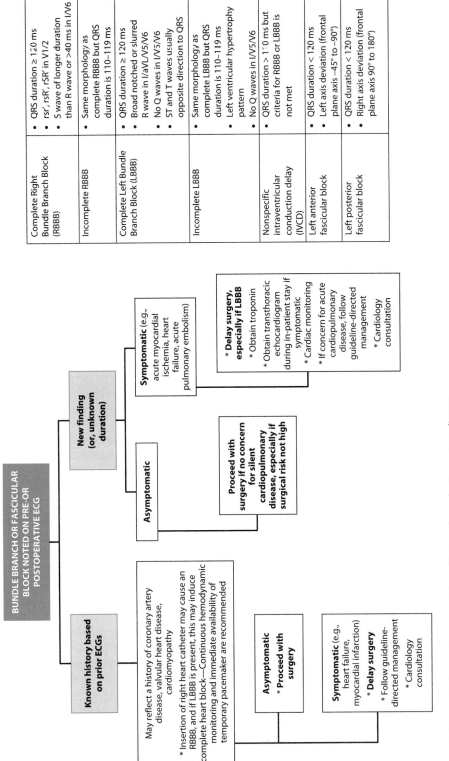

FIGURE 14-4. Perioperative approach to patients with conduction system disease.

TABLE 14-1. Perioperative Considerations for Patients with Cardiovascular Implantable Electronic Devices (CIED)		
PREOPERATIVELY	**INTRAOPERATIVELY**	**POSTOPERATIVELY**
• Establish if the patient has a CIED (History/exam, review of medical records, electrocardiography (ECG), chest x-ray, rhythm monitoring may be used) • Define the type of device (Obtain the manufacturer card from the patient if available or check with patient's cardiologist. A chest x-ray may help distinguish an implantable cardioverter defibrillator (ICD) from pacemaker; an ICD has one or two radio-opaque shock coils on the right ventricle lead. The chest x-ray also may reveal the device manufacturer symbol on the pacemaker or ICD generator) • Determine if the patient is CIED-dependent • Determine device function (done by an electrophysiologist or CIED specialist) within 6 months for ICDs and 12 months for pacemakers • Determine if electromagnetic interference is likely during the planned procedure. (If the patient requires magnetic resonance imaging (MRI) perioperatively, it should be determined if the CIED is MRI-safe, and if not, an electrophysiologist or CIED specialist should be involved in the care of the patient)	• ECG monitoring and monitoring of pulse or pulse waveform should be performed and electromagnetic interference should be minimized when possible • Advanced life-support capabilities should be present • All ICDs should be inactivated if there is concern for electromagnetic interference and the patient should be continuously monitored • ICDs in pacemaker-dependent patients need to be reprogrammed to an asynchronous pacing mode • Electromagnetic interference, such as by use of unipolar cautery, may lead to inappropriate pacing inhibition and asystole or delivery of ICD shock therapy. Bipolar (instead of unipolar) cautery should be considered whenever possible	• The cardiac rhythm and rate should be monitored continuously in the immediate postoperative period with availability of cardioversion-defibrillation equipment and backup pacing • CIED generally should be interrogated after the procedure, but this is not uniformly followed

an ICD from a pacemaker; an ICD has one or two radio-opaque shock coils on the right ventricle lead. The chest x-ray may reveal the device manufacturer symbol on the pacemaker or ICD generator. Subcutaneous ICDs have a subcutaneous or substernal lead for shock energy delivery. Leadless permanent pacemakers are independently functioning pacemakers that are screwed into the endocardium and do not require transvenous leads. Pacing the right ventricle, particularly in the setting of underlying left dysfunction, may lead to heart failure and worsening of the left ventricular function, most commonly occurring the setting of AV block. Recently, physiological pacing of the His bundle or the left bundle branch area has been introduced with the goal of decreasing the frequency and severity of right ventricular pacing induced left ventricular dysfunction.

CIEDs should be interrogated preoperatively to determine that the patient has a CIED, the type of device, the model, programmed setting of the CIED, battery life, whether the patient is pacemaker dependent, if the CIED function is normal, and the underlying cardiac rhythm abnormality. This information should be recorded in the patient's chart and readily accessible to the perioperative team. Patients with pacemakers should have a device check within 12 months prior to surgery, and patients with ICDs should have a device check within 6 months prior to surgery. Intraoperative ECG monitoring and monitoring of pulse or pulse waveform should be performed. There should be an assessment of whether electromagnetic interference is likely or not and if it can be minimized. All ICDs should be inactivated if electromagnetic interference is felt to be present and patients should be continuously monitored. Additionally, ICDs in pacemaker-dependent patients need to be reprogrammed to an asynchronous pacing mode. Patients with ICDs in whom tachytherapies are inactivated preoperatively should be monitored closely until the inactivated ICD is reprogrammed to active therapy. Advanced life-support capabilities should be present. The cardiac rhythm and rate should be monitored continuously in the immediate postoperative period with availability of cardioversion-defibrillation equipment and backup pacing.

CIEDs generally should be interrogated after the procedure, but this procedure is not uniformly followed. If the patient requires magnetic resonance imaging (MRI) perioperatively, it should be determined if the CIED is MRI-safe, and if not, an electrophysiologist or CIED specialist should be involved in the care of the patient.

dependent should have their devices reprogrammed to asynchronous mode during procedures in which electromagnetic interference such as through monopolar electrocautery may occur. Routine practice of placing a magnet intraoperatively without attention to CIED evaluation preoperatively is discouraged.

Clinical pearls

- AV nodal blocking agents (e.g., digoxin, verapamil) that may reduce the refractoriness of the accessory pathway in patients with WPW with atrial fibrillation or flutter should not be given as these patients may progress to ventricular fibrillation. Instead, intravenous amiodarone or procainamide can be given.

- Placement of transcutaneous pacer pads may be reasonable in patients at high risk of intraoperative or perioperative bradyarrhythmia.

- There is no established minimum heart rate or pause duration where permanent pacing is recommended for SND. Establishing temporal correlation between symptoms and bradycardia is important when determining whether permanent pacing is needed.

- Asymptomatic bifascicular block, with or without first-degree AV block, is not an indication for temporary pacing, but an external pacemaker for transcutaneous pacing should be readily available.

- Electromagnetic interference, such as by use of monopolar cautery, may lead to inappropriate pacing inhibition and asystole or delivery of ICD shock therapy. Patients who are pacemaker

REFERENCES

1. Boriani G, Fauchier L, Aguinaga L, et al, ESC Scientific Document Group. European Heart Rhythm Association (EHRA) consensus document on management of arrhythmias and cardiac electronic devices in the critically ill and post-surgery patient, endorsed by Heart Rhythm Society (HRS), Asia Pacific Heart Rhythm Society (APHRS), Card. *Europace*. 2019;21:7-8. PMID: 29905786

2. Thompson A, Fleischmann KE, Smilowitz NR, et al. 2024 AHA/ACC/ACS/ASNC/HRS/SCA/SCCT/SCMR/SVM guideline for perioperative cardiovascular management for noncardiac surgery: a report of the American College of Cardiology/American Heart Association Joint Committee on Clinical Practice Guidelines. *J Am Coll Cardiol*. 2024;84(19):1869-1969. doi:10.1016/j.jacc.2024.06.013. PMID 39320289.

3. Sousa-Uva M, Head SJ, Milojevic M, et al. 2017 EACTS guidelines on perioperative medication in adult cardiac surgery. *Eur J Cardiothorac Surg*. 2018;53:5-33. PMID: 29029110

4. Page RL, Joglar JA, Caldwell MA, et al. 2015 ACC/AHA/HRS guidelines for the management of adult patients with supraventricular tachycardia: a report of the American College of Cardiology/American Heart Association Task Force on Clinical Practice Guidelines and the Heart Rhythm Society. *J Am Coll Cardiol*. 2016;67:e27-e115. PMID: 26409259

5. Brugada J, Katritsis DG, Arbelo E, et al, ESC Scientific Document Group. 2019 ESC guidelines for the management of patients with supraventricular tachycardia: the Task Force for the management of patients with supraventricular tachycardia of the European Society of Cardiology (ESC). *Eur Heart J*. 2020;41:655-720. PMID: 31504425

6. Halvorsen S, Mehilli J, Cassese S, et al, ESC Scientific Document Group. 2022 ESC guidelines on cardiovascular assessment and management of patients undergoing non-cardiac surgery. *Eur Heart J*. 2022;43:3826-3924. PMID: 36017553

7. Al-Khatib SM, Stevenson WG, Ackerman MJ, et al. 2017 AHA/ACC/HRS guideline for management of patients with ventricular arrhythmias and the prevention of sudden cardiac death: a report of the American College of Cardiology/American Heart Association Task Force on Clinical Practice Guidelines and the Heart Rhythm Society. *Hear Rhythm*. 2018;15:e73-e189. PMID: 29097319

8. Zeppenfeld K, Tfelt-Hansen J, de Riva M, et al, ESC Scientific Document Group. 2022 ESC guidelines for the management of patients with ventricular arrhythmias and the prevention of sudden cardiac death. *Eur Heart J*. 2022;43:3997-4126. PMID: 36017572

9. Kusumoto FM, Schoenfeld MH, Barrett C, et al. 2018 ACC/AHA/HRS guideline on the evaluation and management of patients with bradycardia and cardiac conduction delay: a report of the American College of Cardiology/American Heart Association Task Force on Clinical Practice Guidelines and the Heart Rhythm Society. *Circulation*. 2019;140:e382-e482. PMID: 30586772

10. Merli GJ, Weitz HH. Web exclusive. Annals consult guys—new left bundle branch block: should this block surgery? *Ann Intern Med*. 2019;171:CG1. PMID: 31307089

11. Practice Advisory for the Perioperative Management of Patients with Cardiac Implantable Electronic Devices: Pacemakers and Implantable Cardioverter-Defibrillators 2020: an updated report by the American Society of Anesthesiologists Task Force on Perioperative Management of Patients with Cardiac Electronic Implantable Electronic Devices. *Anesthesiology*. 2020;132:225-252. PMID: 31939838

## 15

Hypertension

Alexander I.R. Jackson, BMedSci(Hons), MBChB, MSc and Michael P.W. Grocott, BSc, Msc, MBBS, MD, FRCA, FRCP, FFICM, GChPOM

COMMON CLINICAL QUESTIONS

1. At what blood pressure is it safe to proceed with surgery?
2. How should I manage antihypertensive medications immediately before and after surgery?
3. How does high blood pressure change the risk of surgery?

INTRODUCTION

Background

Hypertension is a common condition identified by the Global Burden of Disease Study to be the leading metabolic risk factor for attributable deaths with 10.8 million deaths attributed annually.[1] In 2010, 1.39 billion people worldwide were estimated to suffer from hypertension, with the burden growing most rapidly in low- and middle-income countries (LMICs).[2] Awareness, treatment, and control remain poor globally. In high-income countries, around one-third of patients with hypertension are unaware and fewer than 30% achieve adequate control, and the metrics are worse in LMICs.[2] It is therefore clear that across the globe patients are highly likely to present for surgery with hypertension, many undiagnosed and most with poor control. It is therefore vital for anesthetists to understand the perioperative implications, evaluation, and management of this globally significant and growing problem.

Long-Term Management

To understand the perioperative management of hypertension, it is helpful to understand the context and aims of long-term hypertension management, particularly as much of the perioperative guidance is extrapolated from the evidence in chronic hypertension. The overall aim is to reduce lifetime cardiovascular risk and both the European Society of Hypertension Guidelines for the Management of Arterial Hypertension,[3] and the American College of Cardiology/American Heart Association (ACC/AHA) Guideline for the Prevention, Detection, Evaluation, and Management of High Blood Pressure in Adults[4] recommend the use of cardiovascular risk calculators to guide treatment. Furthermore, both guidelines share similarities in their initial approach to the measurement of BP, advocating for the use of home/ambulatory monitoring prior to diagnosis. Initial pharmaco-therapeutic approaches include ACE inhibitors, angiotensin receptor blockers, and calcium channel blockers, with monotherapy the recommended first-line strategy before progressing to combination regimes. Where the guidelines differ are in the specifics of their diagnostic cut-off and therapeutic targets. For example, the ACC/AHA defines hypertension as $\geq$130/80 mm Hg, while the ESH defines it as $\geq$140/90 mm Hg. Both guidelines define normal/optimal blood pressure range as <120/80 mm Hg, but the ESH goes into more details regarding the severity of hypertension (Table 15-1A). The

TABLE 15-1A. Categories of Blood Pressure According to the ACC/AHA and ESH

2017 ACC/AHA	2023 ESH
Normal: <120/80	Optimal: <120/80
Elevated: 120–129/< 80	Normal: 120–129/80–84
Stage 1: 130–139/80–89	High-normal: 130–139/85–89
Stage 2: >140/90	Grade 1: 140–159/90–99
	Grade 2: 160–179/100–109
	Grade 3: ≥180/110

ESH, European Society of Hypertension
Source: ACC/AHA, American College of Cardiology/American Heart Association.

TABLE 15-1B. Blood Pressure Targets for Treatment (Long-term) Based on Age

AGE (YEARS)	2017 ACC/AHA	2023 ESH
18–64	<130/80	<130/80
65–79	<130/80	<140/80
		<130/80, if tolerated
≥80	<130/80	140–150/<80

ESH, European Society of Hypertension
Source: ACC/AHA, American College of Cardiology/American Heart Association.

ESH differs from ACC/AHA regarding blood pressure treatment targets (Table 15-1B). Lifestyle modifications, including dietary changes, weight loss, smoking cessation, and alcohol reduction, are advocated,[3,4] and align with the growing body of multi-modal prehabilitation literature in the perioperative setting.

PREOPERATIVE EVALUATION AND RISK

Preoperative Assessment

Preoperative blood pressure readings should form a core part of preoperative assessment for hypertension. However, discrepancies between clinic readings and ambulatory readings are well recognized. Therefore, it is recommended where possible to use ambulatory blood pressure readings, and care should be taken to avoid acting on the basis of isolated clinic readings. Unrepresentative isolated clinical readings risk not only overdiagnosis but also underdiagnosis of hypertension, both of which are linked to adverse outcomes.[5] Preoperative mean arterial blood pressure measurements tend to be approximately 11 mmHg lower than preinduction levels. This difference tended to be greater in patients with lower preoperative blood pressures and less in patients with higher preoperative blood pressures. This needs to be taken into consideration to avoid overtreatment.[6]

In addition to blood pressure measurements, history and examination are essential, with further diagnostic testing, where indicated, to evaluate the risk of hypertension and, importantly, to identify related organ dysfunction or associated conditions. Important components of the history include cause, duration, and severity of hypertension along with medication history, including adherence and resulting control.

Associated comorbidities, such as ischemic heart disease, heart failure, diabetes mellitus, chronic kidney disease, and stroke, should also be considered, evaluated, and optimized. Alongside patient factors, certain surgeries are associated with an increased risk of perioperative hypertension, including coronary artery bypass graft, aortic aneurysm repair, and carotid endarterectomy. Also, being on antihypertensive medication as opposed to no treatment may minimize perioperative blood pressure fluctuations.

Finally, consideration should be given to secondary hypertension, which although considerably less common than essential hypertension, can be of much greater significance to the perioperative care of the patient. Causes such as thyroid dysfunction, renal disease, or pheochromocytoma have profound consequences and necessitate multidisciplinary management beyond the scope of this chapter. Features that may raise the suspicion of secondary hypertension include sudden onset high blood pressure, very high systolic (>180 mmHg) or diastolic (>120 mmHg) pressure, or hypertension resistant to pharmacological therapy.

Perioperative Risk and Hypertension

There remains a paucity of definitive evidence around optimal blood pressure in the preoperative period. Much of the evidence is extrapolated from the nonoperative setting, and most of the perioperative research is observational in nature. One of the largest such studies, a cohort study of over 250,000 patients in the United Kingdom, identified that low (<119/63 mmHg), rather than high, blood pressure exhibited a dose-dependent association with postoperative mortality following noncardiac surgery, although this effect was confined to elderly patients.[7] The adverse effect of hypertension was seen, after adjustment, in diastolic hypertension (>100 mmHg) and absent in systolic hypertension. While this study remains one of the largest, it should be noted it only evaluated mortality and did not consider other outcomes of interest. Recent data from 57,389 elective in-patient cases in the United States suggest that preoperative blood pressures both below and above specific threshold values were independently associated with adverse postoperative events, but do not offer specific strategies for managing patients with perioperative hypo- or hypertension.[8]

When other outcomes such as cardiac, cerebral, and renal morbidity are considered, the observational data appear to suggest an elevated risk in patients with high preoperative arterial pressure, although the magnitude and clinical significance of the effect are debated.[9]

It should be noted that these studies all adjust for numerous other factors, which means that although hypertension is not consistently found to be a strong independent predictor, it should not be ignored. In real-world practice, patients with hypertension are still a higher-risk cohort, due in part to associated comorbidities and risk factors, again emphasizing the importance of a holistic assessment.

PERIOPERATIVE MANAGEMENT

Hypertension and Surgical Delay

Despite the lack of conclusive evidence of harm, elevated blood pressure is frequently cited as a reason for surgical cancellation or delay, which in the absence of a clear rationale may result in physical, psychosocial, and economic harm. The publication of guidelines with specific cut-offs appears to be effective in reducing the rate of such cancellations[10]; however, the development of such guidelines is hampered by the previously discussed limitations of current evidence. This has prompted some to argue against prespecified targets,[5] while other bodies have opted for them,[4,11,12] in part to reduce unwarranted surgical delays. European,[12] American,[4] and British[11] guidelines are consistent in suggesting 180 mmHg systolic and 110 mmHg diastolic, in secondary care, as a threshold for consideration of delaying surgery. Regardless of their recommendations on thresholds, all agree that any decision to cancel or delay surgery should be based on a holistic evaluation of the risk, taking into account all clinical and surgical factors rather than being based on blood pressure values viewed in isolation (see Figure 15-1). It should also be noted that acutely lowering preoperative blood pressure does not appear to make a significant difference to perioperative risk, and there is insufficient evidence to support it as a risk reduction strategy.[5]

Perioperative Medication Management (See Chapter 4)

Antihypertensive agents are cardiovascularly active and have the potential to alter physiological responses to surgery and anesthesia. As such, their management

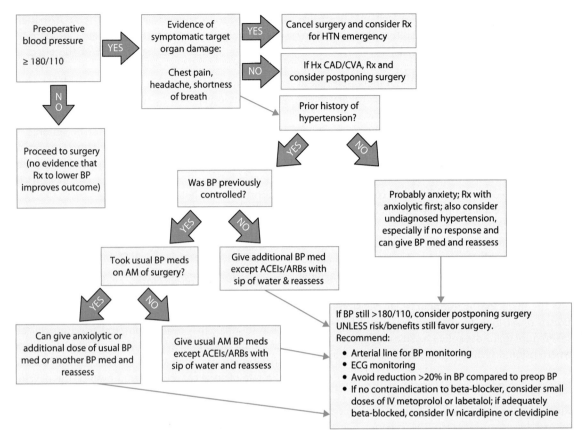

FIGURE 15-1. Approach to Elevated Preoperative Blood Pressure.

in the immediate perioperative period has been the subject of both debate and research. Of note, the recent POISE-3 trial compared hypertensive avoidance and hypotension avoidance strategies using specific protocols for continuing or withholding antihypertensive medications and found no significant difference.[13] There was no benefit of the alternative strategies: intraoperative MAP target of 80 mmHg or greater, discontinuing ACEI or ARB therapy, and administering antihypertensive medications on the basis of patients' SBP, versus intraoperative MAP target of 60 mmHg or greater and continuing all antihypertensive medications.

The initiation of β-blockade has previously been advocated in certain high-risk cohorts to reduce cardiovascular risk. However, the evidence underpinning this recommendation was the subject of significant controversy. Following more definitive randomized controlled

trials and meta-analyses, the consensus is that β-blockade should not be initiated purely to reduce perioperative risk.[4,5] The POISE-1 study found an increase in all-cause mortality, albeit with reduced cardiac injury rates, in patients started on a β-blocker for this purpose.[14] However, patients receiving long-term β-blockade for other indications, including chronic hypertension management, should continue it.[12]

Angiotensin-converting enzyme inhibitors and angiotensin receptor blockers (ACEIs/ARBs) are the subject of ongoing study. They are associated with increased incidence of hypotension during anesthesia,[15] but their effect on outcome is less clear. The VISION study, a landmark cohort study of nearly 15,000 patients, found withholding ACEIs/ARBs was associated with a lower risk of death and postoperative cardiac events.[16] However, a recent randomized controlled trial (the SPACE trial) failed to demonstrate a reduction in myocardial injury from withholding ACEIs/ARBs, but did see a higher rate of hypertensive adverse events,[17] suggesting that this is an area where further research and debate is likely. Additionally, the STOP or NOT trial randomized 2,222 patients to either continue or discontinue their ACEIs/ARBs 3 days before surgery, and although there were more episodes of intraoperative hypotension in the continuation group (55% vs. 41%), there was no difference in perioperative complications or mortality.[18] In contrast to previous recommendations, the most recent published consensus statement from the Perioperative Quality Initiative (POQI) highlights uncertainty in this area and does not advocate for either withholding or continuing such drugs.[19]

The evidence for the optimal management of other agents, including calcium channel blockers, thiazide diuretics, and loop diuretics, is highly limited. In most cases, continuation is a reasonable option, although consideration should be given to the effect of loop diuretics on patient volume and electrolyte status on a case-by-case basis.

Clinical pearls

- Hypertension is associated with worse perioperative outcomes but is not reliably identified as an independent risk predictor. This suggests the risk may be related to comorbidities, organ dysfunction, and other associated factors, such as lifestyle.
- Isolated clinic, office, or hospital-based blood pressure readings should be interpreted with caution. Multiple ambulatory readings over a period of time are a more reliable measure of long-term blood pressure control.
- Secondary hypertension is relatively rare but important to exclude, particularly if red flags such as sudden onset, high absolute values, or treatment-resistant hypertension exist.
- The decision to delay surgery should not be made based on an elevated blood pressure alone but on a holistic evaluation of risk of proceeding versus the risk of delaying surgery. Acutely lowering blood pressure does not appear to alter perioperative risk.

- Most antihypertensive medications can be continued through the perioperative period, but the evidence for ACEIs/ARBs is conflicting and evolving with both withholding on the day of surgery and continuing advocated in different publications.

REFERENCES

1. Murray CJL, Aravkin AY, Zheng P, et al. Global burden of 87 risk factors in 204 countries and territories, 1990–2019: a systematic analysis for the Global Burden of Disease Study 2019. *Lancet*. 2020;396:1223-1249. PMID: 33069327
2. Mills KT, Bundy JD, Kelly TN, et al. Global disparities of hypertension prevalence and control: a systematic analysis of population-based studies from 90 countries. *Circulation*. 2016;134(6):441-450. PMID: 27502908
3. Mancia G, Kreutz R, Brunström M, et al. 2023 ESH guidelines for the management of arterial hypertension: the Task Force for the management of arterial hypertension of the European Society of Hypertension: endorsed by the International Society of Hypertension (ISH) and the European Renal Association (ERA). *J Hypertens*. 2023;41(12):1874-2071. PMID: 37345492
4. Whelton PK, Carey RM, Aronow WS, et al. 2017 ACC/AHA/AAPA/ABC/ACPM/AGS/APhA/ASH/ASPC/NMA/PCNA guideline for the prevention, detection, evaluation, and management of high blood pressure in adults: executive summary: a report of the American College of Cardiology/American Heart Association Task Force on Clinical Practice Guidelines. *Hypertension*. 2018;71(6):1269-1324. PMID: 29133354
5. Sanders RD, Hughes F, Shaw, A, et al. Perioperative quality initiative consensus statement on preoperative blood pressure, risk and outcomes for elective surgery. *Br J Anaesth*. 2019;122:552-562. PMID: 30916006
6. van Klei WA, van Waes JA, Pasma W, et al. Relationship between preoperative evaluation blood pressure and preinduction blood pressure: a cohort study in patients undergoing general anesthesia. *Anesth Analg*. 2017;124(2):431-437. PMID: 27755054
7. Venkatesan S, Myles PR, Manning JH, et al. Cohort study of preoperative blood pressure and risk of 30-day mortality after elective non-cardiac surgery. *Br J Anaesth*. 2017;119:65-77. PMID: 28633374
8. Walco JP, Rengel KF, McEvoy MD, et al. The association between preoperative blood pressures and postoperative adverse events. *Anesthesiology*. 2024 Aug 1;141(2):272-285. PMID: 38558232

9. Howell SJ, Sear JW, Foëx P. Hypertension, hypertensive heart disease and perioperative cardiac risk. *Br J Anaesth.* 2004;92:570-583. PMID: 15013960

10. Soni S, Shah S, Chaggar R, et al. Surgical cancellation rates due to peri-operative hypertension: implementation of multidisciplinary guidelines across primary and secondary care. *Anaesthesia.* 2020;75:1314-1320. PMID: 32488972

11. Hartle A, McCormack T, Carlisle J, et al. The measurement of adult blood pressure and management of hypertension before elective surgery. *Anaesthesia.* 2016;71:326-337. PMID: 26776052

12. Halvorsen S, Mehilli J, Cassese S, et al, ESC Scientific Document Group. 2022 ESC guidelines on cardiovascular assessment and management of patients undergoing non-cardiac surgery. *Eur Heart J.* 2022;43(39): 3826-3924. PMID: 36017553

13. Marcucci M, Painter TW, Conen D, POISE-3 Trial Investigators and Study Groups. Hypotension-avoidance versus hypertension-avoidance strategies in noncardiac surgery: an international randomized controlled trial. *Ann Intern Med.* 2023;176(5):605-614. PMID: 37094336

14. POISE Study Group; Devereaux PJ, Yang H, Yusuf S, et al. Effects of extended-release metoprolol succinate in patients undergoing non-cardiac surgery (POISE trial): a randomised controlled trial. *Lancet.* 2008;371(9627):1839-1847. PMID: 18479744

15. Mets B. Management of hypotension associated with angiotensin-axis blockade and general anesthesia administration. *J Cardiothorac Vasc Anesth.* 2013;27:156-167. PMID: 22854335

16. Roshanov PS, Rochwerg B, Patel A, et al. Withholding versus continuing angiotensin-converting enzyme inhibitors or angiotensin II receptor blockers before noncardiac surgery: an analysis of the vascular events in noncardiac surgery patients cohort evaluation prospective cohort. *Anesthesiology.* 2017;126:16-27. PMID: 27775997

17. Ackland GL, Patel A, Abbott TEF, et al, Stopping Perioperative ACE-inhibitors or Angiotensin-II Receptor Blockers (SPACE) Trial Investigators. Discontinuation vs. continuation of renin-angiotensin system inhibition before non-cardiac surgery: the SPACE trial. *Eur Heart J.* 2024;45(13):1146-1155. PMID: 37935833

18. Legrand M, Falcone J, Cholley B, et al, Stop-or-Not Trial Group. Continuation vs discontinuation of renin-angiotensin system inhibitors before major noncardiac surgery: the stop-or-not randomized clinical trial. *JAMA.* 2024;332(12):970-978. PMID: 39212270

19. Saugel B, Fletcher N, Gan TJ, et al. PeriOperative Quality Initiative (POQI) international consensus statement on perioperative arterial pressure management. *Br J Anaesth.* 2024; Jun 4:S0007-0912(24)00264-2. doi:10.1016/j.bja.2024.04.046. PMID: 38839472

## 16

Pulmonary Disease

Gerald W. Smetana, MD, MACP and Kurt Pfeifer, MD, FACP, SFHM, DFPM

COMMON CLINICAL QUESTIONS

1. How common are postoperative pulmonary complications (PPCs), and how do they impact overall morbidity?

2. What are the most important risk factors for PPCs?

3. Which risk index is the most useful tool to estimate the risk of PPCs?

4. How can I reduce pulmonary risk among high-risk patients?

INTRODUCTION

Postoperative pulmonary complications (PPCs) are common and increase morbidity, length of stay, and mortality. They are even more morbid than postoperative cardiac complications. Among patients who suffer a PPC, 30-day mortality increases from 0.2–3% to 14–30%.[1]

An assessment of the risk of PPCs should be part of every preoperative evaluation. The principal clinically important PPCs are pneumonia, respiratory failure, COPD exacerbation, and atelectasis requiring intervention. In this chapter, we outline preoperative general pulmonary risk assessment and perioperative interventions to mitigate the risk of PPCs. This discussion applies to noncardiothoracic surgery as the risk factors for PPCs differ for cardiac surgery and lung resection surgery. Furthermore, risk assessment and

management for sleep apnea are discussed in a separate chapter.

PREOPERATIVE EVALUATION

It is customary to divide risk factors for PPCs into those that are intrinsic to the procedure itself (procedure-related risk factors) and those due to inherent comorbidities of the patient (patient-related risk factors). Procedure-related risk factors dominate this assessment. In this regard, the preoperative pulmonary evaluation differs from a preoperative cardiac risk assessment where patient-related factors are more important than those intrinsic to the procedure itself.

Patient-Related Risk Factors

While intuitive in some respects, certain patient-related risk factors are more important than others. Table 16-1 lists the most commonly identified risk factors. In contrast to the estimation of cardiac risk, the risk of PPCs due to age holds true even after multivariable adjustment for those conditions that are more common in older persons. The risk is particularly high for patients 70 years of age or older. Therefore, even otherwise healthy older patients should be counseled about PPC risks, and clinicians should consider this factor during the preoperative evaluation.

The other most important patient-related risk factor that persists after adjustment for confounders is the American Society of Anesthesiologists' (ASA) physical status classification (see Chapter 3 on anesthesiology).

TABLE 16-1. Risk Factors for Postoperative Pulmonary Complications

PATIENT-RELATED RISK FACTORS	PROCEDURE-RELATED RISK FACTORS

• Functional dependence (for activities of daily living)
• Age ≥ 60 years
• ASA class 3–5
• Recent respiratory infection (in past month)
• Cigarette use within 8 weeks before surgery
• Abnormal chest x-ray
• Heart failure
• COPD
• Current or recent COVID-19 infection
• Pulmonary hypertension
• Obstructive sleep apnea
	• Surgical site:
	  ○ Upper abdominal
	  ○ Aortic and other intra-abdominal vascular surgery
	  ○ Esophageal
	  ○ Neurosurgery
	  ○ Head and neck
	• General anesthesia (when compared to neuraxial anesthesia)
	• Prolonged surgery (>2 hours)
	• Emergency surgery
	• Intraoperative use of long-acting neuromuscular blockers
	• Routine use of nasogastric tubes after abdominal surgery

ASA, American Society of Anesthesiologists' Physical Status Classification; COPD, chronic obstructive pulmonary disease.

ASA class of 3–5 (on a scale of 1–5) confers increased risk. The ASA classification is based on the estimation of the overall level of chronic illness and comorbid conditions.

Other important patient-related risk factors are heart failure, functional dependence (requiring assistance with activities of daily living), cigarette use, obstructive sleep apnea, pulmonary hypertension, and chronic obstructive pulmonary disease (COPD). Patients with more severe COPD, for example, according to the GOLD (Global Initiative for Chronic Obstructive Lung Disease) classification, are at particularly high risk. Surprisingly, COPD is a weaker risk factor than advanced age or higher ASA classification.

Smoking at any time within the 8 weeks before surgery modestly increases PPC risk. The risk is particularly substantial for active smokers. In addition, current or recent COVID-19 infection increases the risk of PPCs. The duration this risk persists is influenced by the severity of symptoms and vaccination status. Clinicians should follow local protocols for timing of elective surgery after COVID-19 infection[2] (see Chapter 24). Obesity, in the absence of obstructive sleep apnea, has not been consistently identified as an independent risk factor for PPC.

Procedure-Related Risk Factors

Procedure-related risk factors are the most important factors to consider when estimating PPC risk (Table 16-1).[3] Among these, the surgical site is the most important factor. With few exceptions, the risk is greatest for procedures closest to the diaphragm and/or airway. Aortic, other intra-abdominal vascular surgery (e.g., aortobifemoral bypass), esophageal, and upper abdominal surgery confer the highest risk for PPCs. Major orthopedic procedures do not substantially increase PPC rates. Surgical site is a nonmodifiable risk factor other than in instances where a lower-risk procedure (endovascular repair for example) could be performed in lieu of a high-risk procedure (open aortic aneurysm surgery). Prolonged surgery and emergency surgery also increase PPC risk.

The impact of general anesthesia on PPC rates has been well studied and remains controversial. Most authors consider this to be a moderate risk factor, when compared to neuraxial anesthesia (epidural or spinal anesthesia). For example, in a recent review of patients with COPD, regional anesthesia was associated with lower rates of postoperative pneumonia, respiratory failure, and unplanned reintubation compared to general anesthesia.[4]

Preoperative Pulmonary Risk Indices

Similar in concept to preoperative cardiac indices, preoperative risk indices now exist for estimation of PPC rates. These tools have evaluated the risk of PPC in general, as well as specific indices for pneumonia and respiratory failure.

The Assess Respiratory Risk in Surgical Patients in Catalonia index (https://www.mdcalc.com/ariscat-score-postoperative-pulmonary-complications) was derived from a large population of patients in Europe undergoing surgery with either general or neuraxial anesthesia (Table 16-2).[5] This index has the advantage in that information regarding the risk factors is readily available before surgery, and it accurately stratifies risk.

TABLE 16-2. ARISCAT Index for Prediction of Postoperative Pulmonary Complications

RISK FACTOR	RISK SCORE
Age (years)	
• 51–80	3
• >80	16
Preoperative O$_2$ saturation	
• 91–95%	8
• ≤90%	24
Respiratory infection within past month	17
Preoperative hemoglobin <10 g/dL	11
Surgical site	
• Upper abdominal	15
• Intrathoracic	24
Duration of surgery (hours)	
• 2–3	16
• >3	23
Emergency procedure	8

RISK STRATIFICATION	RISK SCORE	RATE OF PPC
Low	<26	1.6–3.4%
Intermediate	26–44	13–13.3%
High	≥45	38–42.1%

Source: Data from Canet J, et al. *Anesthesiology.* 2010;113: 1338-1350.

It is also the most inclusive of different types of PPCs (respiratory failure, atelectasis, aspiration pneumonitis, respiratory infection, pleural effusion, and bronchospasm) and has been externally validated.

Gupta and colleagues have developed risk indices that specifically estimate risk for either pneumonia or respiratory failure (http://www.surgicalriskcalculator.com/home). Both tools are simple to use and include a small number of factors for which information is readily available. However, they do require the use of a downloadable spreadsheet to calculate the risks.

The American College of Surgeons has developed a risk calculator that estimates risks not only for PPCs (pneumonia) but also for multiple other complications and mortality (https://riskcalculator facs org/ RiskCalculator). It is complicated and requires the use of an online tool but may be helpful both for clinicians and patients when considering risks for a number of different postoperative complications.

While each tool has advantages, based on its simplicity and accuracy, for clinicians who wish to use only one risk index, we recommend the ARISCAT index.

PREOPERATIVE TESTING

Chest X-ray

A preoperative chest x-ray usually does not yield unexpected information and should only be ordered selectively. For additional discussion, see Chapter 2 on preoperative testing.

Pulmonary Function Tests

While some studies of pulmonary function testing (PFT) prior to nonthoracic surgery have reported an association between low forced expiratory volume in one second (FEV1) and PPCs, other studies combining PFT with clinical assessment have not identified an additive benefit of PFT beyond the clinical evaluation alone.[6] Therefore, PFT is not recommended for routine preoperative evaluation before nonthoracic surgery unless a patient has an indication regardless of surgery (e.g., unexplained dyspnea or wheezing).

Laboratory Testing

Arterial blood gas (ABG) testing is often considered before surgery in patients with chronic obstructive lung disease. Although hypercapnia may be identified, it usually does not alter management more than clinical assessment alone. A situation where preoperative management would be altered by knowledge of chronic carbon dioxide retention is a patient screened as high risk for sleep apnea. When such patients have an elevated serum bicarbonate, the risk for postoperative complications is particularly high, and perioperative sleep apnea guidelines would recommend delay of nonurgent surgery for further evaluation. See Chapter 17 on sleep apnea for additional information. Low serum albumin levels (<3.5 g/dL) are associated with higher rates of PPCs and postoperative mortality. This may be a marker of comorbidities. We do not recommend routinely measuring serum albumin before surgery, but when a result is already known, it may help to estimate risk.

PERIOPERATIVE RISK REDUCTION (SEE ALGORITHM IN FIGURE 16-1)

Several methods for general pulmonary risk reduction that span the full perioperative period are available for clinicians (Table 16-3).

Anesthesia Techniques

As described earlier in this chapter, some studies have suggested that general anesthesia confers risk for PPC. The majority of recent studies have demonstrated that neuraxial (spinal or epidural) or regional (peripheral nerve block) anesthesia reduces the risk of pulmonary complications when used alone or even in combination with general anesthesia.[7]

When general anesthesia is used, lung-protective ventilation is a potential risk reduction method. Studies have used a variety of methods and found differing results. The preponderance of studies has suggested that use of near-physiologic tidal volumes (i.e., 6–8 cc/kg) with methods to prevent alveolar collapse,

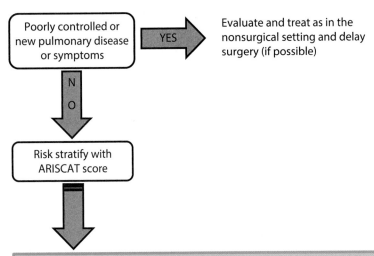

FIGURE 16-1. Algorithm for risk reduction of pulmonary complications.

TABLE 16-3. Pulmonary Risk Reduction Interventions

INTERVENTION	DETAILS
Chronic lung disease optimization	No specific data to support but accepted as best practice
Oral hygiene promotion	Daily to twice daily tooth brushing and oral antiseptic rinse use reduces the risk of aspiration and pneumonia
Smoking cessation	For greatest benefit should be for at least 4–6 weeks before surgery
Chronic pulmonary medication continuation	Only medication to consider withholding may be theophylline (due to potential for arrhythmia)
Preoperative respiratory therapy (pulmonary prehabilitation)	Programs of inspiratory muscle training and pulmonary prehabilitation substantially reduce risk of PPCs in high-risk patients
Regional and neuraxial anesthesia	Reduces PPCs even when combined with general anesthesia
Perioperative CPAP for patients with obstructive sleep apnea	Reduces risk of PPCs, unplanned reintubation, and unwitnessed respiratory arrest (see Chapter 17 for details)
Lung-protective ventilation	Data mixed on best ventilation strategy; overall, literature suggests benefit from using non-supraphysiologic V_T with techniques to prevent atelectasis (PEEP, lung alveolar recruitment maneuvers)
Neuromuscular blockade minimization	Judicious use of NMB, avoidance of long-acting paralysis agents, and close monitoring and assurance of neuromuscular recovery can prevent complications from prolonged NMB
Opioid and sedating medication minimization	Reduces risk for hypoventilation which may lead to atelectasis and other PPCs
Early and frequent mobilization	Encourage patient to get out of bed as much as possible (at least three times daily)
Non-supine positioning while in bed	May prevent aspiration and atelectasis
Postoperative lung expansion	Incentive spirometry, deep breathing techniques, IPPB, and CPAP are all potentially beneficial options

PPCs, postoperative pulmonary complications; IPPB, intermittent positive-pressure breathing; CPAP, continuous positive airway pressure; V_T, tidal volume; PEEP, positive end-expiratory pressure; NMB, neuromuscular blockade.

such as alveolar recruitment maneuvers and positive end-expiratory pressure, is likely superior to supraphysiologic tidal volumes (i.e., ≥ 10 cc/kg) without similar atelectasis-preventing interventions.[8]

Multiple studies have also demonstrated increased PPC risk with the use of neuromuscular blockade (NMB). When NMB must be used, long-acting NMB agents (e.g., pancuronium) should be avoided, and the depth of NMB should be closely monitored, particularly close to the time of extubation.

Goal-directed hemodynamic therapy involves protocol-based optimization of cardiovascular parameters, and in addition to surgical site infections and other outcomes, its use is associated with lower rates of pneumonia and acute respiratory distress syndrome.

Non-anesthesiology clinicians should be aware of these intraoperative risk reduction measures but should not provide specific recommendations for intraoperative care. Instead, non-anesthesiologists performing the preoperative evaluation should make sure the anesthesia team is aware of patients with increased pulmonary risk so that the anesthetist can factor this into their intraoperative care plan.

Analgesia Techniques

Sedation leads to hypoventilation, which can precipitate atelectasis. For this reason, the use of opioid-sparing strategies reduces PPCs. Provision of opioids via epidural catheter and patient-controlled analgesia can reduce systemic opioid use and PPCs.[9] Nonpharmacologic analgesic techniques such as ice or heating pad application should be utilized as well as acetaminophen and nonsteroidal anti-inflammatory drugs (NSAIDs).

Lung Expansion Methods

Postoperative lung expansion methods may help prevent and treat early atelectasis and subsequent PPCs like respiratory failure and pneumonia. The most recent Cochrane review of incentive spirometry (IS) suggested no benefit from routine postoperative use, but these negative results may relate to the variable study methods and the relatively low risk of many included patients. Protocols incorporating IS have shown reductions in PPCs.[10] Some studies of postoperative intermittent positive-pressure breathing and continuous positive airway pressure (CPAP) ventilation have also shown benefit for reducing PPCs.

Preoperative Respiratory Therapy

Preoperative respiratory therapy interventions (pulmonary prehabilitation) incorporate methods to improve inspiratory muscle strength and lung capacity. Substantial reductions in PPCs have been demonstrated with both inspiratory muscle training (IMT) and cardiopulmonary rehabilitation before major abdominal and cardiac surgery.[11] In most studies, IMT was employed for at least 1–2 weeks before surgery with the use of an inspiratory threshold device as trained by a respiratory therapist. The benefit extends to reductions both in respiratory failure and pneumonia rates. Many surgical programs have employed preoperative deep breathing exercises or IS as part of their prehabilitation programs.

Smoking Cessation

Smoking cessation modestly reduces the risk of PPCs. A single older study suggested increased risk from quitting smoking shortly before surgery, but recent studies have not demonstrated the same association. For the greatest reduction in PPCs, smoking cessation should be accomplished at least 4–6 weeks before surgery.[12] However, even shorter durations of cessation have other benefits, and counseling patients in the preoperative setting to quit smoking is associated with increased rates of long-term abstinence.[13] Therefore, patients should be counseled to quit smoking regardless of the timeline to surgery.

Risk Reduction Bundles

Bundles of risk reduction strategies, usually part of standardized order sets, can reduce risk in high-risk patients and are increasingly being used for this purpose. One such bundle is the I-COUGH program.[10]

Clinical pearls

- Preoperative pulmonary complications are morbid and increase length of stay and mortality.
- Procedure-related risk factors are more important than patient-related factors; the most important risk factor is the type of surgery (surgical site). General anesthesia also increases risk.
- Important patient-related risk factors include age $\geq$ 60 years old, functional dependence, COPD, heart failure, recent COVID-19 infection, and obstructive sleep apnea.
- Preoperative tests add little to the risk prediction available through a careful clinical evaluation.
- Preoperative IMT, lung protective ventilation, and postoperative lung expansion maneuvers reduce rates of PPCs.
- Smoking cessation before surgery reduces PPCs. The optimal duration is at least 4–6 weeks.

REFERENCES

1. Miskovic A, Lumb AB. Postoperative pulmonary complications. *Br J Anaesth.* 2017;118:317-334. PMID: 28186222
2. Le ST, Kipnis P, Cohn B, Liu VX. COVID-19 vaccination and the timing of surgery following COVID-19 infection. *Ann Surg.* 2022;276(5):e265-e272. PMID: 35837898
3. Smetana GW, Lawrence VA, Cornell JE. Preoperative pulmonary risk stratification for noncardiothoracic surgery: systematic review for the American College of Physicians. *Ann Intern Med.* 2006;144:581-595. PMID: 16618956

4. Hausman MS Jr, Jewell ES, Engoren M. Regional versus general anesthesia in surgical patients with chronic obstructive pulmonary disease: does avoiding general anesthesia reduce the risk of postoperative complications? *Anesth Analg.* 2015;120(6):1405-1412. PMID: 25526396

5. Canet J, Gallart L, Gomar C, et al. Prediction of postoperative pulmonary complications in a population-based surgical cohort. *Anesthesiology.* 2010;113:1338-1350. PMID: 21045639

6. Dankert A, Neumann-Schirmbeck B, Dohrmann T, et al. Preoperative spirometry in patients with known or suspected chronic obstructive pulmonary disease undergoing major surgery: the prospective observational PREDICT study. *Anesth Analg.* 2023;137:806-818. PMID: 36730893

7. Smith LM, Cozowicz C, Uda Y, et al. Neuraxial and combined neuraxial/general anesthesia compared to general anesthesia for major truncal and lower limb surgery: a systematic review and meta-analysis. *Anesth Analg.* 2017;125(6):1931-1945. PMID: 28537970

8. Buonanno P, Marra A, Iacovazzo C, et al. Impact of ventilation strategies on pulmonary and cardiovascular complications in patients undergoing general anaesthesia for elective surgery: a systematic review and meta-analysis. *Br J Anaesth.* 2023;131(6):1093-1101. PMID: 37839932

9. Guay J, Kopp S. Epidural pain relief versus systemic opioid-based pain relief for abdominal aortic surgery. *Cochrane Database Syst Rev.* 2016;2016(1):CD005059. PMID: 26731032

10. Cassidy MR, Rosenkranz P, McCabe K, et al. I COUGH: reducing postoperative pulmonary complications with a multidisciplinary patient care program. *JAMA Surg.* 2013;148(8):740-745. PMID: 23740240

11. Katsura M, Kuriyama A, Takeshima T, et al. Preoperative inspiratory muscle training for postoperative pulmonary complications in adults undergoing cardiac and major abdominal surgery. *Cochrane Database Syst Rev.* 2015 Oct 5;2015(10):CD010356. PMID: 26436600

12. Wong J, An D, Urman RD, et al. Society for Perioperative Assessment and Quality Improvement (SPAQI) consensus statement on perioperative smoking cessation. *Anesth Analg.* 2020;131(3):955-968. PMID: 31764157

13. Lee SM, Landry J, Jones PM, et al. Long-term quit rates after a perioperative smoking cessation randomized controlled trial. *Anesth Analg.* 2015;120(3):582-587. PMID: 25695576

Sleep Apnea and Airway Management

Kurt Pfeifer, MD, FACP, SFHM, DFPM and Frances Chung, MD, MBBS, SAMBAf, FRCPC

COMMON CLINICAL QUESTIONS

1. What is the best method to screen for undiagnosed sleep apnea?
2. Do all patients with suspected sleep apnea require sleep medicine evaluation before elective surgery?
3. What are the best methods for assessment of airway and mask ventilation difficulty?
4. What are risk reduction interventions for patients with diagnosed or suspected sleep apnea?

INTRODUCTION

Current studies estimate at least 25 million people in the United States have obstructive sleep apnea (OSA), and in the surgical population, the incidence of moderate or severe sleep apnea (defined as a respiratory event index [REI] or apnea-hypopnea index [AHI] $\geq$ 15 events per hour) is approximately 30%.[1] OSA is associated with 1.5 times increased risk in postoperative cardiovascular complications and a twofold increase in respiratory complications, hospital, and ICU readmission.[2] These risks are likely higher among patients with undiagnosed sleep apnea.[3] Although OSA is often the primary focus of clinicians, it is important to note that central sleep apnea is also a major source of morbidity and mortality.

A concomitant problem in many OSA patients (but also in those without sleep apnea) is challenging airway management. Potentially difficult bag-mask ventilation and endotracheal intubation should be identified in advance of surgery to allow for appropriate perioperative care planning.

PREOPERATIVE EVALUATION (SEE ALGORITHM IN FIGURE 17-1)

Sleep Apnea

Previously Diagnosed Sleep Apnea. Surgical patients with known sleep apnea require a thorough history and physical exam to document their management requirements and identify evidence suggestive of inadequate treatment. Previous sleep study reports should be obtained, and key findings documented for the perioperative care team (Table 17-1). The number of central sleep apneas and variation in AHI by sleep position (supine) and sleep stage (rapid eye movement [REM]) should also be noted since these may influence perioperative management.[4] For patients using noninvasive ventilatory treatment, the ventilation type (positive airway pressure: automatic [APAP], continuous [CPAP], or bilevel [BiPAP]; or adaptive-servo ventilation [ASV]) and settings, compliance with therapy, and need for oxygen supplementation should be determined. Signs and symptoms of sleep apnea, including daytime sleepiness, snoring/gasping during sleep,

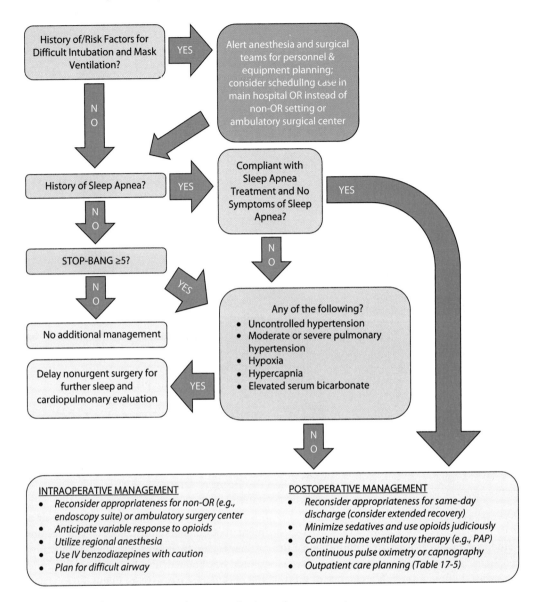

FIGURE 17-1. Algorithm for perioperative pulmonary evaluation and management.

morning headaches, and poorly controlled hypertension, should be sought even in patients with good treatment compliance since these may indicate a need for therapy adjustment prior to nonurgent surgery.

Suspected Sleep Apnea. Guidelines from the Society of Anesthesia and Sleep Medicine (SASM) recommend that all surgical patients without diagnosed sleep apnea should be screened for this condition using a standardized tool.[5] Although several tools are available, the STOP-BANG questionnaire is the most studied in the perioperative setting and predicts risk of complications (Table 17-2).[6] A STOP-BANG score of 5 or higher suggests increased risk for postoperative complications. The SASM guideline recommends informing all suspected sleep apnea patients of the increased risk for postoperative

TABLE 17-1. Sleep Study Parameters Associated with Postoperative Complications[1,3]

PARAMETER	COMMENTS
AHI ≥ 5	Risk increases with increasing AHI; measured in polysomnography
REI > 30	Measured in home sleep apnea testing
ODI ≥ 5	Risk increased with increasing ODI
CT90 > 0	Risk of complications doubled at CT90 > 7%

AHI, apnea-hypopnea index; REI, respiratory event index; ODI, oxygen desaturation index; CT90, cumulative time during sleep with oxygen saturation < 90%.

TABLE 17-2. STOP-BANG Questionnaire for Screening for Sleep Apnea

Snoring?

Do you *snore loudly* (loud enough to be heard through closed doors or your bed-partner elbows you for snoring at night)?

Tired?

Do you often feel *tired, fatigued,* or *sleepy* during the daytime (such as falling asleep during driving)?

Observed Apneas?

Has anyone *observed* you *stop breathing* or *choking/gasping* during your sleep?

High Blood Pressure

Do you have or are being treated for *high blood pressure*?

BMI >35 kg/m²?

Age older than 50 years?

Neck size large?

For male, shirt collar ≥ 17 in./43 cm?

For female, shirt collar ≥ 16 in./41 cm?

Gender is male?

Reproduced with permission from University Health Network; 2020.

complications but only advises delay of nonurgent surgery for further testing if there is evidence of an associated significant or uncontrolled systemic disease (e.g., pulmonary hypertension) or abnormal gas exchange (i.e., hypoxia, hypercapnia, or elevated serum bicarbonate).[5]

Difficult Airways

Evaluation of Patients with Known Difficult Airways. Clinicians performing a preoperative evaluation should review available anesthesia records for information regarding the patient's previous airway management. This is particularly important for those patients who have a history of difficult intubation as related by them or through the medical record. Information to seek includes the degree of difficulty of mask ventilation, number of attempts at endotracheal intubation, final successful approach to intubation (direct laryngoscopy, video laryngoscopy, laryngeal mask airway), grade of laryngoscopic view, use of glottic view improvement maneuvers (e.g., cricoid pressure), and size of endotracheal tube or laryngeal mask airway. For patients with difficult (requiring two practitioners) mask ventilation, multiple intubation attempts, no visualization of the glottis on laryngoscopy (grade 3 or 4 view), or other documentation suggestive of a difficult airway, the anesthesia team should be notified well in advance of surgery to allow time for perioperative care planning.

Difficult Airway Screening. In addition to identifying a history of OSA or difficult intubation/ventilation, a focused airway examination should be performed on all patients scheduled for possible general anesthesia. A variety of different examination methods have been developed for the prediction of difficult intubation (Table 17-3).[7] The Mallampati classification assesses the view of the oropharynx during maximal mouth opening and tongue protrusion (but not phonation). In a Mallampati class III airway, only the base of the uvula can be visualized, and in a class IV airway, none of the soft palate. The upper lip bite test evaluates how far a patient can bite her lower teeth over the upper lip. Inability to bite past the upper lip's vermillion border has the highest positive likelihood ratio of any of the available methods of difficult intubation prediction.[7]

TABLE 17-3. Methods of Prediction of Difficult Intubation[6]

ASSESSMENT	SENSITIVITY	SPECIFICITY
Upper lip bite test class 2–3	60%	96%
Wilson score ≥ 2	43%	95%
Hyomental distance < 3 cm	20%	97%
Mallampati class III–IV	55%	87%
Inter-incisor gap < 2 cm	36%	90%
Decreased neck range of motion	28%	93%
Thyromental distance < 4 cm	45%	86%

TABLE 17-4. DIFFMASK Score for Predicting Difficult Mask Ventilation[7]

FACTOR		POINTS
Age	45–59 years	2
	≥ 60 years	3
Male gender		1
BMI	25–35	2
	>35	3
Previous difficult intubation		1
Thyromental distance	6.0–6.5 cm	1
	<6.0 cm	2
Mallampati score	3	1
	4	2
Full beard		2
Snoring		1
Sleep apnea		1
Neck radiation skin changes		2

SCORE	SENSITIVITY	SPECIFICITY
≥4	93.1%	45.1%
≥5	85.1%	58.8%
≥6	71.1%	73.0%
≥7	54.9%	85.0%
≥8	41.8%	92.2%
≥9	27.7%	96.3%
≥10	14.7%	98.6%

Several different risk factors can also predict difficult mask ventilation, and the recently validated DIFFMASK score provides a standardized approach for stratifying risk (Table 17-4).[8]

PERIOPERATIVE MANAGEMENT

General Measures

All patients with sleep apnea should receive oxygen therapy as needed to maintain baseline pulse oximetry values.[9] Non-supine positioning should also be maintained (unless contraindicated by surgical factors) to reduce obstruction and aspiration risk.[9]

Minimize Sedation

A key to perioperative risk mitigation in all patients with known or suspected sleep apnea is to minimize sedation, which can precipitate upper airway obstruction and exacerbate sleep-disordered breathing. In addition to avoiding the use of benzodiazepines and other sedative medications, opioid-sparing methods should be employed, including regional anesthesia/analgesia, provision of the lowest effective opioid doses, and maximum use of nonpharmacologic analgesia (e.g., cold/heat packs) and non-opioid analgesics

(e.g., nonsteroidal anti-inflammatory medications, scheduled acetaminophen).[9,10] Clinicians should also anticipate variable responses to opioids in patients with sleep apnea.[10]

PAP and Other Sleep Apnea Treatments

Patients who use ventilatory support (e.g., PAP) at home should bring their device to the hospital and continue its use perioperatively unless there is a surgical contraindication such as after craniotomy or sinus surgery.[9,10] If the patient's device is not available, a hospital device can be applied using the settings from their sleep study. Alternatively, if no information is available about their settings, APAP can be utilized, but clinicians should note this therapy is usually insufficient for patients who utilize BiPAP or ASV at home. For patients with suspected sleep apnea, empiric use of PAP is not recommended since it has not been clearly shown to improve clinical outcomes and may be difficult for patients to adapt to in the postoperative setting.[5] Instead, it should be reserved for patients demonstrating severe obstruction, hypoxia, or CO_2 retention.[9]

A recent systematic review and meta-analysis analyzed the impact of PAP therapy on postoperative outcomes in OSA patients undergoing noncardiac and cardiac surgery. In patients with OSA undergoing noncardiac surgery, PAP therapy was associated with a 28% reduction in the risk of postoperative respiratory complications (RR 0.72) and 56% reduction in the risk of unplanned ICU admission (RR 0.44).[11] In patients with OSA undergoing cardiac surgery, PAP therapy was associated with a decreased risk of postoperative cardiac complications by 37% (RR 0.63) and atrial fibrillation by 41% (RR 0.59).[11] This review suggests that there may be some benefits to having PAP therapy before surgery.

Some patients with mild sleep apnea may use mandibular advancement devices at home. Use of these devices should be continued postoperatively unless the surgical site makes this difficult.

Upper airway stimulation devices (Inspire®) are another treatment option for patients with OSA. These devices deliver electrical stimuli to upper airway muscles to keep the upper airway open during sleep. The device is activated with the use of a remote control, which patients should bring with them to the hospital. The anesthesiology team should be alerted so they can determine if the device should be activated during the procedure. Postoperatively, these devices can be used as usual unless there is concern for the device causing electromagnetic interference with other necessary devices.

Continuous Respiratory Monitoring

A small percentage of surgical patients with OSA who receive postoperative oxygen therapy may have significant CO_2 retention despite increased SpO_2. The ability of pulse oximetry to detect significant desaturations and hypoventilation may be masked during oxygen therapy. This may result in a delayed response to prolonged hypoventilation, resulting in CO_2 narcosis, or cardiopulmonary arrest.[12] Hospitalized patients with known or suspected sleep apnea should receive continuously monitored pulse oximetry (or capnography) after discharge from the postanesthesia care unit.[9] Such monitoring should not be done through unmonitored bedside devices. Instead, it should be accomplished with a system incorporating trained observers (telemetry) or utilizing alert systems governed by response policies (connection to room/bed alarm system).

Appropriate Operative Location and Postoperative Triage

Patients with known or suspected sleep apnea require careful contemplation regarding operative location and postoperative triage. The Society for Ambulatory Anesthesia (SAMBA) guidelines recommend that outpatient surgery for patients with known sleep apnea be limited to those with optimized comorbid conditions and able to use their home ventilatory support after surgery.[13] For patients with suspected sleep apnea, SAMBA recommends that outpatient surgery be restricted to patients with optimized comorbid conditions whose pain will be predominantly treated with non-opioid methods.[13] Surgery should be pursued in a hospital setting for patients with additional risk factors. If home ventilatory therapy cannot be continued due to surgical contraindications, upgrading postoperative triage should be considered (e.g., admission instead of same-day discharge), particularly if the patient has severe or complex (mixed obstructive and central) sleep apnea or sleep-disordered breathing that is much worse during REM sleep. Sleep apnea is worsened in the postoperative period, and sleep-disordered breathing peaks on postoperative day 3 due to "REM rebound."[14] As a result, patients with sleep apnea and additional perioperative risk factors may need additional planning for safe recovery at home (Table 17-5).

Difficult Airways

The anesthesiology team must be given advance notification of patients with known or risk factors for

TABLE 17-5. Discharge Care Planning for Patients with Known or Suspected Sleep Apnea

Sleep with head elevated
Avoid over-the-counter and prescribed sleep medications
Avoid alcohol
If opioids are prescribed, provide naloxone as well
If unable to use home ventilatory therapy due to surgical contraindication, speak to sleep medicine provider about alternative treatments (e.g., nocturnal oxygen)
If severe sleep apnea or additional perioperative risk factors, consider arranging for family or friends to stay with patient or check in for the first few days after surgery

difficult intubation or mask ventilation. This information can be used to assure that specialized intubation equipment is available and appropriate personnel are assigned to the case. Furthermore, patients with these issues may not be appropriate for surgery with more than minimal sedation at ambulatory surgical centers or in nonoperative settings (e.g., endoscopy suite), so the preoperative clinician should discuss this with anesthesiology and the surgeon.

Clinical pearls

- Sleep apnea is associated with an increased risk of multiple perioperative complications and should be screened for in all surgical patients.

- Nonurgent surgery should be delayed for patients with STOP-BANG scores of 5 or higher plus uncontrolled comorbidities, hypoxia, hypercapnia, or elevated serum bicarbonate.

- Ambulatory surgery should be reconsidered for patients with severe or complex sleep apnea or with additional risk factors for perioperative complications.

- Postoperative management of sleep apnea focuses on minimizing sedation, continuing previous sleep apnea treatment, and close respiratory monitoring in an appropriate setting.

REFERENCES

1. Chan MTV, Wang CY, Seet E, et al. Association of unrecognized obstructive sleep apnea with postoperative cardiovascular events in patients undergoing major noncardiac surgery. *JAMA.* 2019;321(18):1788-1798. PMID: 31087023
2. Pivetta B, Sun Y, Nagappa M, et al. Postoperative outcomes in surgical patients with obstructive sleep apnoea diagnosed by sleep studies: a meta-analysis and trial sequential analysis. *Anaesthesia.* 2022;77(7):818-828. PMID: 35332537
3. Fernandez-Bustamante A, Bartels K, Clavijo C, et al. Preoperatively screened obstructive sleep apnea is associated with worse postoperative outcomes than previously diagnosed obstructive sleep apnea. *Anesth Analg.* 2017;125(2):593-602. PMID: 28682951
4. Suen C, Ryan CM, Mubashir T, et al. Sleep study and oximetry parameters for predicting postoperative complications in patients with OSA. *Chest.* 2019;155(4):855-867. PMID: 30359618
5. Chung F, Memtsoudis SG, Ramachandran SK, et al. Society of Anesthesia and Sleep Medicine guidelines on preoperative screening and assessment of adult patients with obstructive sleep apnea. *Anesth Analg.* 2016;123(2):452-473. PMID: 27442772
6. Chung F, Subramanyam R, Liao P, et al. High STOP-BANG score indicates a high probability of obstructive sleep apnoea. *Br J Anaesth.* 2012;108(5):768-775. PMID: 22401881
7. Detsky ME, Jivraj N, Adhikari NK, et al. Will this patient be difficult to intubate? The rationale clinical examination systematic review. *JAMA.* 2019;321(5):493-503. PMID: 30721300
8. Lundstrøm LH, Rosenstock CV, Wetterslev J, Nørskov AK. The DIFFMASK score for predicting difficult face-mask ventilation: a cohort study of 46,804 patients. *Anaesthesia.* 2019;74(10):1267-1276. PMID: 31106851
9. American Society of Anesthesiologists Task Force on perioperative management of patients with obstructive sleep apnea. Practice guidelines for the perioperative management of patients with obstructive sleep apnea: an updated report by the American Society of Anesthesiologists Task Force on perioperative management of patients with obstructive sleep apnea. *Anesthesiology.* 2014;120(2):268-286. PMID: 24346178
10. Memtsoudis SG, Cozowicz C, Nagappa M, et al. Society of Anesthesia and Sleep Medicine guideline on intraoperative management of adult patients with obstructive sleep apnea. *Anesth Analg.* 2018;127(4):967-987. PMID: 29944522

11. Berezin L, Nagappa M, Poorzargar K. The effectiveness of positive airway pressure therapy in reducing postoperative adverse outcomes in surgical patients with obstructive sleep apnea: a systematic review and meta-analysis. *J Clin Anesth*. 2023;84:110993. PMID: 36347195

12. Ruan B, Nagappa M, Rashid-Kolvear M, et al. The effectiveness of supplemental oxygen and high-flow nasal cannula therapy in patients with obstructive sleep apnea in different clinical settings: a systematic review and meta-analysis. *J Clin Anesth*. 2023;88:111144. PMID: 37172556

13. Joshi GP, Ankichetty SP, Gan TJ, Chung F. Society for Ambulatory Anesthesia consensus statement on preoperative selection of adult patients with obstructive sleep apnea scheduled for ambulatory surgery. *Anesth Analg*. 2012;115(5):1060-1068. PMID: 22886843

14. Chung F, Liao P, Elsaid H, et al. Factors associated with postoperative exacerbation of sleep-disordered breathing. *Anesthesiology*. 2014;120(2):299-311. PMID: 24158050

Pulmonary Hypertension

Kurt Pfeifer, MD, FACP, SFHM, DFPM and Angela Roberts Selzer, MD, FASA, DFPM

COMMON CLINICAL QUESTIONS

1. How does pulmonary hypertension (PH) impact anesthesia management?
2. What is the recommended preoperative evaluation for a patient with previously undiagnosed PH?
3. What is the best perioperative management of medications used to treat PH?
4. What perioperative risk mitigation measures should be employed for patients with PH?

INTRODUCTION

In a healthy patient, the ability of the thin-walled right ventricle (RV) to increase its cardiac output during stress and exercise while maintaining mean pressures around 14 mmHg is remarkable. The RV achieves this by pumping blood into the very low resistance, high capacitance system of the pulmonary vasculature. Pulmonary hypertension (PH) is a pathologic disorder of increased pressure within the pulmonary arteries. The sixth World Symposium on Pulmonary Hypertension (WSPH) formally defines PH as a mean pulmonary artery pressure (mPAP) $\geq$ 20 mmHg measured via right heart catheterization.[1]

Increasing use of echocardiography and heightened awareness of PH have increased the overall incidence of diagnosed disease. The prevalence of PH is approximately 1% in the global population, 5% of individuals living at high altitude, and up to 10% of individuals over 65 years of age.[2] The WSPH classifies patients into five groups based on the underlying etiology of disease (Table 18-1).[1]

Group 1, or pulmonary arterial hypertension (PAH), arises from remodeling of the distal pulmonary vasculature, primarily affecting precapillary vessels. PAH is rare, affecting approximately 25 people per 1 million in developed nations.[2] PAH is essentially a disease of endothelial hyperproliferation and vasoconstriction.[3] Pharmacotherapy for PAH patients increases vasodilation and reduces endothelial proliferation through three essential pathways: the nitric oxide, endothelin-1, and prostacyclin pathways (Table 18-2).

Approximately 75% of PH patients fall under the Group 2 classification, or PH secondary to left heart disease.[4] These patients benefit from treatment and optimization of their underlying heart disease. These patients should be optimized further with their cardiologist, and most do not require regular invasive measurements of right-sided pressures or evaluation by a PH specialist unless right-side pressure elevations persist despite optimization of heart disease.

Group 3 PH patients have elevated pulmonary pressures secondary to chronic hypoxia and/or lung disease.

Group 4 PH results from clotting or other obstructions in the pulmonary vasculature, or chronic thromboembolic PH (CTEPH). This is a particularly difficult type of PH, requiring treatment at a specialized center.

TABLE 18-1. Pulmonary Hypertension (PH) Classification Based on Pathophysiology[1]

GROUP	PATHOPHYSIOLOGY
1	Pulmonary arterial hypertension (PAH)
2	PH due to left heart disease
3	PH due to chronic lung disease and/or hypoxia
4	PH due to pulmonary artery obstructions such as chronic thromboembolic PH (CTEPH)
5	PH due to multisystemic disorders or multiple/unknown mechanisms

There is currently only one PH medication that reduces mortality in CTEPH patients, riociguat.

Group 5 PH patients do not fall under any of the above groups and have multisystemic disease, such as connective tissue disorders or rheumatologic diseases.

Regardless of the etiology of PH, exposure of the RV to sustained increases in afterload causes physiologic changes in RV structure and function over time. Initially, the RV can compensate for the PH with hypertrophic changes, but ultimately, long-standing PH can result in asymmetric hypertrophy, RV dilation, and reduced function. PH patients with decompensated RVs are particularly difficult to manage intraoperatively. Conditions present during surgery stress the struggling RV further, and in contrast to the more muscular left ventricle, the RV responds poorly to

TABLE 18-2. Pharmacotherapy Specific for Pulmonary Arterial Hypertension (PAH)[3]

CLASS	MEDICATIONS (ROUTE OF ADMINISTRATION)	MECHANISM OF ACTION	SPECIAL FEATURES
Calcium channel blockers	Amlodipine (PO) Diltiazem (PO) Nifedipine (PO)	Vasodilation	Only ~10% of PAH patients are responders to calcium channel blockers
Endothelin receptor antagonists	Ambrisentan (PO) Bosentan (PO) Macitentan (PO)	Endothelin receptors blockade → smooth muscle cell relaxation → vasodilation	Ambrisentan selectively blocks the endothelin type-A receptor and has a better side effect profile than bosentan or macicentan (both nonselective blockers)
Guanylate cyclase stimulator	Riociguat (PO)	Stimulates soluble GC, the enzyme target of NO	Only agent also approved for group 4 PH; may increase bleeding risk
PDE-5 inhibitors	Sildenafil (PO) Tadalafil (PO)	Preventing PDE-5 breakdown → increased cGMP → increased NO → smooth muscle cell relaxation → vasodilation	
Prostacyclin analogs and receptor agonists	Epoprostenol (IV, SQ) Iloprost (INH) Selexipag (PO) Treprostinil (INH, IV, PO, SQ)	Prostacyclin synthase expression impaired in PH → prostacyclin is potent arterial vasodilator	Continuous infusion (SQ/IV) used for severe disease— can have severe rebound vasoconstriction with abrupt discontinuation

PO, by mouth; INH, inhalation; SQ, subcutaneous injection; IV, intravenous infusion; PDE-5, phosphodiesterase-5; GC, guanylate cyclase; NO, nitric oxide; RHC, right heart catheterization; cGMP, cyclic guanosine monophosphate.

TABLE 18-3. Perioperative Factors Associated with Poor Outcomes in PH Patients[5]		
PERIOPERATIVE FACTORS ASSOCIATED WITH POOR OUTCOMES IN PULMONARY HYPERTENSION PATIENTS HAVING NONCARDIAC SURGERY		
RISK FACTOR	INCITING FACTOR	SURGERY OR ANESTHESIA TYPE
Hypercapnia	Insufflation	Laparo- or thoracoscopic surgery
	Hypoventilation	MAC anesthesia
Elevation in Venous Pressure	Insufflation	Laparo- or thoracoscopic surgery
	Trendelenburg positioning	Gynecologic or urologic surgery
	Positive pressure ventilation (PPV)	General anesthesia
	Vasopressor use	General anesthesia
Preload Reduction	Vasodilatory effects of anesthesia	General or neuraxial anesthesia
	SIRS	Emergency Surgery
	Hemorrhage	High risk operations
Venous Emboli	Air emboli	Vascular surgery
	Amniotic fluid emboli	Caesarean section
	Carbon dioxide emboli	Laparo- or thoracoscopic surgery
	Cement emboli	Orthopedic surgery
	Fat emboli	Orthopedic surgery
Reduction in lung volume	Single lung ventilation	Thoracic surgery, lung lavage
	Lung resection	Thoracic surgery
High risk surgery	Hemorrhage, vasopressor use, PPV, insufflation	Major abdominal, thoracic, vascular or neurosurgeries
Emergency surgery	Hemorrhage, SIRS, PPV	
Prolonged surgical time	Surgery time > 3 hours	

MAC, monitored anesthesia care; SIRS, systemic inflammatory response syndrome.

inotropic support.[5] Operative factors associated with morbidity in patients with PH are listed in Table 18-3, most of which are nonmodifiable. Maintenance of euvolemia and avoidance of hypercapnia and hypoxia are modifiable factors that anesthesiologists are adept at managing. Recent data show decreases in PH-associated perioperative complications, but morbidity and mortality estimates remain high in noncardiac surgery: 6–42% and 4–26%, respectively.[6]

PREOPERATIVE EVALUATION (SEE ALGORITHM IN FIGURE 18-1)

Formally Diagnosed PH

Preoperative evaluation of patients with previously diagnosed PH should begin with a thorough history of the patient's symptoms, such as dyspnea, cough, peripheral edema, chest pain, syncope, and

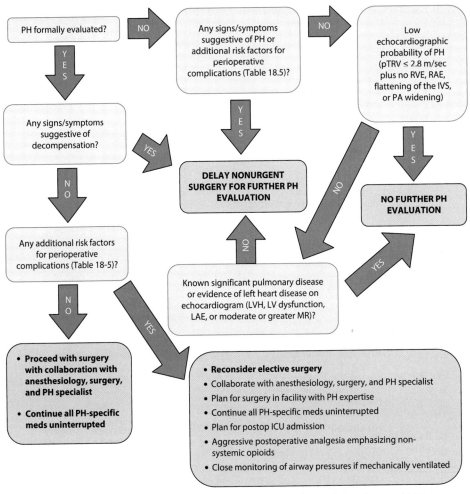

PH, pulmonary hypertension; pTRV, peak tricuspid regurgitant velocity; RVE, right ventricular enlargement; RAE, right atrial enlargement; IVS, interventricular septum; PA, pulmonary artery; LV, left ventricle; LVH, left ventricular hypertrophy; LAE, left atrial enlargement; MR, mitral regurgitation.

FIGURE 18-1. Algorithm for perioperative evaluation and management of pulmonary hypertension.

lightheadedness. Elucidating a patient's functional capacity is especially important in these patients for accurate risk assessment and placement in the correct class (I–IV) of the World Health Organization Functional Classification (WHO-FC)[1] (Table 18-4). Additionally, clinicians should examine the patient closely for signs of decompensation, including hypotension, hypoxia, elevated jugular venous pressure, third heart sound, and peripheral edema. Nonurgent surgery for patients with new or worsened signs or symptoms related to PH should be delayed for further evaluation by a PH specialist.

All previous diagnostic testing related to PH, including cardiac imaging, right heart catheterization, pulmonary function testing, sleep study reports, and chest radiography reports, should be obtained and documented for the perioperative care team. All other patients with known PH should have regular assessment of pulmonary artery systolic pressure (PASP) and RV function. The American College of Cardiology/American Heart Association perioperative guidelines also recommend preoperative evaluation by a PH specialist if possible, within the necessary surgical timeline.[7]

TABLE 18-4. World Health Organization Functional Classification System for Patients with Pulmonary Hypertension[1]

WORLD HEALTH ORGANIZATION FUNCTIONAL CLASSIFICATION SYSTEM

	CLASS I	CLASS II	CLASS III	CLASS IV
Symptoms with activity	None	Ordinary physical activity causes dyspnea, fatigue, chest pain, or near syncope	Less than ordinary physical activity causes dyspnea, fatigue, chest pain, or near syncope	Dyspnea or fatigue at rest or signs of right heart failure
Functional limitations	None	Slight	Marked limitations	Severe
Comfort level at rest	Comfortable at rest	Comfortable at rest	Comfortable at rest	Symptomatic at rest

TABLE 18-5. Risk Factors for Perioperative Complications in Patients with Pulmonary Hypertension[6]

Pulmonary arterial hypertension (Group 1 PH)

WHO functional class ≥ 2

6-minute walk distance < 300 meters

ASA class ≥ 3

RVSP > 70 mmHg on echocardiogram

mPAP > 50 mmHg

RV dilation and/or dysfunction

Sleep apnea

Left ventricular dysfunction

History of pulmonary embolism

Chronic kidney disease

Coronary artery disease

PH, pulmonary hypertension; WHO, World Health Organization; ASA, American Society of Anesthesiologists; RVSP, right ventricular systolic pressure; mPAP, mean pulmonary artery pressure; RV, right ventricle.

Shared decision-making discussions with the patient should fully disclose the potential risks related to PH in the setting of the proposed surgery. Several factors indicate particularly high perioperative risk for patients with PH (Table 18-5). Preoperative decision making for patients with PH should include discussion of potential nonsurgical or lower-risk invasive treatments or a modified surgical technique. Close collaboration with anesthesiology and PH specialists is essential to assure appropriate perioperative management. For patients with PH and other risk factors for complications, surgery should be performed in a facility with medical and anesthetic expertise in managing PH.[7]

PH Without Formal Diagnostic Evaluation

Incidental notation of PH on echocardiograms obtained for other purposes is common. Frequently, this finding does not result in a specific evaluation of PH. Preoperative evaluation can be challenging for patients presenting for surgery with such findings. Many authors recommend delay of nonurgent surgery for complete assessment of the current status and underlying causes of PH, but there are no published recommendations for what severity or likely type of PH should prompt surgical delay. Certainly, patients with symptoms potentially related to PH or additional risk factors noted in Table 18-5 should not undergo nonurgent surgery without further evaluation. Guidelines for the evaluation of PH in the general setting also provide some guidance on patients who may not warrant further investigation.[1] Patients with low echocardiographic probability of PH (peak tricuspid regurgitant velocity ≤ 2.8 m/s and no right ventricular enlargement, right atrial dilatation, flattening of the interventricular septum, or pulmonary artery widening) likely need no further evaluation. Also, if the patient has known significant pulmonary disease or evidence of left heart disease on echocardiogram (left ventricular hypertrophy, left ventricular dysfunction, left atrial enlargement, or moderate or greater mitral regurgitation) and does not have evidence of RV dysfunction or estimated PASP > 70 mmHg, further evaluation is not required.[8] If the surgical timeline allows, all other patients should be further evaluated using established guidelines.

PERIOPERATIVE MANAGEMENT

Preoperative

PH should be medically optimized as much as possible before surgery in consultation with PH specialists and/or cardiologists. This includes achieving a stable euvolemic state and full treatment of underlying medical diseases. All PH-specific medications should be continued uninterrupted through noncardiac surgery unless there are specific contraindications, which would be determined in consultation with the surgeon and anesthesiologist.

Perioperative cardiac risk assessment tools, such as the Revised Cardiac Risk Index, may underestimate perioperative risk in patients with PH without a diagnosis of heart failure or ischemic heart disease. However, there are validated risk assessment tools for patients with PAH (Group 1 PH), which can help surgeons, anesthesiologists, and patients better understand individual mortality risk. The Compera 2.0 tool incorporates only three variables: a patient's WHO-FC, their distance during a 6-minute walk test, and a recent BNP or NT-proBNP value in order to stratify patients into four categories: low risk, intermediate-low risk, intermediate-high risk, and high risk.[1,9] These four categories correspond to a 1-year overall mortality risk of 0–3%, 2–7%, 9–19%, and >20%, respectively. Risk stratification tools can help give pause when deciding whether to proceed with surgery in a higher risk patient, but they have not yet been validated for use in the perioperative setting.

Intraoperative

Evidence-based literature is lacking for the intraoperative management of patients with PH, and discussion of specific anesthesia, hemodynamic, and fluid management is beyond the scope of this book. Suffice to say, the preoperative clinician must involve anesthesiology in perioperative care planning as far in advance as possible. The anesthesia team can then provide recommendations for additional preoperative testing and plan for appropriate resources and personnel for the day of surgery.

Postoperative

Patients with PH plus additional perioperative risk factors (Table 18-5) should initially be monitored in the intensive care unit after surgery due to the increased risk for sudden clinical deterioration.[6] Aggressive pain control balanced with maximization of regional analgesia (e.g., nerve blocks) and non-opioid therapies is crucial because inadequate analgesia worsens pulmonary vasoconstriction, whereas the effects of opioids on respiratory depression can increase pulmonary vascular resistance (PVR) through hypercapnia and hypoxia. Intravascular volume status requires close monitoring (though not necessarily through invasive means) to prevent both hypo- and hypervolemia. If providing mechanical ventilation, airway pressures should be monitored to prevent PH exacerbation due to barotrauma. Hypoxia and acidosis should also be identified and treated rapidly to prevent decompensation. All PH-targeted medications should be continued without interruption, and the postoperative care team should continue to work in close collaboration with PH specialists to assure best management.

Clinical pearls

- PH is associated with significant perioperative morbidity and mortality.

- Elective surgery should be reconsidered in patients with group 1 PH, severe PH (echocardiographically estimated right ventricular systolic pressure [RVSP] > 70 mmHg), mPAP > 50 mmHg, right ventricular dysfunction, or substantial physical limitations due to PH (e.g., 6-minute walk distance < 300 m, WHO-FC class ≥ 2).

- When surgery is pursued in patients with high-risk PH, it should be performed in a facility with PH expertise with plans for postoperative ICU admission.

■ Collaboration between perioperative care providers (including anesthesiologists, preoperative evaluation clinicians, and postoperative care providers) and PH specialists is essential.

REFERENCES

1. Hubert M, Kovacs G, Hoeper MM, et al. 2022 ESC/ERS guidelines for the diagnosis and treatment of pulmonary hypertension. *Eur Respir J.* 2023;61(1):2200879. PMID: 36028254

2. Hoeper MM, Humbert M, Souza R, et al. A global view of pulmonary hypertension. *Lancet Respir Med.* 2016;4(4):306-322. PMID: 26975810

3. Hassoun PM. Pulmonary arterial hypertension. *N Engl J Med.* 2021;385(25):2361-2376. PMID: 34910865

4. Rajagopal S, Ruetzler K, Ghadimi K, et al. Evaluation and management of pulmonary hypertension in noncardiac surgery: a scientific statement from the American Heart Association. *Circulation.* 2023;147(17):1317-1343. PMID: 36924225

5. Jha AK, Jha N, Malik V. Perioperative decision-making in pulmonary hypertension. *Heart Lung Circ.* 2023;32(4):454-466. PMID: 36841637

6. Pilkington SA, Taboada D, Martinez G. Pulmonary hypertension and its management in patients undergoing noncardiac surgery. *Anaesthesia.* 2015;70(1):56-70. PMID: 25267493

7. Fleisher LA, Fleischmann KE, Auerbach AD, et al. 2014 ACC/AHA guideline on perioperative cardiovascular evaluation and management of patients undergoing noncardiac surgery: executive summary. *Circulation.* 2014;130(24):2215-2245. PMID: 25085962

8. Minai OA, Yared JP, Kaw R, Subramaniam K, Hill NS. Perioperative risk and management in patients with pulmonary hypertension. *Chest.* 2013;144(1):329-340. PMID: 23880683

9. Hoeper MM, Pausch C, Olsson KM, et al. COMPERA 2.0: a refined four-stratum risk assessment model for pulmonary arterial hypertension. *Eur Respir J.* 2022;60(1):2102311. PMID: 34737226

Diabetes Mellitus

Leonard S. Feldman, MD, FACP, FAAP, MHM and Guillermo E. Umpierrez, MD, CDCES, FACE, MACP

COMMON CLINICAL QUESTIONS

1. What should I do with the patient's home medications before surgery?
2. How do I manage insulin in the hospital?
3. Is there a preoperative HbA1c or plasma glucose result that should lead me to cancel surgery?
4. What are the perioperative concerns regarding GLP-1 agonists and SGLT2 inhibitors?

INTRODUCTION

According to the 2023 National Diabetes Statistics Report, 38.4 million Americans, 11.6% of the adult population, have diabetes mellitus (DM). Adults 65 years old and older make up as much as 43% of the DM cases, and adults 46–64 years old constitute 41%, depending on the definition. Moreover, we estimate that another 97.6 million Americans age 18 years or older have prediabetes (38% of the adult population). Perioperative hyperglycemia, defined as a blood glucose (BG) > 140 mg/dL, is common and reported in 20–40% of persons undergoing general surgery and 80% of individuals after cardiac surgery.[1] Up to 30% of patients with postoperative hyperglycemia have no prior history of DM. Their hyperglycemia is due to undiagnosed DM or the effects of the counter regulatory stress hormones (glucagon, catecholamines, cortisol, and growth hormone). In addition, the stress of surgery results in the release of inflammatory cytokines and a cascade of effects that result in a state of insulin resistance. This chapter will review preoperative evaluation and perioperative management of the patients with DM undergoing noncardiac surgery.

HOW TO DIAGNOSE DIABETES

Diabetes is diagnosed using glycosylated hemoglobin (HbA1c), fasting plasma glucose (FPG), oral glucose tolerance test, or classic hyperglycemic symptoms with the values listed in Table 19-1.[2] HbA1c reflects the average BG over the last 3 months but cannot differentiate whether the glucose control has improved, worsened, fluctuated, or stayed the same immediately before or during the perioperative period. The HbA1c can result in false negatives in persons with increased red blood cell turnover, such as in patients with hemoglobinopathies like sickle cell disease, G6PD deficiency, end-stage kidney disease, or chronic blood loss. HIV patients, end-stage kidney disease and hemodialysis patients, or patients who receive erythropoietin therapy can also have misleading results. In these populations, FPG or the 2-hour value during a 75-gram oral glucose tolerance test may confirm the diagnosis of DM.

PREOPERATIVE EVALUATION HISTORY

Caring for patients with diabetes requires performing an appropriate history and physical examination (Table 19-2). The history should focus

TABLE 19-1. DM Diagnosis

HbA1c	Normal: <5.7%
	Prediabetes: 5.7–6.4%
	DM: ≥6.5%
Fasting blood glucose (no caloric intake for >8 hours)	Normal: <100 mg/dL
	Prediabetes: 100–125 mg/dL
	DM: ≥126 mg/dL
Classic DM symptom	Polyuria and polydipsia with BG ≥ 200 mg/dL

TABLE 19-2. Preoperative DM-Focused History

DISEASE AND SURGERY-SPECIFIC HISTORY	EXPLANATION
Provider who manages the DM	PCP, endocrinologist, or another provider
Type of DM	Type 1 or type 2, including history of diabetic ketoacidosis
Last HbA1c	When it was last tested and the result
Medication	Dose, frequency, and route of noninsulin medications and insulin; length of time on insulin; non-DM medications that may impact care of DM
Medication adverse effects	Frequency and severity of hypoglycemia
Macrovascular target organ damage	Stroke, TIA, myocardial infarction, angina, heart failure, peripheral vascular disease
Microvascular target organ damage (including lab data)	Nephropathy, retinopathy, hepatic dysfunction, gastroparesis, peripheral neuropathy, orthostatic symptoms
Type of surgery	Including length of surgery
Presurgical NPO status	Influences management of DM before surgery
Type of anesthesia	

on disease-specific information, including the duration of DM, medical treatment (insulin or noninsulin agents), adverse consequences of the medications, including hypoglycemia, and long-term complications of DM. The history should also include surgery-specific details that might affect DM management.

PREOPERATIVE EVALUATION AND HbA1c

The ADA recommends measuring HbA1c on admission in people with a known history of DM or hyperglycemia (glucose > 140 mg/dL) if not performed within the 3 months before admission. Hyperglycemia on admission and elevated HbA1c values are associated with longer length of stay, increased risk of perioperative complications, and mortality.[3] Screening patients for DM identifies people at risk of perioperative complications. Clinical guidelines encourage DM screening in overweight and obese patients over the age of 35. Most importantly, the level of HbA1c on admission can influence inpatient and discharge management plans.[1]

HbA1c Threshold for Surgery

Regardless of whether the patient's upcoming surgery is emergent, time-sensitive, urgent, or elective, no definitive data guide what HbA1c threshold should lead to the cancellation of surgery. The recent Endocrine Society guidelines for managing inpatient hyperglycemia and diabetes recommend targeting an HbA1c level < 8% for persons undergoing elective surgery.[4] However, many surgeons choose arbitrary lower cut-offs like 7%. Studies have not found that preoperative glucose control independently affects intraoperative or postoperative noncardiac surgery outcomes. If anything, preoperative glucose control predicts postoperative glucose control, especially for ambulatory surgery and the convalescent period after discharge. One study reported that improvement of glucose control and reduced HbA1c prior to orthopedic surgery results in good postoperative glycemic control.[5] Some surgeons and preoperative clinic providers have turned away from HbA1c testing to fructosamine testing. Unlike HbA1c that reflects the average BG control over the last 3 months, fructosamine reflects BG control over the last 2–3 weeks. One study reported that fructosamine better predicted adverse outcomes after total knee arthroplasty than HbA1c.[6] Since fructosamine reflects BG from the last 3 weeks, patients may be able to show they have gained control of their DM in a shorter period than if they had to wait 3 months for follow-up HbA1c testing. However, fructosamine levels can be falsely low or high in the presence of altered protein and albumin metabolism in patients with low albumin state or increased protein turnover due to chronic inflammation or chronic kidney disease.[7,8]

PERIOPERATIVE CARE

Preoperative Glucose Control

Preoperative glucose control has multiple determinants: admission and preoperative glucose concentration, preoperative medication plan, and acute medical/surgical issues. How to manage preoperative hyperglycemia depends on the cause and severity. First, cancel elective surgery if the patient has symptoms of severe hyperglycemia or diabetic ketoacidosis, elevated ketone value > 3 mmol/L, or significant dehydration. Second, cancel elective surgery for an obvious source of sepsis or severe infection, a previously unknown pregnancy, or an acute malady like acute myocardial ischemia. In the absence of high HbA1c on admission in a person with a markedly elevated glucose on admission, assess conditions that may artificially decrease HbA1c. There is no specific BG or HbA1c mandating cancellation of surgery. For a BG less than 400 mg/dL, treat with subcutaneous rapid-acting insulin. A subcutaneous dose of rapid-acting insulin analogs (lispro, aspart, glulisine) is preferred over the IV route. The administration of 0.1 U/kg of a rapid-acting insulin analog usually reduces plasma glucose between 75 and 125 mg/dL in 1–2 hours. A BG greater than 400 mg/dL may necessitate delaying or canceling the surgical procedure until metabolic control is achieved. Surgeons should be more conservative with surgeries associated with high risk of complications like major adverse cardiac events, postoperative pulmonary complications, and surgical site infections. Low-risk surgeries like cataract surgery will have different preoperative glucose cut offs than high-risk neurosurgery procedures.

Postoperative Glucose Control

Numerous publications in the literature demonstrate a correlation between hyperglycemia and adverse outcomes in noncardiac, cardiac, and intensive care unit (ICU) patients, such as prolonged length of hospital stay, surgical site infection, and mortality.[3] The severity of hyperglycemia on admission and during the hospital stay correlates with increased rates of infection and mortality rate.

Van den Berghe et al. published a major trial on intensive insulin treatment (IIT) in a surgical ICU setting in 2001.[9] The researchers randomized 1,548 mostly postoperative CABG patients to IIT with a BG goal of 80–110 mg/dL versus a conventional treatment arm with a BG target of 180–200 mg/dL. The trial found a statistically significant difference of 3.4% inhospital survival that favored the IIT arm. They also found that the IIT arm patients experienced more severe hypoglycemia (BG < 40 mg/dL) than did the conventional arm, although that did not affect the mortality rate. Numerous publications followed that did not always duplicate the positive results of IIT found in the van den Berghe trial. In 2009, the Nice-Sugar Study Investigators published a 6,104-person randomized controlled trial of mixed surgical and medical ICU patients (63% postoperative).[10] The IIT arm targeted a BG of 81–108 mg/dL, while the conventional arm aimed for a BG of 144–180 mg/dL. The primary endpoint, "death from any cause within 90 days after randomization," occurred more often in the intensive treatment arm (27.5%) than in the conventional arm (24.9%), with an odds ratio of 1.14; $p = 0.02$. A Cochrane systematic review and meta-analysis in 2023 found that IIT did not improve outcomes for perioperative patients. Moreover, IIT caused more hypoglycemia. More recently, a large randomized clinical trial of more than 9,000 medicine and surgery patients in the ICU confirmed that intensive glucose control (80–110 mg/dL) or relaxed (180–215 mg/dL) glucose control did not improve length of stay, infections, or mortality.[11]

During the perioperative period, correcting severe hyperglycemia and preventing hypoglycemia are crucial for reducing perioperative complications. Several organizations have released guidelines for BG targets in hospitalized patients.

Operationalizing Conventional BG Control (Table 19-3)

Consult a specialized diabetes management team when available. Treating DM and hyperglycemia in the perioperative setting usually involves the administration of insulin. Most guidelines recommend stopping noninsulin medications on admission; however, noninsulin medications such as DPP-4 inhibitors are safe and effective in improving glycemic control in persons with mild hyperglycemia (glucose < 180–200 mg/dL).[3]

Ideally, insulin should be administered in a physiological regimen, including a combination of long-acting "basal" insulin given once or twice a day plus short-acting insulin analogs given before meals. The details of perioperative DM management depend on the setting of the surgery: ambulatory, ward, or critical care.

Ambulatory Surgery. Most patients should be instructed to hold noninsulin DM medications on the day of surgery, particularly medications that can result in hypoglycemia, like sulfonylureas (see Chapter 4). In ambulatory surgery, the oral medications can be restarted after surgery. The widening use of glucagon-like peptide 1 (GLP-1) agonists has brought to light concerns over delayed gastric emptying in patients receiving a GLP-1. Delayed gastric emptying can result in aspiration. A multi-society clinical practice guidance document for the safe use of GLP-1 agonists in the perioperative period recommends holding the GLP-1 dose on the day of surgery for those taking a daily GLP-1 and holding the dose a week prior for those taking a weekly GLP-1.[12] It is unknown whether holding doses a day or a week before is enough time to prevent aspiration. It is unknown whether holding them longer would improve outcomes or may worsen glycemic control, increasing the rate of hyperglycemia-associated complications. The American Gastroenterological Association (AGA) recommends considering transabdominal ultrasonography to evaluate for retained stomach substances.[13]

TABLE 19-3. Perioperative Blood Glucose Control

American Association of Endocrinologists/American Diabetes Association (AACE/ADA)	
Critically ill	100–180 mg/dL. Start IV insulin infusion therapy for persistent BG ≥ 180 mg/dL
Noncritically ill	100–180 mg/dL
American College of Physicians (ACP)	
Critically ill	140–200 mg/dL
Noncritically ill	No intensive insulin therapy No target range defined
Society of Thoracic Surgeons (STS)	
Adults undergoing cardiac surgery	<180 mg/dL during surgery Continuous infusion preferred over intermittent or subcutaneous
Society for Ambulatory Anesthesia (SAMBA)	
Intraoperative blood glucose levels	<180 mg/dL using subcutaneous rapid-acting insulin (for ambulatory surgery)

Sodium-glucose transport protein 2 (SGLT2) inhibitors may be associated with an increased risk of diabetic ketoacidosis (often euglycemic) in persons with poor oral intake for several days. The FDA recommends stopping an SGLT2 inhibitor 3 days before scheduled surgery (4 days for ertugliflozin).[14]

Patients on long-acting basal insulin glargine and degludec are generally advised to reduce their daily dose before surgery by 20–25%,[15] but that reduction may result in a predictable trade-off. Patients who take their total dose of long-acting insulin while fasting for surgery experience hypoglycemia more often than their counterparts who take a reduced dose. Patients who reduce daily doses of long-acting insulin by 50% or more often experience hyperglycemia during the perioperative period.[15] After arriving at the ambulatory surgery center, the team will test the patient's BG and will generally use short-acting insulin analogs to achieve a BG of <180 mg/dL.[1] Patients can restart full-dose long-acting, short-acting, and noninsulin medications once they start eating again. To reduce the risk of hypoglycemia, the dose of rapid-acting insulin should be held during fasting, except for correcting hyperglycemia. In the short term, hypoglycemia can have deadlier results than hyperglycemia, so we usually recommend daily adjustment of insulin doses.

Hospitalized (Figure 19-1). Insulin is the preferred agent to control hyperglycemia and diabetes during the perioperative period. The total daily dose (TDD) of insulin is determined in two ways:

1. Calculate the TDD for patients on insulin therapy before admission, adding both long-acting and short-acting insulin doses. Do not include noninsulin medications in this calculation.
2. Calculation can also be weight based. For patients without a known DM history who present with postoperative hyperglycemia or those with poorly controlled DM, calculate the TDD using the patient's weight in kilograms (kg). Multiply the weight in kg times an insulin sensitivity factor ranging from 0.3 to 0.5 to determine the TDD. For patients with more sensitivity to insulin (newly diagnosed DM, age > 70, BMI < 25 GFR < 45), use the lower range (0.3), and for those more resistant to insulin (outpatient insulin requirement > 80 U/day, BMI > 35, or steroid use > 20 mg prednisone/day), use the higher factor (0.5).

Once the TDD of insulin is determined, divide the dose in half between long-acting (basal) and short-acting (nutritional or bolus) insulin. Then, divide the short-acting nutritional bolus insulin equally between the three meals. Do not start short-acting insulin if the patient cannot or will not eat. For those on tube feeds, divide the TDD as 20% basal and 80% nutritional with the nutritional, then divide into six equal amounts of short-acting insulin.

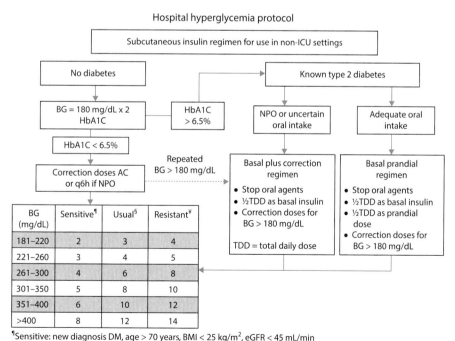

FIGURE 19-1. Inhospital management of DM and hyperglycemia.
Reproduced with permission from Duggan EW, Klopman MA, Berry AJ, Umpierrez G. The Emory university perioperative algorithm for the management of hyperglycemia and diabetes in non-cardiac surgery patients. *Curr Diab Rep.* 2016;16(3):34.

Studies have evaluated insulin therapy for hyperglycemia in surgical patients in general wards.[16] Using basal, bolus nutritional, plus correctional, or basal plus correctional regimens generally produces good results. Basal plus correctional regimens may result in slightly less tight control but reduce the likelihood of hypoglycemia. Most guidelines recommend against using sliding scale insulin regimens as the sole treatment of DM patients. Data do not show that sliding scales improve care. Patients receiving minimal non-insulin home medications may do well in the hospital just on correctional insulin.

The calculated TDD of insulin represents a starting point, and daily adjustments may be needed based on the BG results from point-of-care (POC) testing. Finally, if patients and their BG show stability and no hypoglycemia, consider limiting the number of POC glucose tests. Duggan et al. provide an excellent resource on this topic.[1]

Critical Care. Critically ill persons in the ICU are generally treated with IV insulin infusion to control hyperglycemia.[17] Computer-directed algorithms often provide a safer way to administer IV infusion. Experts have encouraged providers to avoid hyperglycemia and hypoglycemia and minimize glucose fluctuations. Continuous glucose monitoring (CGM) with validated computer algorithms may help to achieve glycemic goals.

Insulin Pump. Patients on an insulin pump generally have type 1 DM, but endocrinologists have started a growing number of type 2 DM on insulin pumps. Insulin pump provides continuous insulin administration; thus, do not stop the pump without replacing the basal insulin. Consider consulting an endocrinologist or inpatient specialized diabetes team for patients on an insulin pump. Often, the insulin pump's basal rate can run continuously throughout surgery if the surgical field does not include the pump and the anesthesia team feels comfortable operating the pump. The BG is monitored hourly until the patient can reliably manage the pump again. As described previously, provide correction doses of rapid-acting insulin if the patient's BG surpasses 180–200 mg/dL and stop the infusion if the BG falls below 100 mg/dL. Follow the BG closely to determine when to turn the pump back on. If the anesthesia team decides not to use the pump, they should replace it with an insulin drip or a basal-bolus regimen (pump holiday) and restart the pump after surgery. For patients admitted after surgery, consult the inpatient diabetes team unless the patient is awake, alert, and able to manage the pump. All institutions should have a policy regarding the use of insulin pumps.

Noninsulin Medications in Hospitalized Patients. The medications that may prove safe for hospitalized patients include metformin, the GLP-1 agonists, and possibly the DPP-4 inhibitors (DPP4I).[1] These medications often allow for a reduction in insulin dosage without increasing the risk of low BG. The ADA acknowledges that multiple trials have shown the safety of using GLP-1 agonists and DPP4I.[14] Be aware of the potential for gastrointestinal symptoms and delayed gastric emptying with GLP-1 agonists, which may decrease oral intake and increase the risk of hypoglycemia if the patient receives bolus nutritional insulin. SGLT2 inhibitors have not received as much scrutiny and should not be prescribed perioperatively in patients who will remain NPO or will have poor oral intake for more than 24–48 hours. For patients with type 2 DM hospitalized with heart failure, the American Diabetes Association recommends "SGLT2 inhibitors be initiated or continued during hospitalization and upon discharge if there are no contraindications and after recovery from the acute illness."[14] Urinary tract infections and euglycemic diabetic ketoacidosis may occur with SGLT2I treatment. Do not use sulfonylureas in the hospital (see Table 19-4).

Safely Discharging Patients with DM or Postoperative Hyperglycemia. All patients with known DM or with "new onset" hyperglycemia should have an HbA1c measured if not done during the previous 3 months. The target HbA1c after discharge depends on the individual patient. Patients with fewer comorbidities should have a lower HbA1c target. The ACP recommends an HbA1c of 7–8% for most patients,[18] while the ADA advocates for a target of <7% for most non-pregnant adults.[19] Knowing the patient's HbA1c and the target can allow us to create a discharge plan for our perioperative patients.[20] For patients with an HbA1c of <7%, do not change their home regimen. For patients with an HbA1c of 7–8%, consider discussing the patient's regimen with the primary care physician or DM consult team, especially in the postoperative

TABLE 19-4.   Preoperative Management of Diabetic Medications

MEDICATION USE ON THE *DAY PRIOR* TO SURGERY

ORAL AGENTS*		GLARGINE OR DETEMIR		NPH OR 70/30 INSULIN		LISPRO, ASPART, GLULISINE, REGULAR		NONINSULIN INJECTABLES[†]	
AM dose	PM dose	AM dose	PM dose	AM dose	PM dose	AM dose	PM dose	AM dose	PM dose
Usual dose	Usual dose	Usual dose	80% of usual dose	Usual dose	80% of usual dose	Usual dose	Usual dose	Usual dose	Usual dose

MEDICATION USE ON THE *DAY OF* SURGERY

ORAL AGENTS	GLARGINE OR DETEMIR	NPH INSULIN	LISPRO, ASPART, GLULISINE, REGULAR	NONINSULIN INJECTABLES[†]
Hold	80% of usual dose	50% of usual dose if BG > 120 mg/dL	Hold if NPO	Hold

*Stop SGLT2 inhibitors 3 days before scheduled surgeries and 4 days in the case of ertugliflozin.

[†]Stop daily dosing GLP-1 agonists on the day of the procedure/surgery and weekly dosing a week prior to the procedure/surgery.
Source: Reproduced with permission from Duggan EW, Klopman MA, Berry AJ, Umpierrez G. The Emory university perioperative algorithm for the management of hyperglycemia and diabetes in non-cardiac surgery patients. *Curr Diab Rep*. 2016;16(3):34.

period. Finally, an HbA1c of >8% means that most patients' home regimens need adjustment. Discuss changes with the patient's primary care physician or diabetes management team.

Glucose Monitoring. It's important to monitor BG levels accurately, regardless of whether patients are being cared for in the ambulatory setting, in the hospital wards, or in the ICU. POC capillary glucose testing using glucometers can produce inaccurate results of more than 20%, especially for patients with lower glucose values. This means that a POC BG of 60 mg/dL could range from as low as 48 mg/dL to as high as 72 mg/dL. POC testing problems usually arise with significant tissue edema, hypoperfusion, and severe anemia. Plasma glucose readings lose accuracy when contaminated with IV solutions. In the ICU, blood gas analyzers can accurately and quickly provide BG results. CGM has spread rapidly throughout the United States. The American Diabetes Association recommends using CGM if it is clinically appropriate for patients who already use CGM at home. Furthermore, providers should confirm CGM results with POC glucose testing for results that will change management, including hypoglycemia assessment.[14]

SUMMARY

Build protocols to ensure preoperative diagnosis of type 2 DM and assessment of admission BG control in the past 3 months with HbA1c. A combination of long-acting basal, short-acting bolus nutritional, and correctional insulin is the preferred regimen for managing hyperglycemia in people with diabetes. Calculate the TDD of insulin using the weight-based method unless a patient on home insulin has good BG control. Hold most noninsulin medications, although metformin, GLP1RA, and DPP4I medications are likely safe. Use IV insulin infusions for ICU patients. Target a BG level of 100–200 mg/dL for all inpatients with type 2 DM or stress hyperglycemia.[14] Make decisions on patients' discharge medications based on their BG control as summarized by the HbA1c. Consult the diabetes management team, general medicine consultants, or endocrinologists for help.

Clinical pearls

- Be cautious of patients on large amounts of home insulin (>0.5 × weight in kg), especially if their HbA1c is >8%. The question is whether they need that much insulin or are just not taking it at home. Consider using the weight-based method to determine their TDD and start with lower dosing, then adjust as needed.

- Patients taking NPH should reduce their dose by 50% when fasting. Patients taking a premixed insulin formulation should reduce the TDD to prevent hypoglycemia. Reduce the dose of the long-acting basal insulin by 20–25% on the day of surgery.

- Use the lower insulin sensitivity factors (0.3) for calculating insulin TDD in elderly patients and patients with reduced GFRs.

- If a patient with known type 2 DM has an HbA1c of <6%, discuss the patient's regimen with the primary care physician and/or the endocrine consult service and consider down-titrating the regimen, especially if the patient has developed episodes of hypoglycemia in the recent past.

- Patients on insulin treatment prior to admission usually require insulin administration during the perioperative period.

REFERENCES

1. Duggan EW, Carlson K, Umpierrez GE. Perioperative hyperglycemia management: an update. *Anesthesiology.* 2017;126:547-560. PMID: 28121636

2. American Diabetes Association Professional Practice C. 2. Diagnosis and classification of diabetes: standards of care in diabetes—2024. *Diabetes Care.* 2024;47:S20-S42. PMID: 38078589

3. Pasquel FJ, Lansang MC, Dhatariya K, Umpierrez GE. Management of diabetes and hyperglycaemia in the hospital. *Lancet Diabetes Endocrinol.* 2021;9:174-188. PMID: 33515493

4. Korytkowski MT, Muniyappa R, Antinori-Lent K, et al. Management of hyperglycemia in hospitalized adult patients in non-critical care settings: an Endocrine Society Clinical Practice Guideline. *J Clin Endocrinol Metab.* 2022;107:2101-2128. PMID: 35690958

5. Giori NJ, Ellerbe LS, Bowe T, Gupta S, Harris AH. Many diabetic total joint arthroplasty candidates are unable to achieve a preoperative hemoglobin A1c goal of 7% or less. *J Bone Joint Surg Am.* 2014;96:500-504. PMID: 24647507

6. Shohat N, Tarabichi M, Tan TL, et al. 2019 John Insall Award: fructosamine is a better glycaemic marker compared with glycated haemoglobin (HbA1C) in predicting adverse outcomes following total knee arthroplasty: a prospective multicentre study. *Bone Joint J.* 2019; 101-B:3-9. PMID: 31256656

7. Ling J, Ng JKC, Chan JCN, Chow E. Use of continuous glucose monitoring in the assessment and management of patients with diabetes and chronic kidney disease. *Front Endocrinol (Lausanne).* 2022;13:869899. PMID: 35528010

8. Kaminski CY, Galindo RJ, Navarrete JE, et al. Assessment of glycemic control by continuous glucose monitoring, hemoglobin A1c, fructosamine, and glycated albumin in patients with end-stage kidney disease and burnt-out diabetes. *Diabetes Care.* 2024;47:267-271. PMID: 38085705

9. van den Berghe G, Wouters P, Weekers F, et al. Intensive insulin therapy in critically ill patients. *N Engl J Med.* 2001;345:1359-1367. PMID: 11794168

10. Investigators N-SS, Finfer S, Chittock DR, et al. Intensive versus conventional glucose control in critically ill patients. *N Engl J Med.* 2009;360:1283-1297. PMID: 19318384

11. Gunst J, Debaveye Y, Guiza F, et al. Tight blood-glucose control without early parenteral nutrition in the ICU. *N Engl J Med.* 2023;389:1180-1190. PMID: 37754283

12. Kindel TL, Wang AY, Wadhwa A, et al. epresenting the American Gastroenterological Association, American Society for Metabolic and Bariatric Surgery, American Society of Anesthesiologists, International Society of Perioperative Care of Patients with Obesity, and the Society of American Gastrointestinal and Endoscopic Surgeons. Multi-society clinical practice guidance for the safe use of glucagon-like peptide-1 receptor agonists in the perioperative period. *Surg Endosc.* 2025;39(1):180-183. PMID: 39370500.

13. Hashash JG, Thompson CC, Wang AY. AGA rapid clinical practice update on the management of patients taking GLP-1 receptor agonists prior to endoscopy: communication. *Clin Gastroenterol Hepatol.* 2024;22:705-707. PMID: 37944573

14. American Diabetes Association Professional Practice C. 16. Diabetes care in the hospital: standards of care in diabetes—2024. *Diabetes Care.* 2024;47:S295-S306. PMID: 38078585

15. Demma LJ, Carlson KT, Duggan EW, Morrow JG 3rd, Umpierrez G. Effect of basal insulin dosage on blood glucose concentration in ambulatory surgery patients with type 2 diabetes. *J Clin Anesth*. 2017;36:184-188. PMID. 28183363

16. Umpierrez GE, Smiley D, Hermayer K, et al. Randomized study comparing a basal-bolus with a basal plus correction insulin regimen for the hospital management of medical and surgical patients with type 2 diabetes: basal plus trial. *Diabetes Care*. 2013;36: 2169-2174. PMID: 23435159

17. Gunst J, De Bruyn A, Van den Berghe G. Glucose control in the ICU. *Curr Opin Anaesthesiol*. 2019;32: 156-162. PMID: 30817388

18. Qaseem A, Wilt TJ, Kansagara D, et al. Hemoglobin A1c targets for glycemic control with pharmacologic therapy for nonpregnant adults with type 2 diabetes mellitus: a guidance statement update from the American College of Physicians. *Ann Intern Med*. 2018;168:569-576. PMID: 29507945

19. American Diabetes Association Professional Practice C. 6. Glycemic goals and hypoglycemia: standards of care in diabetes—2024. *Diabetes Care*. 2024;47:S111-S125. PMID: 38078586

20. Umpierrez GE, Reyes D, Smiley D, et al. Hospital discharge algorithm based on admission HbA1c for the management of patients with type 2 diabetes. *Diabetes Care*. 2014;37:2934-2939. PMID: 25168125

## 20

Thyroid Disease

Christopher M. Whinney, MD, FACP, SFHM

COMMON CLINICAL QUESTIONS

1. Does mild to moderate hypothyroidism increase the risk of postoperative complications?
2. Is there a TSH level above which surgery should be postponed?
3. How do you manage a patient with hyperthyroidism preoperatively?

INTRODUCTION

Thyroid dysfunction is ubiquitous in the general population, with approximately 4–21% of females and 3–16% of males having abnormal thyrotropin (thyroid-stimulating hormone or TSH) values.[1] Thyroid hormones affect several systemic functions that impact the perioperative period. While routine testing of thyroid parameters in patients with known stable disease is not necessary, clinical assessment of patients with known or suspected thyroid dysfunction and optimization of these conditions are essential to mitigating adverse perioperative outcomes. In addition, both subclinical and overt hyperthyroidism and hypothyroidism are present in millions of patients, so a higher index of suspicion is warranted to recognize these subclinical variants and determine if management changes in the perioperative period are warranted.

HYPOTHYROIDISM

Preoperative Evaluation and Risk Assessment

Hypothyroidism affects many body systems including cardiac, pulmonary, hematologic, gastrointestinal, and free water and electrolyte balance.[2] Retrospective studies report intraoperative hypotension, sensitivity to opioids and sedatives, ileus, and altered mentation and delirium as significant side effects. In the absence of randomized trial data, experts historically have recommended that patients achieve clinical and laboratory parameters of a euthyroid state prior to surgery. However, retrospective data do not support this blanket recommendation.[3-6] It should be noted that the definitions of severity of hypothyroidism vary between studies and are often inconsistent.

A retrospective case-control study of 59 hypothyroid patients and 59 euthyroid-matched controls undergoing surgery at Mayo Clinic found no significant differences in perioperative outcomes, complications, or length of hospital stay. No differences were noted based on serum thyroxine level; however, only seven patients were severely hypothyroid as defined with a thyroxine level of <1 mcg/dL. The authors concluded that it is safe to proceed with elective surgery in patients with mild to moderately severe hypothyroidism; no definitive conclusion could be made regarding severely hypothyroid patients.[3]

Another study of 40 hypothyroid surgical patients compared with 80 matched controls noted a higher rate of intraoperative hypotension, gastrointestinal, and neuropsychiatric complications in hypothyroid patients as well as an increased rate of heart failure in cardiac surgery patients. No differences were noted in perioperative blood loss, length of stay, arrhythmia, anesthesia recovery, pulmonary complications, or death. No clear association was noted between clinical and biochemical features of hypothyroidism to define patients at risk.[4]

A large study of 800 patients undergoing non-cardiac surgery at Cleveland Clinic who were biochemically hypothyroid (TSH > 5.5) and 5,612 biochemically euthyroid patients (TSH < 5.5) found no differences in postoperative mortality, wound, or cardiovascular outcomes, leading the authors to suggest that postponing surgery to initiate therapy in an asymptomatic patient is likely not necessary. The same group did an analysis of cardiac surgical patients evaluating cardiac complications (myocardial infarction [MI], cardiac arrest, and atrial fibrillation), vasopressor use, and wound infections and found hypothyroid patients actually had a lower rate of atrial fibrillation than euthyroid patients, and corrected hypothyroid patients had a shorter hospital length of stay than euthyroid patients.[5,6]

A study from Beijing retrospectively compared 545 coronary artery bypass graft patients with subclinical hypothyroidism with 545 propensity score-matched euthyroid controls, and found no difference in the incidence of postoperative atrial fibrillation, but did note longer mechanical ventilation times, durations of inotropic support, and increased incidence of impaired wound healing.[7]

A prospective study of 398 patients with subclinical hypothyroidism undergoing total knee arthroplasty in China found a higher incidence of both medical and surgical complications and hospital readmissions, especially when TSH was >10 mu/L, when anti-TPO was positive, and when thyroid hormone was not supplemented.[8]

A retrospective review of nationwide inpatient sample data from 2004 to 2014 for over 4 million hypothyroid patients undergoing spinal fusion found a higher rate of hematologic complications, but a decrease in hospital mortality and perioperative MI. It is unclear what the mechanism of protection is for this mortality and MI difference.[9]

A review of Medicare claims data for hypothyroid patients undergoing lumbar fusion found that they had longer lengths of hospital stay and higher rates of readmissions, complications, and costs. However, both of these studies are limited in terms of drawing clinical conclusions from administrative database research as well as the lack of assessment of potential confounders.[10,11]

Based on the above data, the authors recommend that it is safe to proceed to surgery with mild to moderate hypothyroidism but maintain vigilance regarding minor complications.

Severe hypothyroidism may have diverse manifestations.[12,13] Myxedema coma is the "end stage" of hypothyroidism, characterized by profound hypothermia and impaired consciousness or coma. Less severe presentations may manifest as disorientation, depression, paranoia, or hallucinations. Neurologic findings including cerebellar findings, memory loss and seizures, respiratory depression, cardiac arrhythmias, and depressed myocardial contractility can lead to hypoventilation, hypoxia, and hypotension intraoperatively and postoperatively.

Relative adrenal insufficiency also may be present related to hypopituitarism, Hashimoto disease, or accelerated metabolism of cortisol following T4 therapy. Table 20-1 highlights clinical features of hypothyroidism and the perioperative relevance of these findings.

Perioperative Management and Risk Reduction

Patients with stable disease based on either clinical or laboratory parameters and no symptoms referable to hypothyroidism do not need repeat TSH testing and can proceed to surgery without delay.[2,14,15] Patients who are symptomatic (Table 20-1) should have a TSH level drawn, and if elevated, then T4 and T3 should be obtained. It is important to note that dose changes require 6–8 weeks to take effect; if a patient's dose was changed in less than that time, rechecking in a shorter timespan may not provide time for an appropriate response to the dose adjustment. Although there is no absolute level of TSH at which surgery is prohibited, elevated levels should be used to more closely evaluate symptoms of hypothyroidism and, if time permits, decide whether subsequent evaluation and treatment is required before surgery. The most common agent

TABLE 20-1. Clinical Features of Hypothyroidism and Perioperative Impact

ORGAN SYSTEM	CLINICAL PICTURE	PERIOPERATIVE IMPACT
Cardiovascular	Diminished cardiac output ($\downarrow$HR, $\downarrow$SV); increased PVR from RAAS suppression from HTN; increased serum cholesterol	Hypotension and organ hypoperfusion with anesthesia induction and blood loss; increased risk of CV events
Pulmonary	Diminished hypoxic and hypercapnic respiratory drive; respiratory muscle weakness; pleural effusions; higher OSA prevalence	Difficulty with mechanical ventilation; postoperative respiratory failure (pneumonia, atelectasis)
Renal	Diminished renal perfusion; SIADH, free water retention, and hyponatremia; decreased clearance of medications and anesthetics	Protracted anesthetic effect and respiratory failure, postoperative renal insufficiency with hypoperfusion from vasodilation from anesthesia and from blood loss; worsening mentation from hyponatremia
Gastrointestinal	Delayed gastric emptying, gut motility	Postoperative ileus, nausea and vomiting, especially with GI surgeries, risk of postoperative aspiration and respiratory failure
Immunologic	Impaired febrile response to infection or inflammation	Delayed diagnosis of sepsis
Metabolic	Decreased medication clearance; hypoglycemia	Increased sensitivity to anesthetics, opioids, sedatives
Hematologic	Anemia, diminished factor VIII activity, prolonged aPTT, acquired vWD	Increased risk of bleeding, hemodynamic instability
Psychiatric	Coma, psychosis, diminished mental status (also from hyponatremia); depression, memory loss	Prolonged vent wean, risk of respiratory failure

used for management of hypothyroidism is levothyroxine which is the recommended therapy from the American Thyroid Association 2014 Guidelines on Treatment of Hypothyroidism.[16] If starting the drug de novo, they suggest roughly 1.6 µg/kg body weight for marked elevations in TSH or 25–50 µg per day for milder elevations, for elderly patients with decreased absorption (to avoid iatrogenic thyrotoxicosis), and for patients with coronary artery disease to mitigate any precipitation of ischemia. If time allows, rechecking the TSH in 6–8 weeks is appropriate prior to elective surgery; however, most preoperative assessments are done more proximately to surgery. Levothyroxine should be taken on the day of surgery; however,

because it has a half-life of approximately 7 days, one to two missed doses will not substantially affect thyroxine levels. Parenteral formulations at 75% of the oral dose can be started if oral intake is not feasible postoperatively, then the oral drug can resume postoperatively once tolerating oral intake.[2,14,15]

For severely hypothyroid patients with myxedematous symptoms, delay of elective surgery is warranted, and prompt replacement of thyroid hormone is appropriate, with consideration of formal endocrinology consultation.[13,17] Loading doses of 200–400 µg of levothyroxine intravenously should be given, with subsequent daily doses of 1.6 µg/kg of body weight; note that this dose should be reduced to 75% when administering the intravenous formulation due to a greater bioavailability. Empiric glucocorticoids should be administered in stress doses; liothyronine (T3) in low doses may also be considered.[12] Myxedema coma has a mortality as high as 80%; therefore, management is best done in a critical care setting with respiratory and hemodynamic support due to the risks for congestive heart failure, myocardial ischemia, and arrhythmias. If emergent surgery is warranted, thyroid hormone replacement and stress-dose glucocorticoids should be administered due to the risk of relative adrenal insufficiency related to hypopituitarism, Hashimoto disease (Schmidt syndrome), or accelerated metabolism of cortisol following T4 therapy.[12,13] Coordination of care with the surgeon, anesthesiologist, and endocrinologist should be done to optimize evidence-based therapies and improve outcomes. Figure 20-1 highlights the suggested perioperative management strategy of patients with hypothyroidism.

HYPERTHYROIDISM

Preoperative Evaluation and Risk Assessment

Hyperthyroidism is less common in the population than hypothyroidism. The term "hyperthyroidism" refers to the biochemical presence of excess thyroid hormone produced by the thyroid gland, whereas "thyrotoxicosis" refers to the clinical manifestations of excess thyroid hormone, irrespective of the source (extrathyroidal sources may include struma ovarii or functional thyroid cancer metastases).[18] The majority of patients with hyperthyroidism have autoimmune thyroiditis or Graves' disease. Uncontrolled or untreated hyperthyroidism can lead to tachyarrhythmias such as atrial fibrillation, decompensated heart failure, and cardiac ischemia from increased myocardial oxygen demand, leading to a higher risk of perioperative myocardial infarction. The extreme state of thyrotoxicosis, thyroid storm, or thyrotoxic storm may manifest as fever and diaphoresis, tachycardia, dyspnea or tachypnea, and gastrointestinal symptoms (nausea, vomiting, diarrhea, and jaundice), and can progress to an encephalopathic picture, seizures, or stroke. This is primarily a clinical diagnosis, as the laboratory findings may not help to differentiate this from uncomplicated hyperthyroidism.[13] As with hypothyroidism, there is no absolute level of TSH at which surgery is prohibited; one should use this level as an indicator to more closely evaluate symptoms of hyperthyroidism and, if time permits, pursue subsequent evaluation and therapies. T3 levels may even be normal as the underlying precipitating illness may lead to reduced T4 to T3 conversion. A semiquantitative scale exists to aid in the timely diagnosis of

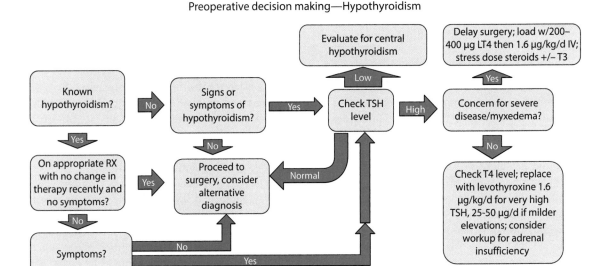

FIGURE 20-1. Preoperative decision making—hypothyroidism.

TABLE 20-2. Clinical Features of Hyperthyroidism and Perioperative Impact

ORGAN SYSTEM	CLINICAL PICTURE	PERIOPERATIVE IMPACT
Cardiovascular	Tachyarrhythmias especially atrial fibrillation (most common finding); systolic hypertension and increased pulse pressure; high output congestive heart failure, pulmonary hypertension; angina and cardiac ischemia	Increased risk of perioperative MI, congestive heart failure and end organ hypoperfusion
Pulmonary	Increased oxygen consumption, CO_2 production, dyspnea, respiratory and skeletal muscle weakness, diminished lung volumes	Postoperative respiratory failure
Gastrointestinal	Gut hypermotility with malabsorption; unexplained weight loss	Malnutrition, poor wound healing
Immunologic	Fever, diaphoresis	Concern for ongoing sepsis, antibiotic therapy, and consequent resistance
Metabolic	Increased metabolic rate and drug metabolism	Higher doses required for anesthetics, opioids, sedatives
Endocrine	Concomitant adrenal insufficiency	Addisonian crisis with surgical stress, hypotension, shock
Psychiatric	Delirium, psychosis; hyperreflexia and tremor, mania/depression;	Impaired compliance with treatment regimen, requirement for sedation, and antipsychotics for behavioral control

thyrotoxicosis. Table 20-2 highlights the clinical features of hyperthyroidism relevant to the perioperative period.

Perioperative Management and Risk Reduction

Patients with stable hyperthyroidism on thionamide therapy and no symptoms can proceed to surgery without additional laboratory or diagnostic testing.[14,15,17] Symptomatic patients should have a serum TSH level determined, and if this is low, serum-free T4 and T3 levels to assess if subclinical versus overt hyperthyroidism is present. Further steps in evaluation include radioactive iodine uptake, ultrasonography, or measurement of TSH receptor antibodies (TRAb, also referred to as thyroid-stimulating immunoglobulins or antibodies).[19] Diffusely high radioiodine uptake, an enlarged thyroid on ultrasound without nodules, and/or positive TRAb confirm Graves' disease; medical management with thionamides is appropriate here. Focal or asymmetric radioiodine uptake or nodular

goiter on ultrasound with negative TRAb suggests toxic multinodular goiter or a solitary functioning adenoma. If radioiodine uptake is low and/or ultrasound is inconsistent, then consider other etiologies including thyroiditis, iodine induced, drug induced, excess exogenous hormone (iatrogenic or factitious), or an ectopic source of thyroid hormone including struma ovarii or functional thyroid cancer metastases.

If time does not allow for this workup in the setting of urgent or emergent surgery, then it is appropriate to manage the consequences of hyperthyroidism with thyroid hormone suppression with antithyroid drugs (ATDs) and end organ management with ATDs and beta-blocker therapy.[13,18,19] Radioactive iodine ablation and surgery may not be valid treatment options in these circumstances. ATDs are helpful to restore a clinically euthyroid state. Methimazole is preferred currently to propylthiouracil in the United States due to better efficacy, longer half-life, longer duration of action, once daily dosing, and fewer side effects including

Preoperative decision making—Hyperthyroidism

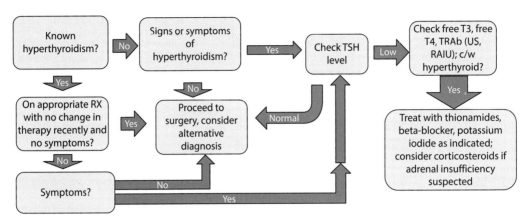

FIGURE 20-2. Preoperative decision making—hyperthyroidism.

the concern for liver damage with propylthiouracil. Starting doses of methimazole are 10–15 mg daily for mild disease and smaller patients, and 20–40 mg daily are appropriate for more severe disease and larger patients. Administration of potassium iodide solution (to block T4 and T3 release from the thyroid gland) is also done after thionamide administration (as iodide prior to thionamide therapy may exacerbate hyperthyroidism). Beta-blocker therapy is appropriate to manage the peripheral effects of excess thyroid hormone.[16] Thyroid storm has a mortality estimated between 8% and 25%; therefore, a critical care setting for optimization for emergent or urgent surgery is appropriate, with coordination of care with the surgeon, anesthesiologist, and endocrinologist. Figure 20-2 highlights the suggested perioperative management strategy of patients with hyperthyroidism.

CONCLUSION

The perioperative management of thyroid disease in stable patients does not require significant testing or interventions. However, clinician awareness of the clinical manifestations of both myxedema and thyrotoxicosis is critical to institute appropriate therapies and optimize perioperative outcomes.

Clinical pearls

- Do not routinely perform lab testing on patients with stable thyroid disease in the absence of signs or symptoms of decompensated thyroid function.

- There is no absolute level of TSH at which surgery is prohibited; one should use this level as an indicator to more closely evaluate symptoms of hypothyroidism (and hyperthyroidism) and, if time permits, pursue subsequent evaluation and therapies.

- Proceed to surgery in patients with mild or subclinical thyroid dysfunction as outcomes are not impacted in the perioperative period.

- Postpone elective surgery in patients with severe symptomatic hypothyroidism or hyperthyroidism for treatment and medical optimization.

- Patients who require emergent or urgent surgery with severe hypothyroidism or hyperthyroidism should be treated expeditiously and closely monitored perioperatively, preferably in a critical care setting.

REFERENCES

1. Vanderpump MPJ. The epidemiology of thyroid disease. *Br Med Bull.* 2011;99(1):39-51. PMID: 21893493

2. Schiff RL, Welsh GA. Perioperative evaluation and management of the patient with endocrine dysfunction. *Med Clin North Am.* 2003;87(1):175-192. PMID: 12575889

3. Weinberg AD, Brennan MD, Gorman CA, et al. Outcome of anesthesia and surgery in hypothyroid patients. *Arch Intern Med.* 1983;143(5):893-897. PMID: 6679233

4. Ladenson PW, Levin AA, Ridgway EC, et al. Complications of surgery in hypothyroid patients. *Am J Med.* 1984;77(2):261-266. PMID: 6465175

5. Komatsu R, Karimi N, Zimmerman NM, et al. Biochemically diagnosed hypothyroidism and postoperative complications after cardiac surgery: a retrospective cohort analysis. *J Anesth.* 2018;32(5):663-672. PMID: 30014234

6. Komatsu R, You J, Mascha EJ, et al. The effect of hypothyroidism on a composite of mortality, cardiovascular and wound complications after noncardiac surgery: a retrospective cohort analysis. *Anesth Analg.* 2015;121(3):716-726. PMID: 26287300

7. Zhao D, Xu F, Yuan X, Feng W. Impact of subclinical hypothyroidism on outcomes of coronary bypass surgery. *J Card Surg.* 2021;36(4):1431-1438. PMID: 33567099

8. Jing W, Long G, Yan Z, et al. Subclinical hypothyroidism affects postoperative outcome of patients undergoing total knee arthroplasty. *Orthop Surg.* 2021;13(3):932-941. PMID: 33817980

9. Luther E, Perez-Roman RJ, McCarthy DJ, et al. Incidence and clinical outcomes of hypothyroidism in patients undergoing spinal fusion. *Cureus.* 2021;13(8):e17099. PMID: 34527485

10. Vakharia RM, Ehiorobo JO, Mahmood B, et al. Does hypothyroidism increase complications, lengths of stay, readmissions, and costs following primary 1- to 2-level lumbar fusion? *Clin Spine Surg.* 2020;33(10):E559-E562. PMID: 32341326

11. Bajaj A, Shah RM, Kurapaty S, et al. Hypothyroidism and spine surgery: a review of current findings. *Curr Rev Musculoskelet Med.* 2023;16(1):33-37. PMID: 32341326

12. Wartofsky L. Myxedema coma. *Endocrinol Metab Clin North Am.* 2006;35(4):687-698. PMID: 17127141

13. Klubo-Gwiezdzinska J, Wartofsky L. Thyroid emergencies. *Med Clin North Am.* 2012;96(2):385-403. PMID: 22443982

14. Stathatos N, Wartofsky L. Perioperative management of patients with hypothyroidism. *Endocrinol Metab Clin North Am.* 2003;32(2):503-518. PMID: 12800543

15. Kohl BA, Schwartz S. Surgery in the patient with endocrine dysfunction. *Med Clin North Am.* 2009;93(5):1031-1047. PMID: 19665618

16. Jonklaas J, Bianco AC, Bauer AJ, et al. Guidelines for the treatment of hypothyroidism: prepared by the American Thyroid Association Task Force on thyroid hormone replacement. *Thyroid.* 2014;24(12):1670-1751. PMID: 25266247

17. Palace MR. Perioperative management of thyroid dysfunction. *Health Serv Insights.* 2017;10:1178632916689677. PMID: 28469454

18. De Leo S, Lee SY, Braverman LE. Hyperthyroidism. *Lancet.* 2016;388(10047):906-918. PMID: 27038492

19. Ross DS, Burch HB, Cooper DS, et al. 2016 American Thyroid Association guidelines for diagnosis and management of hyperthyroidism and other causes of thyrotoxicosis. *Thyroid.* 2016;26(10):1343-1421. PMID: 27521067

## 21

Adrenal Disease (Including Pheochromocytoma)

Christopher M. Whinney, MD, FACP, SFHM and Sunil K. Sahai, MD, FAAP, FACP, SFHM

COMMON CLINICAL QUESTIONS

1. Which patients are at risk for perioperative adrenal insufficiency?

2. When are stress dose steroids indicated?

3. What preoperative management is recommended for a patient with pheochromocytoma?

ADRENAL INSUFFICIENCY (AI): INTRODUCTION

Adrenal function is critical to stability in the surgical milieu in order to maintain hemodynamic stability and end-organ perfusion.[1-3] The stress of surgery, trauma, and critical illness, and the vasodilation associated with anesthesia, in conjunction with blood loss and fluid shifts, can lead to hypotension and shock in the setting of inadequate adrenal reserves. A systematic review of 71 trials of 2,953 patients looking at the invasiveness of surgery and cortisol release found that peak cortisol output was two to four times higher than healthy, unstressed individuals within the first 24 hours after surgery; this was proportional to the invasiveness of surgery as noted by blood loss. Cortisol levels peak within 24 hours of surgery and return to baseline in 7 days or less.[4]

There are two distinct populations of relevance in this regard: patients with established and confirmed primary or secondary AI (from cortisol or adrenocorticotropic hormone (ACTH) deficiency, respectively), and patients with suspected tertiary AI related to use of exogenous glucocorticoid therapy that suppresses the hypothalamic-pituitary-adrenal (HPA) axis and ACTH release from the hypothalamus.

Primary AI most commonly results from autoimmune destruction of the adrenal glands.[1] Other causes include adrenalectomy, adrenal infarction or hemorrhage, granulomatous disease, infiltrative diseases, tumors, and HIV. Patients with primary AI taking therapeutic replacement steroids will generally require additional supplementation when undergoing a procedure involving significant blood loss, fluid shifts, and anesthesia time. In contrast to patients taking exogenous steroids, patients with primary/secondary AI do not have the ability to mount an appropriate adrenal response to stress and therefore require additional supplementation.

For patients with tertiary AI from exogenous corticosteroids, suppression of the HPA axis is quite variable depending on dose, duration of treatment, and patient-related factors including age, weight, hepatic function, concomitant drugs metabolized by the P450 system, and concurrent illnesses. However, a reduced response to ACTH (cosyntropin) stimulation testing is reported to last for 5 days after a similar duration of 25 mg prednisone therapy.[5]

PREOPERATIVE EVALUATION AND RISK ASSESSMENT

Clinicians evaluating patients with known primary AI in the preoperative setting should clarify the etiology of the AI. Some patients may have a clear history of adrenalectomy, tuberculosis, sarcoid, or other etiology, evident by history, examination, imaging, or laboratory assessment including morning cortisol determinations and/or ACTH (cosyntropin) stimulation testing (CST). Others may not have convincing evidence of AI and may have been told that they are "dependent" on steroids, when in fact they have tertiary AI from exogenous corticosteroid use. Conferring with other treating physicians can help to clarify this issue. Corticosteroid dose, frequency (i.e., daily or alternate day dosing), and duration of therapy are key historical elements to help inform decision making. Physical examination is often limited in utility but may demonstrate Cushingoid facies, abdominal and flank striae, and centripetal obesity as manifestations or glucocorticoid excess from exogenous supplementation.

A low morning cortisol level and/or a positive ACTH (cosyntropin) stimulation test (defined as an increase in serum cortisol by less than 7 mg/dL or an absolute cortisol level less than 18 mg/dL 1 hour after the administration of 1 mcg ACTH) helps to confirm the diagnosis; this does not need to be repeated in the perioperative setting unless the diagnosis is in question or if the patient is already taking exogenous corticosteroids, thereby limiting the utility of the test. Other experts have suggested the use of ACTH (cosyntropin) stimulation tests for risk stratification, but there have been no studies to correlate the results of this testing with intraoperative or postoperative adrenal crisis.[6] Therefore, we do not recommend this testing prior to surgery unless there is a specific indication to make the diagnosis regardless of the indication for surgery, such as when corticosteroids are tapered and discontinued preoperatively to mitigate postoperative complications such as impaired wound healing and hyperglycemia.[5]

PERIOPERATIVE MANAGEMENT AND RISK REDUCTION

Patients with confirmed AI require corticosteroid supplementation. In the absence of a robust cohort of randomized trials, there are several expert opinions recommending additional "coverage" in the immediate intraoperative and postoperative timeframes with a rapid taper back to the patient's home dose, unless there are other indications to maintain a higher dose of corticosteroids for therapeutic benefit.[1,7] Patients with secondary AI from exogenous steroids likely have some residual adrenal reserve, but this is dependent on the length of time they have been on corticosteroids and the dose they received over that time. Recent guidelines from the United Kingdom recommend a more aggressive approach with 100 mg of hydrocortisone preoperatively for most patients undergoing moderate-to-high-risk surgeries, with a rapid taper back to baseline dosage.[8] Table 21-1 provides this guidance for dosing of patients with confirmed or suspected AI of any etiology.

Patients on Exogenous Corticosteroids

The genesis of the principle of perioperative stress-dose steroids is from two case reports from the 1950s of patients who developed circulatory shock after surgery associated with withdrawal of their usual cortisone therapy.[9,10] One of these authors recommended substantial glucocorticoid support for patients beyond what is produced by the adrenal gland. However, glucocorticoids have a plethora of adverse clinical consequences including glucose intolerance, infection risk, impaired wound healing, and osteoporosis.[3,5] A retrospective study of 432 patients with Rheumatoid Arthritis (RA) who underwent THA and TKA found a higher rate of hyperglycemia and complications with higher glucocorticoid exposure, with no association between lower GC dose and hypotension; the risk of short-term complications was increased by 8.4% for every 10-mg increase in GC dose.[11]

Several systematic reviews find that most replacement doses of glucocorticoids are likely excessive, that continuing the patient on their current dose of corticosteroid through surgery is likely appropriate, and that risk of adrenal stress is likely related to the duration and severity of the surgery.[5,12] A systematic review of two randomized controlled trials and seven cohort studies found no evidence of adrenal crisis except for two patients in the cohort studies who had their usual doses stopped prior to surgery and developed unexplained hypotension.[6] The UK guidelines noted previously suggest 100 mg of hydrocortisone

TABLE 21-1. Perioperative Corticosteroid Dosing			
	PRIMARY AI KNOWN HYPOTHALAMIC-PITUITARY-ADRENAL (HPA) AXIS SUPPRESSION	**SECONDARY AI** UNCERTAIN HPA AXIS SUPPRESSION	NO HPA AXIS SUPPRESSION
Clinical picture:	≥ 20 mg prednisone daily or equivalent Cushingoid appearance Confirmed biochemical HPA axis suppression	5–20 mg prednisone daily or equivalent for 3 weeks in last year	<5 mg prednisone daily Alternate day dosing Any dosing < 3 weeks
Low surgical risk	Give usual daily dose (no stress dosing) OR give 25 mg hydrocortisone IV or equivalent prior to induction of anesthesia	Give usual daily dose (no stress dosing)	Give usual daily dose (no stress dosing)
Moderate surgical risk	• 50 mg IV hydrocortisone or equivalent prior to induction of anesthesia • 25 mg IV hydrocortisone every 8 hours × 24–48 hours • Then resume usual daily dose	Give supplemental steroids: • 50 mg IV hydrocortisone or equivalent prior to induction of anesthesia • 25 mg IV hydrocortisone every 8 hours × 24–48 hours, then resume usual daily dose • ACTH test results are not correlated with postoperative adrenal crisis	Give usual daily dose (no stress dosing)
High surgical risk	• 50–100 mg IV hydrocortisone or equivalent prior to induction of anesthesia • 25–50 mg IV hydrocortisone every 8 hours × 48–72 hours • Then resume usual daily dose	Give supplemental steroids: • 50–100 mg IV hydrocortisone or equivalent prior to induction of anesthesia • 25–50 mg IV hydrocortisone every 8 hours × 48–72 hours, then resume usual daily dose • ACTH test results are not correlated with postoperative adrenal crisis	Give usual daily dose (no stress dosing)

Source: Data from Schiff and Welsh. *Med Clin N Amer*. 2003;87:175-192; Kohl and Schwartz. *Med Clin N Am*. 2009;93:1031-1047; Chen Cardenas et al. *J Endo Society*. 2023;7:1-16.

for both minor and major procedures;[6] after several letters to the editor questioned this recommendation, the authors suggested that minor procedures may not require this dose.[13] The American College of Rheumatology/American Association of Hip and Knee Surgeons updated guidelines from 2022 suggest continuing home dosage of steroids for hip and knee replacements.[14] Thus, for low-risk surgeries (from a duration and severity standpoint), it is appropriate to continue the current chronic dosage of steroids through the perioperative period. However, for moderate-to-high risk surgeries, especially if significant blood loss, fluid shifts, and prolonged anesthesia time are anticipated, stress-dosage administration of steroids is reasonable as noted in Table 21-1.

Of note, dexamethasone is now commonly used for prevention of postoperative nausea and vomiting as well as for pain control.[15] In most cases, this is sufficient as a stress dose for patients taking exogenous glucocorticoids, but it is not sufficient for patients with confirmed AI due to the lack of mineralocorticoid effect. In these cases, the addition of hydrocortisone or fludrocortisone is required. If patients have discontinued glucocorticoids in advance of surgery for other clinical reasons (reducing infection risk, wound healing optimization, etc.), it is recommended that the HPA axis be assessed with ACTH (cosyntropin) stimulation testing, and treated based on degree of surgical stress if CST is abnormal.[5]

HYPERCORTISOLISM AND NONENDOCRINE SURGERY

Hypercortisolism outside of exogenous corticosteroid use can be due to Cushing's disease, manifested by a pituitary tumor with autonomous ACTH production leading to a hypercortisol state, or Cushing's syndrome, with primary adrenal gland disease from an adrenal adenoma.[16] Perioperative risks include hyperglycemia, impaired wound healing, hypertension, and hypokalemia, and these should be addressed and managed appropriately. Therapies such as steroidogenesis inhibitors including metyrapone or mitotane are generally safe to use in the perioperative period. Ketoconazole has also been used but has numerous drug interactions and risk for hepatotoxicity. Etomidate can be used, but it is an anesthetic and requires an intensive care unit (ICU) setting for titration to avoid excessive sedation. Centrally acting agents including cabergoline, pasireotide, and temozolomide are therapeutic options; glucose monitoring is required for pasireotide and temozolomide, but no specific contraindications exist for these agents. Mifepristone is also used as a glucocorticoid receptor antagonist and is approved for patients with Cushing's who are not candidates for surgery. If patients require nonendocrine surgery in this state, then suppression of the endocrine excess in coordination with the patient's endocrinologist is appropriate, and these agents are essentially safe to continue in the perioperative period. There are little data on management of hypercortisol states in the nonendocrine surgeries; however, a retrospective analysis of a prospective database at a single large academic center showed that bilateral adrenal incidentalomas had a 21% rate of subclinical hypercortisolism but had good outcomes.[17,18] Patients undergoing nonendocrine surgery can proceed without further intervention if they are on appropriate therapy and end-organ manifestations such as hypertension, hyperglycemia, and hypokalemia are absent.

CONCLUSION

Corticosteroid use and the consideration of the need for "stress-dose steroids" in the perioperative period is a conundrum facing surgeons, anesthesiologists, and perioperative specialists. The true incidence of adrenal suppression from exogenous steroids is likely very low based on existing data. Although the risk of adrenal crisis with hypotension is low, it is a potentially serious problem. On the other hand, adverse consequences of corticosteroid therapy do occur but are usually less significant. Clinicians must balance these risks and benefits in deciding whether to prescribe "stress-dose steroids." If they are prescribed, a clear plan of expeditious tapering and returning to the patient's home dose must be clearly articulated to surgery and anesthesia teams.

PHEOCHROMOCYTOMA AND PARAGANGLIOMAS: INTRODUCTION

Pheochromocytomas and paragangliomas (PPGL) are rare tumors, with a prevalence between 0.2% and 0.6% in the general population.[19] Once diagnosed, most patients are referred to academic or cancer centers for further evaluation and management. However, these patients may present for nontumor-related procedures, and therefore the perioperative clinician needs to be aware of medical management strategies.

In practice, the terms pheochromocytoma and paraganglioma are often used interchangeably as they both arise from catecholamine (epinephrine, norepinephrine, and dopamine) producing chromaffin cells. Paragangliomas that arise in the adrenal medulla are known as pheochromocytomas, and those outside the adrenal gland are called paragangliomas. Paragangliomas are usually found in the sympathetic and parasympathetic paravertebral ganglia of the thorax, abdomen, and pelvis. Most PPGLs are functional, synthesizing and secreting catecholamines, and thus causing symptoms. About 10% of patients with PPGL have metastatic and malignant disease, defined as the presence of chromaffin cells in nonchromaffin organs.[20] Patients with metastatic PPGL rarely undergo primary resection of tumor but may present with other issues requiring surgical intervention (pregnancy, orthopedic procedures, trauma).

PREOPERATIVE EVALUATION

The majority of diagnosed PPGL patients are followed by multidisciplinary teams consisting of endocrinologists and surgeons. The major perioperative concern is hemodynamic instability during and immediately following surgery, usually manifested by extreme blood pressure lability. This process is mediated by a catecholamine surge of epinephrine and norepinephrine from metabolically active tissues during anesthesia induction and during surgery, leading to critical cardiovascular complications. In addition, clinicians unfamiliar with PPGL management should refrain from prescribing medications that might trigger a catecholamine crisis such as certain anesthetics (succinylcholine, pancuronium, halothane, ketamine), antidepressants (amitriptyline, nortriptyline bupropion, duloxetin, paroxetine, fluoxetine), unopposed ß-blockers (propranolol, metoprolol), dopamine-2 antagonists (metoclopramide, haloperidol, olanzapine, chlorpromazine), opioid analgesics (morphine, tramadol), peptide hormones glucagon), and sympathomimetics (ephedrine, amphetamine, sibutramine, phentermine)".[21]

The preoperative evaluation of the patient with PPGL should include a thorough history and physical exam, basic metabolic panel, and complete blood count. Cardiac evaluation should include an echocardiogram to assess for cardiac sequela from excessive catecholamine release (LV dysfunction, cardiomyopathy, primary cardiac pheochromocytoma) and electrocardiogram that may reveal left ventricular hypertrophy and ischemic ST-T changes due to catecholamine-induced coronary artery vasoconstriction. In addition, other medical comorbid conditions from prolonged hypertension, such as renal insufficiency and hypertensive encephalopathy, need to be assessed. "Routine" ischemic workup with cardiac stress testing is not recommended unless other indications are present.

PERIOPERATIVE MANAGEMENT

Preoperative Hemodynamic Control Regimens (Figure 21-1)

In the weeks leading up to surgery, it is important to control hemodynamic instability. In 2014, the Endocrine Society published perioperative medication guidelines.[19] The goal is to reach a resting systolic blood pressure close to 130/80 mmHg and prevent orthostatic drops below 90 mmHg systolic. Sitting pulse should be in 60s to 70s, with orthostatic standing pulse no more than 90.

The recommendation is to start *alpha-blockade* with phenoxybenzamine 10 mg BID and titrate the dose up to 1 mg/kg/day. Alternatively, doxazosin 2 mg/day titrated up to 32 mg/day can be used. If adequate blood pressure management is not achieved with maximum doses of the alpha-blockers, then the calcium channel blockers can be started. Nifedipine can be started at 30 mg/day and titrated up to 60 mg/day. Amlodipine can be started at 5 mg/day and doubled to a maximum dose of 10 mg/day. Once alpha-blockers and/or calcium channel blockers are onboard, 3–4 days later, *beta-blockade* can commence. Propranolol 20 mg TID titrated to a max dose of 40 mg TID and atenolol 25 mg/day titrated to 50 mg/day are the drugs of choice.

It is important to note that *beta-blockers should only be added after adequate alpha-blockade* has been achieved to prevent hypertensive crisis due to unopposed stimulation of alpha-adrenergic receptors. Patients should achieve a steady state before proceeding to the operating room. Of note, combined ↑- and ↓-adrenoceptor antagonists such as labetalol and carvedilol should not be used because of fixed ratios of alpha- to beta-blockade. These fixed ratios prevent adequate titration of blood pressure and may induce a hypertensive crisis.[22] PPGL patients tend to be intravascularly depleted due to peripheral vasoconstriction, and as such, preoperative evaluation should also focus on restoring and maintaining euvolemia by a high sodium diet and generous oral fluid intake. Volume resuscitation should start a few days after alpha-blockade is started.

It is recognized that patients may not be able to reach the goal blood pressure and pulse ranges, and as such, the decision to proceed to surgery rests on clinical judgment and relative stability of blood pressure, pulse, and restoration of volume status.

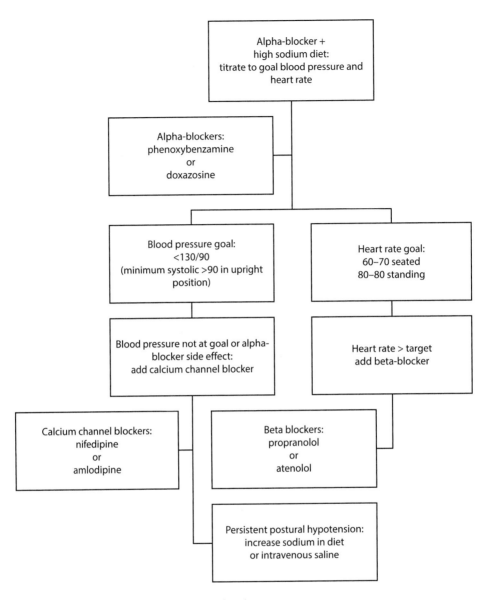

FIGURE 21-1. Preoperative hemodynamic management in pheochromocytoma.

As anxiety may provoke a catecholamine surge, some centers recommend the use of a long-acting anxiolytic starting the day before surgery. The recommendation continues in the preop holding area where anxiolytics such as midazolam may be administered intravenously prior to heading to the operating room.

Intraoperative Management

In order to minimize catecholamine release during induction, the use of propofol and etomidate is recommended. Additionally, the use of intraarterial cardiovascular monitoring is mandatory in all patients with PPGL as blood pressure may be highly labile.[23]

Patients may experience a "roller coaster" of blood pressure ranges during an operation; therefore, short-acting agents are preferred to manage any blood pressure lability. Recommended agents are sodium nitroprusside, esmolol, phentolamine, and magnesium sulfate ($MgSO_4$). For acute hypotension that may occur following tumor resection, the vasopressors of choice are norepinephrine, followed by vasopressin. Calcium may be used if magnesium was previously administered. Resection of the tumor may precipitate hypotension due to relative hypovolemia from the aforementioned peripheral vasoconstriction, and as such, large bore IV access is also mandated for rapid fluid resuscitation.

Postoperative Management

In the immediate postoperative period, the patient may require steroids if undergoing bilateral adrenalectomy. Additionally, postsurgical PPGL patients should be managed in the ICU as they may continue to experience hemodynamic instability along with AI, hypoglycemia, and hyperglycemia. The involvement of a multidisciplinary team experienced in treating PPGL is a must.

Clinical pearls

- Patients on corticosteroids for any reason can continue *only* their home dose on the day of the procedure for low-or moderate-risk procedures.

- Consider giving patients stress-dose corticosteroids who are undergoing high-risk procedures with known or suspected HPA axis suppression, in doses congruent with the duration and severity of the procedure or surgery.

- HPA axis testing in the preoperative setting has little predictive value for perioperative adrenal crisis.

- Alpha-blockade before beta-blockade is critical in preparing patients with PPGL for surgery.

- The hallmark of PPGL is hemodynamic instability, manifested by labile blood pressures.

- There is a perioperative catecholamine surge due to preoperative anxiety, anesthesia induction, and tumor resection in PPGL.

- Multidisciplinary team involvement with endocrinology is highly recommended to manage PPGL.

REFERENCES

1. Kohl BA, Schwartz S. Surgery in the patient with endocrine dysfunction. *Med Clin North Am.* 2009;93:1031-1047. PMID: 19665618
2. Schiff RL, Welsh GA. Perioperative evaluation and management of the patient with endocrine dysfunction. *Med Clin North Am.* 2003;87:175-192. PMID: 12575889
3. Seo KH. Perioperative glucocorticoid management based on current evidence. *Anesth Pain Med (Seoul).* 2021;16:8-15. PMID: 33445232
4. Prete A, Yan Q, Al-Tarrah K, et al. The cortisol stress response induced by surgery: a systematic review and meta-analysis. *Clin. Endocrinol (Oxf).* 2018;89:554-567. PMID: 30047158
5. Chen Cardenas SM, Santhanam P, Morris-Wiseman L, et al. Perioperative evaluation and management of patients on glucocorticoids. *J Endocr Soc.* 2022;7:bvac185. PMID: 36545644
6. Marik PE, Varon J. Requirement of perioperative stress doses of corticosteroids: a systematic review of the literature. *Arch Surg.* 2008;143:1222-1226. PMID: 19075176
7. Coursin DB, Wood KE. Corticosteroid supplementation for adrenal insufficiency. *JAMA.* 2002;287:236-240. PMID: 11779267
8. Woodcock T, Barker P, Daniel S, et al. Guidelines for the management of glucocorticoids during the perioperative period for patients with adrenal insufficiency: guidelines from the Association of Anaesthetists, the Royal College of Physicians and the Society for Endocrinology UK. *Anaesthesia.* 2020;75:654-663. PMID: 32017012
9. Fraser CG, Preuss FS, Bigford WD. Adrenal atrophy and irreversible shock associated with cortisone therapy. *J Am Med Assoc.* 1952;149:1542-1543. PMID: 14945970
10. Lewis L, Robinson RF, Yee J, et al. Fatal adrenal cortical insufficiency precipitated by surgery during prolonged continuous cortisone treatment. *Ann Intern Med.* 1953;39:116-126. PMID: 13065993
11. Chukir T, Goodman SM, Tornberg H, et al. Perioperative glucocorticoids in patients with rheumatoid arthritis having total joint replacements: help or harm? *ACR Open Rheumatol.* 2021;3:654-659. PMID: 34288590
12. Salem M, Tainsh RE Jr, Bromberg J, et al. Perioperative glucocorticoid coverage: a reassessment 42 years after

emergence of a problem. *Ann Surg*. 1994;219:416-425. PMID: 8161268

13. Vercueil A, Working P. Guidelines for the management of glucocorticoids during the peri-operative period for patients with adrenal insufficiency: a reply. *Anaesthesia*. 2020;75:1398-1399. PMID: 32621301

14. Goodman SM, Springer BD, Chen AF, et al. 2022 American College of Rheumatology/American Association of Hip and Knee Surgeons Guideline for the perioperative management of antirheumatic medication in patients with rheumatic diseases undergoing elective total hip or total knee arthroplasty. *Arthritis Rheumatol*. 2022;74:1464-1473. PMID: 35722708

15. Gan TJ, Belani KG, Bergese S, et al. Fourth consensus guidelines for the management of postoperative nausea and vomiting. *Anesth Analg*. 2020;131:411-448. PMID: 32467512

16. Tritos NA, Biller BMK. Current management of Cushing's disease. *J Intern Med*. 2019;286:526-541. PMID: 31512305

17. Pasternak JD, Seib CD, Seiser N, et al. Differences between bilateral adrenal incidentalomas and unilateral lesions. *JAMA Surg*. 2015;150:974-978. PMID: 26200882

18. Yip L, Carty SE. Nonoperative management of bilateral adrenal incidentalomas: the value of restraint. *JAMA Surg*. 2015;150:978. PMID: 26200261

19. Lenders JW, Duh QY, Eisenhofer G, et al. Pheochromocytoma and paraganglioma: an endocrine society clinical practice guideline. *J Clin Endocrinol Metab*. 2014;99:1915-1942. PMID: 24893135

20. Nomura K, Kimura H, Shimizu S, et al. Survival of patients with metastatic malignant pheochromocytoma and efficacy of combined cyclophosphamide, vincristine, and dacarbazine chemotherapy. *J Clin Endocrinol Metab*. 2009;94:2850-2856. PMID: 19470630

21. Fagundes GFC, Almeida MQ. Perioperative management of pheochromocytomas and sympathetic paragangliomas. *J Endocr Soc*. 2022;6:bvac004. PMID: 35128297

22. Pacak K. Preoperative management of the pheochromocytoma patient. *J Clin Endocrinol Metab*. 2007;92:4069-4079. PMID: 17989126

23. Ramakrishna H. Pheochromocytoma resection: current concepts in anesthetic management. *J Anaesthesiol Clin Pharmacol*. 2015;31:317-323. PMID: 26330708

Anemia and Transfusion Medicine

Barbara Slawski, MD, MS, SFHM and Moises Auron, MD, FAAP, FACP, SFHM, FRCP (Lon), FRCPCH

COMMON CLINICAL QUESTIONS

1. What is the impact of untreated anemia in surgical patients?
2. What are the recommended screening and evaluation tests for anemia in surgical patients?
3. What are the current non-transfusional treatment strategies to optimize anemia in surgical patients?

INTRODUCTION

Anemia is a significant risk for morbidity and mortality in surgical patients. That risk depends on the patient's comorbidities, type of surgery planned, and the severity, stability, and etiology of the anemia. The prevalence of baseline anemia ranges from 36% up to 75%, with a higher prevalence in women and elderly. Its prevalence also varies in different surgical populations: gynecologic (64%), colorectal cancer (58%), cardiac surgery (40%), orthopedic surgery (elective—26%; acute hip fracture repair—75%).[1,2] Even mild anemia, with an approximate hemoglobin of <13 g/dL in men and <12 g/dL in women, is associated with adverse perioperative outcomes.[3] In addition to the risk of mortality, perioperative anemia is associated with an increased risk of pulmonary, wound, and thromboembolic complications.

A restrictive approach to anemia, aiming to avoid transfusion of packed red blood cells (PRBCs), is preferred to avoid complications associated with allogeneic PRBC transfusion, which include transfusion-related acute lung injury, acute hemolytic transfusion reactions, increased risk of infections, allergic reactions, transfusion-related immunomodulation, and transfusion-associated circulatory overload.[4,5] Another risk of increased exposure to allogeneic blood transfusions is antibody production, which can make subsequent transfusion or transplantation more difficult. Transfusion is also associated with mortality. In a study of cardiac surgical patients, transfusion of red cells was associated with an odds ratio for mortality of 1.18 (95% confidence interval [CI], 1.14–1.22) per unit of blood transfused.[6] Transfusion is also associated with increased cost of care.[4]

When the timeframe to surgery permits, a preoperative blood management protocol in which evaluation and treatment of anemia is implemented can decrease the risks associated with anemia and perioperative transfusion and enhance overall patient outcomes.[1,2]

PREOPERATIVE EVALUATION/ RISK FACTORS

Patient risk factors for anemia and excessive bleeding should be considered during the preoperative evaluation. These include anemia history, liver disease, age, and other hematologic disorders.[7]

Preoperative Testing

Preoperative evaluation with respect to anemia and blood management should include a review of medical records/laboratories, a patient interview and physical exam, and ordering of additional required tests. Specific history that is useful includes history or symptoms of anemia, previous blood transfusions, coagulopathies (heritable or drug-induced), thrombotic history, and risks for organ ischemia (coronary artery disease, renal disease, etc.).

Criteria for Testing

Testing for abnormal hemoglobin levels in preoperative patients should be targeted to identify patients at risk of anemia and blood loss, while decreasing wasteful testing in patients at lower risk. For patients who receive selected testing, over half have abnormal findings, while significantly fewer are abnormal when routine or unselected testing is performed.[7] Preoperative hemoglobin levels are indicated for patients scheduled to undergo procedures with expected significant blood loss or where history or physical exam suggests a likelihood of anemia, as well as in groups with a higher prevalence of underlying anemia.[1] Hemoglobin measurements are not indicated in young, healthy patients and those undergoing low-bleeding-risk procedures.

Ideally, a hemoglobin level can be obtained well in advance of surgery so that if additional evaluation or intervention is needed, there is time to improve the hemoglobin level to decrease the risk of perioperative transfusion without a potential surgical delay. This strategy is primarily effective in elective cases.

Laboratory Evaluation of Anemia

A structured approach to the preoperative evaluation of anemia is demonstrated in Figure 22-1 and Table 22-1.

In preoperative patients with all anemias, it is important to identify the source of the deficiency if possible. For example, if the source of iron deficiency is an undiagnosed bleeding source, the patient may experience increased and excessive bleeding in the postoperative period if anticoagulants or antiplatelet agents are used, or patients with underlying vitamin B_{12} deficiency can develop neurotoxicity if nitric oxide is used in anesthesia.

Indications for Type and Crossmatch

A high-value approach to type and crossmatch testing allows its appropriate use in specific groups: patients with anticipated significant blood loss, patients in whom significant anemia could not be corrected preoperatively, and those who may not tolerate blood loss due to comorbidities. A maximal surgical blood ordering schedule (MSBOS) is a list of surgical procedures, along with the maximum number of blood units being crossmatched preoperatively for each procedure. MSBOS implementation, specific for an individual hospital, allows appropriate allocation and use of blood bank resources.[5,8]

PERIOPERATIVE MANAGEMENT

Treatment of Anemia

In some surgical groups, treatment of preoperative anemia has been shown to decrease transfusion and adverse outcomes.[8-11] At least 6 to 8 weeks of treatment are usually required to see an appropriate response to treatment with an increase in hemoglobin levels.[1-4]

Preoperative Interventions to Decrease the Risk of Transfusion and Adverse Perioperative Outcomes Associated with Anemia

Optimization of contributing and complicating chronic illnesses, including cardiovascular disease, lung disease, and disorders that increase bleeding risk, may improve perioperative outcomes in anemic patients. The elements that can be most readily optimized are the hematinic or nutrient substrate deficiencies (e.g., iron, vitamin B_{12}, folate).[1,2]

- *Correct iron deficiency*—The most common nutritional deficiency that causes anemia is iron deficiency, which can be associated with multiple causes including malabsorption, blood loss, and hemolysis. Treatment of iron deficiency anemia before surgery may reduce the rate of PRBC transfusion, although available evidence conflicts.[8] In a meta-analysis of major noncardiac surgical patients, perioperative iron therapy was associated with a reduction in transfusion and mortality, without a substantial effect on hemoglobin.[9] In a recent systemic review, preoperative oral and IV iron therapy did not reduce blood transfusions.[12] The PREVENTT study in abdominal surgery patients

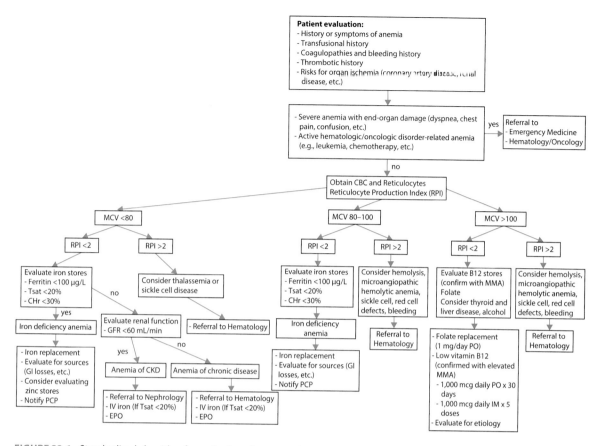

FIGURE 22-1. Standardized algorithm for evaluation of preoperative anemia.
Hgb, hemoglobin; CBC, complete blood count; MCV, mean corpuscular volume; IDA, iron deficiency anemia; IV, intravenous; IM, Internal Medicine; RPI, reticulocyte production index.
Adapted from Warner MA, Shore-Lesseson L, Shander A, Patel SY, Perelman SI, Guinn NR. Perioperative anemia: prevention, diagnosis, and management throughout the spectrum of perioperative care. *Anesth Analg.* 2020 May;130(5):1364–1380. PMID: 32167979; Slawski B. Ch 21. Anemia and transfusion medicine. In Cohn S. *Decision making in perioperative medicine: clinical pearls.* McGraw Hill. 2021.

TABLE 22-1. Differentiating Anemias Based on Lab Testing			
LAB TEST	IRON DEFICIENCY ANEMIA	ANEMIA OF INFLAMMATION	COMBINED IRON DEFICIENCY/ ANEMIA OF INFLAMMATION
Iron level	Decreased	Decreased	Decreased
Total iron binding capacity	Increased	Decreased or normal	Decreased
Transferrin saturation	Decreased <20%	Decreased	Decreased
Ferritin	Decreased <100 ng/mL	Normal or increased	Reduced to normal
Reticulocyte hemoglobin content (CHr)	Decreased <30%	Normal	Normal

with anemia demonstrated that one dose of IV iron approximately 2 weeks before surgery did not reduce perioperative transfusion or mortality when compared to placebo.[13] If time to surgery is sufficient, iron therapy may improve the preoperative hemoglobin and/or decrease the risk of perioperative transfusion.

■ *Oral iron*—Although oral iron can be effective, its utility in the preoperative period is somewhat limited by a long timeframe to efficacy, poor oral absorption in some patients, and side effects. Oral iron formulations include ferrous sulfate, ferrous gluconate, and ferrous fumarate. Iron absorption in the gastrointestinal tract is limited. Approximately 20–25% of an oral iron dose is absorbed, and higher doses result in increased side effects, especially constipation, without substantial incremental benefit. Elemental iron doses of 15–30 mg daily are adequate to replete iron stores with a better side effect profile. However, serum hepcidin levels rise for 24 hours after an oral iron dosing, with subsequent impaired absorption of additional iron supplements given later on the same or next day. Therefore, to enhance iron absorption from supplements, it is best to administer once daily on alternate days. It takes about 4–8 weeks to see a 2-g hemoglobin increase with oral dosing,

assuming no ongoing blood loss. Oral iron is better absorbed in an acidic environment, so it may be given along with oral ascorbic acid. We recommend a dose of 500 mg vitamin C for a dose of 60 mg of elemental iron.[1]

■ *Intravenous (IV) iron therapy* is indicated in patients who cannot absorb oral iron or require a rapid response to therapy. IV iron preparations include ferric carboxymaltose, ferric gluconate, iron sucrose, and iron dextran. IV iron is more expensive than oral iron, and dextran preparations have been associated with anaphylaxis. However, in general, IV iron is safe. In a study of 13,509 iron infusions, there was a 1.4% incidence of infusion reactions. In patients with Fishbane reaction (transient flushing, truncal myalgias) or mild reaction (localized cutaneous manifestations, non-hives), the infusion was safely recommenced or switched to a different iron preparation.[14] Typically, IV iron will also increase the hemoglobin level more rapidly than oral iron and may be useful in patients with a shorter interval to surgery for whom the procedure cannot be delayed. IV iron dosing and frequency vary by preparation (Table 22-2).

■ *Vitamin B$_{12}$ deficiency* can be repleted orally or parenterally. High-dose oral B$_{12}$ therapy (2,000 mcg/day) has been demonstrated in some studies

TABLE 22-2. Intravenous Iron Preparations

IRON FORMULATION	DOSE/ INFUSION	FREQUENCY/NUMBER OF DOSES	NOTES
Iron dextran	100–1,000 mg IV	Can be given daily until calculated dose is reached, or A 1,000 mg single dose can be given	Risk of hypersensitivity reactions/ anaphylaxis more prevalent in high molecular weight than low molecular weight formulations; requires a test dose
Sodium ferric gluconate	62.5–125 mg	Four to eight daily doses	
Iron sucrose	100–200 mg	Five doses over 14 days	Has the safest profile
Ferumoxytol	510 mg	Two doses separated by 3–8 days	Number of doses is low over a short period
Ferric carboxymaltose	750 mg	Two doses separated by at least 7 days	Number of doses is low over a short period. Increased risk of hypophosphatemia
Ferric derisomaltose	1,000 mg	Single dose	Less risk of hypophosphatemia

to be equally effective to parental therapy in producing a hematologic response. However, parental therapy is preferred in patients with suspicion for malabsorption or pernicious anemia. Patients generally have a brisk increase in reticulocyte count within a week and total recovery of anemia at 6–8 weeks.

- *Folate deficiency* is a rare cause of anemia in people with adequate oral intake because foods commonly contain folate supplements. In patients with suspected or confirmed folate deficiency, 1–5 mg/day orally usually corrects anemia, and parental therapy is reserved for patients with malabsorption.

- *Erythropoiesis-stimulating agents (ESAs)* may reduce the risk of transfusion in patients with renal insufficiency, anemia of chronic inflammation, and potentially those who decline transfusion; however, like the use of preoperative iron therapy, there is conflicting evidence.[5] In a recent systematic review and meta-analysis, use of ESAs in surgical patients resulted in a significant decrease in allogeneic blood transfusion in all patients, cardiac, and elective orthopedic surgery patients.[10] ESAs may be effective with coadministration of iron in patients with anemia or chronic inflammation and anemia associated with kidney disease.[5,11] A recent systemic review of anemic noncardiac surgery patients showed that preoperative ESA and iron therapy increased hemoglobin concentrations and decreased the need for red cell transfusion; however, there was not a substantial impact on the number of units transfused or mortality.[15] Although there is concern about VTE events in patients using ESAs, two recent meta-analyses in surgical patients have not demonstrated a difference in thromboembolic complications.[10,11] ESAs have also been associated with increased risks of hypertension and cancer progression in patients with malignancies. Expert consensus recommendations and guidelines vary in whether ESAs should be used preoperatively.[5,8]

- *Anemia of inflammation* is a functional iron deficiency anemia in which iron stores are normal with low serum iron levels. This is common in patients with malignancy, renal insufficiency, chronic infections (e.g., osteomyelitis), and critical illness. Concomitant absolute iron deficiency should also be considered in patients with renal insufficiency. The best approach in these patients is to treat the underlying illness if possible; however, in many patients, iron supplementation and ESAs are used because underlying diseases cannot be reversed.

Intraoperative considerations, in detail, are beyond the scope of this chapter and include fluid management, temperature control, intraoperative blood conservation, and use of fibrinolytic agents, as well as acute normovolemic hemodilution.[5]

Transfusion

Blood management protocols can decrease the use of allogeneic blood and include multimodal protocols, specific transfusion criteria, and maximal surgical blood order schedules.[5,8]

Autologous donation of PRBCs in preoperative patients has been used as a method of decreasing the risk of postoperative allogeneic PRBC transfusion; however, this is not usually an effective venture, given that it takes weeks for optimal red cell regeneration, and as the pre-donation hemoglobin value may not be achieved, patients may present to surgery with iatrogenic anemia. Additionally, due to the cost of collecting and storing autologous blood, which is often wasted, healthcare facilities are increasingly limiting this process.[16]

Indications for Transfusion in the Postoperative Period

Multiple trials have demonstrated that when compared to higher transfusion thresholds (hemoglobin >10 g/dL), transfusing postoperative patients at hemoglobin thresholds of 7–8 g/dL or if symptomatic is not associated with a difference in mortality and complications. This has been demonstrated in cardiac and noncardiac surgery patients, as well as patients with underlying cardiovascular disease. Specific guidelines for transfusion thresholds include[4]:

- <7 g/dL for most hospitalized patients who are hemodynamically stable, including critically ill patients, rather than a hemoglobin of 10 g/dL.
- <7.5 g/dL is recommended for cardiac surgery patients.
- <8 g/dL is recommended for orthopedic surgery patients.

A threshold of <7 g/dL is likely comparable to 8 g/dL; however, randomized controlled trial evidence is still lacking.

Special Populations. Several patient populations have unique considerations when considering transfusion.

- Transplant patients may require leukocyte-reduced or cytomegalovirus-negative blood products.

- Antibodies may make type and crossmatch challenging. Careful review of medical records will reveal some patients in whom previous crossmatching was difficult and/or prolonged due to antibodies. These patients need crossmatching in advance of the surgical day to increase the ability to provide matched blood products.

- Sickle cell anemia patients have unique preoperative considerations, and perioperative clinicians can collaborate with their hematologist to guide care. Surgery can increase anemia, and surgical stress can lead to additional sickle cell formation. A multicenter study demonstrated that patients with sickle disease have improved outcomes with a preoperative hemoglobin of 10 g/dL. Simple transfusion, as opposed to strategies such as exchange transfusion, is recommended preoperatively. Hematology consultation may also be considered.[1]

Consent

Patients being considered for transfusion should receive informed consent. Some patients may decline transfusion based on religious or other personal beliefs. This should be carefully discussed and documented in the record including which, if any, blood products would be acceptable.

CONCLUSIONS

Perioperative anemia is associated with adverse outcomes. Targeted preoperative evaluation can identify patients with anemia and permit intervention that improves patient outcomes. Transfusions are associated with risks and costs that can be reduced by alternative treatment of anemia and targeted transfusion thresholds.

Clinical pearls

- Preoperative hemoglobin levels are indicated for patients scheduled to undergo procedures with expected significant blood loss or where history or physical exam suggest a likelihood of anemia, not in young, healthy patients and those undergoing low-bleeding-risk procedures.

- Oral iron has limited absorption, and elemental iron doses beyond 30 mg daily cause increased side effects without clinical benefit. Hemoglobin levels are expected to increase by 2 g/dL every 4–8 weeks with oral iron supplementation and more rapidly with IV replacement.

- A restrictive strategy with a transfusion threshold of 7 g/dL is appropriate in most surgical patients.

REFERENCES

1. Gómez-Ramírez S, Jericó C, Muñoz M. Perioperative anemia: prevalence, consequences and pathophysiology. *Transfus Apher Sci*. 2019;58(4):369-374. PMID: 31416710

2. Warner MA, Shore-Lesserson L, Shander A, et al. Perioperative anemia: prevention, diagnosis, and management throughout the spectrum of perioperative care. *Anesth Analg*. 2020;130(5):1364-1380. PMID: 32167979

3. Musallam KM, Tamim HM, Richards T, et al. Preoperative anaemia and postoperative outcomes in non-cardiac surgery: a retrospective cohort study. *Lancet*. 2011;378(9800):1396-1407. PMID: 21982521

4. Carson JL, Stanworth SJ, Guyatt G, et al. Red blood cell transfusion: 2023 AABB international guidelines. *JAMA*. 2023;330(19):1892-1902. PMID: 37824153

5. American Society of Anesthesiologists Task Force on Perioperative Blood Management. Practice guidelines for perioperative blood management: an updated report by the American Society of Anesthesiologists Task Force on perioperative blood management. *Anesthesiology*. 2015;122(2):241-275. PMID: 25545654

6. Ming Y, Med M, Liu J, et al. Transfusion of red blood cells, fresh frozen plasma, or platelets is associated with mortality and infection after cardiac surgery in a dose-dependent manner. *Anesth Analg*. 2020;130(2):488-497. PMID: 31702696

7. American Society of Anesthesiologists Task Force on Preanesthesia Evaluation. Practice advisory for

preanesthesia evaluation: an updated report by the American Society of Anesthesiologists Task Force on preanesthesia evaluation. *Anesthesiology.* 2012;116(3):522-538. PMID: 22273990

8. Mueller MM, Van Remoortel H, Meybohm P, et al. Patient blood management: recommendations from the 2018 Frankfurt Consensus Conference. *JAMA.* 2019;321(10):983-997. PMID: 30860564

9. Schack A, Berkfors AA, Ekeloef S, et al. The effect of perioperative iron therapy in acute major non-cardiac surgery on allogenic blood transfusion and postoperative haemoglobin levels: a systematic review and meta-analysis. *World J Surg.* 2019;43(7):1677-1691. PMID: 30824959

10. Cho BC, Serini J, Zorrilla-Vaca A, et al. Impact of preoperative erythropoietin on allogeneic blood transfusions in surgical patients: results from a systematic review and meta-analysis. *Anesth Analg.* 2019;128(5):981-992. PMID: 30649068

11. Kei T, Mistry N, Curley G, et al. Efficacy and safety of erythropoietin and iron therapy to reduce red blood cell transfusion in surgical patients: a systematic review and meta-analysis. *Can J Anaesth.* 2019;66(6):716-731. PMID: 30924000

12. Ng O, Keeler BD, Mishra A, et al. Iron therapy for preoperative anaemia. *Cochrane Database Syst Rev.* 2019;12(12):CD011588. PMID: 31811820

13. Richards T, Baikady R, Clevenger B, et al. Preoperative intravenous iron to treat anaemia before major abdominal surgery (PREVENTT): a randomised, double-blind, controlled trial. *Lancet.* 2020;396(10259):1353-1361. PMID: 32896294

14. Stojanovic S, Graudins LV, Aung AK, et al. Safety of intravenous iron following infusion reactions. *J Allergy Clin Immunol Pract.* 2021;9(4):1660-1666. PMID: 33248279

15. Kaufner L, von Heymann C, Henkelman A, et al. Erythropoietin plus iron versus control treatment including placebo or iron for preoperative anaemic adults undergoing non-cardiac surgery. *Cochrane Database Syst Rev.* 2020;13(8):CD012451. PMID: 32790892

16. Vassallo R, Goldman M, Germain M, Lozano M, BEST Collaborative. Preoperative autologous blood donation: waning indications in an era of improved blood safety. *Transfus Med Rev.* 2015;29(4):268-275. PMID: 26006319

## 23

Coagulation Disorders

Kurt Pfeifer, MD, FACP, SFHM, DFPM

COMMON CLINICAL QUESTIONS

1. Are coagulation and hematologic laboratory studies required to screen surgical patients for undiagnosed bleeding disorders?

2. What is the appropriate workup for a patient with abnormalities in coagulation studies?

3. What are key considerations in the management of patients with hereditary bleeding disorders?

INTRODUCTION

Disorders of coagulation challenge normal hemostasis, increasing the risk of bleeding complications and the need for transfusion of blood products. Thrombotic coagulation disorders can be associated with increased risk of perioperative arterial and venous thromboembolic events.

Bleeding disorders can be categorized by disorders of platelets and the coagulation system proteins including clotting factors. Mild disorders often do not require hemostatic intervention to allow for surgery. More severe bleeding disorders can typically be treated with medications, factor concentrates, and transfusions to allow for surgery to be successfully completed.

Thrombotic disorders can be inherited or acquired. This chapter will review inherited thrombophilias and the antiphospholipid antibody (APLA) syndrome. Other acquired thrombophilic conditions, including liver disease, malignancy, kidney disease, and rheumatic diseases, are reviewed in other chapters. Perioperative management of antiplatelet and anticoagulants is also covered elsewhere within this textbook (see Chapters 4, 5, and 11).

PREOPERATIVE EVALUATION

All patients undergoing planned surgical treatment warrant preoperative evaluation for a bleeding disorder. Despite advances in ease and reliability of blood counts, coagulation studies, and thrombophilia tests, an accurate history and physical examination remain the most effective screening tools for bleeding and clotting disorders. Multiple meta-analyses have demonstrated routine use of "screening" coagulation tests in asymptomatic patients leads to inappropriate delay of procedures and unnecessary concern for patients with abnormal results.[1] Instead, a focused history should evaluate for personal or family history of bleeding and clotting symptoms, previous procedural complications, obstetric/gynecologic history, and medications. Physical examination findings that may suggest an underlying bleeding disorder and warrant further evaluation include petechiae, ecchymosis, joint hypermobility, telangiectasias, joint hypermobility, jaundice, and other stigmata of liver disease.

If the history or physical exam is suggestive of a possible bleeding disorder, laboratory evaluation is warranted. Initial laboratory evaluation should include a complete blood count (CBC), prothrombin time (PT), and partial thromboplastin time (PTT).

A. Abnormal PT/INR /PTT Evaluation

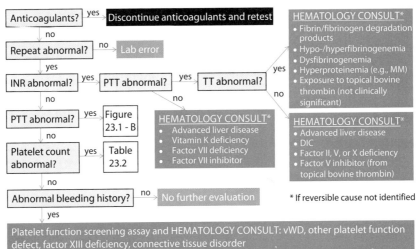

B. Isolated PTT Elevation

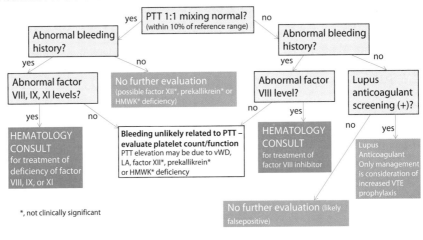

Adapted from Tcherniantchouk O et al. Am J Hematol. 2013;88:82-85.

FIGURE 23-1. Diagnostic approach to the patient with an abnormal PT/INR and/or PTT.
Reproduced with permission from Pfeifer K. www.preopevalguide.com.
HMWK, high-molecular-weight kininogen; LA, lupus anticoagulant; vWD, von Willebrand disease.

Additional diagnostic testing including liver and kidney function, peripheral blood smear, coagulation factors (factor VIII, IX, XI, fibrinogen, von Willebrand factors [vWF]), and platelet function assays should be performed based on both clinical suspicion of possible bleeding disorder and screening labs.

Table 23-1 reviews causes of prolongation of PT and PTT, and Figure 23-1 includes algorithms on the diagnostic approach to evaluation of the patient with an abnormal PT/INR and/or PTT. Table 23-2 reviews common causes of thrombocytopenia. If diagnosis is uncertain, preoperative evaluation by a hematologist

TABLE 23-1. Causes of Bleeding Associated with Prolongation of PT/INR and PTT

TEST		CAUSE OF BLEEDING
PT/INR	PTT	
Prolonged	Normal	Inherited: Factor VII deficiency
		Acquired: Warfarin use, mild vitamin K deficiency
Normal	Prolonged	Inherited: Factor VIII, Factor IX, or Factor XI deficiency (hemophilia); Factor XII deficiency (not associated with bleeding)
		Acquired: Heparin, some DOACs, lupus anticoagulant (associated with thrombosis), inhibitor to factor VIII, IX, XI
Prolonged	Prolonged	Inherited: Factor II, V, or X deficiency; dysfibrinogenemia
		Acquired: Liver disease, DIC, severe vitamin K deficiency, supratherapeutic warfarin, acquired factor X or V deficiency
Normal	Normal	Inherited: vWD, platelet function defect, congenital thrombocytopenia
		Acquired: Antiplatelet medication, acquired vWD

PT, prothrombin time; PTT, partial thromboplastin time; DOACs, direct oral anticoagulants; DIC, disseminated intravascular coagulation; vWD, von Willebrand disease.

TABLE 23-2. Common Causes of Thrombocytopenia

	CAUSES OF THROMBOCYTOPENIA
Pseudothrombocytopenia	In vitro clumping of platelets related to agglutination from EDTA; not a cause of true thrombocytopenia
Primary immune thrombocytopenia	
Drugs	Sulfonamides, quinine, NSAIDs, penicillins, linezolid, vancomycin, GP II b/IIIa inhibitors, antiepileptics, alcohol, immunosuppression
Infections	HIV, hepatitis C, Epstein-Barr virus, cytomegalovirus, *H. pylori*, ehrlichiosis, babesiosis
Liver Disease	Impaired thrombopoietin production, splenic sequestration
Nutritional	Deficiency of vitamin B_{12}, folic acid, copper
Rheumatologic	Rheumatoid arthritis, systemic lupus erythematosus, antiphospholipid antibody syndrome
Malignancy	Lymphoproliferative neoplasms, myelodysplastic syndrome, other hematologic malignancy, myelofibrosis, bone marrow metastases
Bone Marrow Failure Syndromes	Aplastic anemia, paroxysmal nocturnal hemoglobinuria, Fanconi's anemia
Thrombotic Microangiopathies	TTP, HUS, DIC, HELLP syndrome, malignant hypertension
Hereditary	von Willebrand disease type 2B, Wiskott-Aldrich syndrome, May Heglin anomaly, Bernard-Soulier syndrome

TTP, thrombotic thrombocytopenia purpura; HUS, hemolytic uremic syndrome; DIC, disseminated intravascular anticoagulation.

is appropriate to establish a diagnosis and determine an appropriate treatment plan. Regular use of whole blood and point of care assays including bleeding time (BT), platelet function analyzer (PFA-100), and thromboelastography (TEG) have not been reliable at predicting perioperative bleeding.

Preoperative evaluation of inherited thrombophilias rarely impacts perioperative management and should not regularly be performed unless it is likely to affect recommendations for perioperative thromboprophylaxis.

PERIOPERATIVE MANAGEMENT

Coagulation disorders often require specialized perioperative management to reduce bleeding and thrombotic risk. Treatment of bleeding disorders typically involves transient replacement or improvement of defects in platelets or coagulation factors rather than using a global prohemostatic agent. Appropriate use of specific therapies attempts to minimize risk of thrombosis, hypervolemia, allergy, alloimmunization, and infection from hemostatic agents. Cooperation with hematology, transfusion medicine, anesthesiology, and pharmacy is essential for perioperative management of bleeding disorders. Regardless of the type of coagulation abnormality, blood product needs should be anticipated, and an appropriate number of units made available.

Thrombocytopenia

A normal platelet count is typically 150–350,000/μL subject to variations in laboratory and physiologic state (e.g., pregnancy). Reduction in platelet count to <100,000/μL has been associated with a nearly doubled risk of postoperative death, as well as increased risk of sepsis, renal and pulmonary injury, and possibly bleeding.[2] Perioperative thrombocytopenia has been historically categorized into mild (100–149,000/μL), moderate (50–99,000/μL), and severe (<50,000/μL). The clinical utility of this categorization is of uncertain benefit. The relationship between platelet count and bleeding risk is not linear and depends on platelet function, other hemostatic defects, and patient-specific variables. Data from large studies suggest that the risk of spontaneous bleeding is difficult to predict until platelet count decreases to extremely low values, below approximately 7,000–10,000/μL. Few studies

TABLE 23-3. Target Platelet Count for Procedures

PLATELET COUNT TARGET	PROCEDURE/ SITUATION	SOCIETY
>100,000/μL	Neuro or posterior eye surgery	BCSH
>50,000/μL	Major nonneuraxial surgery	AABB
>50,000/μL	Therapeutic enteroscopy	ASGE
>50,000/μL	Liver, renal, or transbronchial biopsy	JPAC
>20,000/μL	Central vascular access device	AABB
>20,000/μL	Diagnostic enteroscopy	ASGE
>20,000/μL	Bronchoscopic lavage	BTS
>10,000/μL	Prophylaxis against spontaneous bleeding	AABB

BCSH, British Committee for Standardization in Hematology; AABB, American Association of Blood Banking; ASGE, American Society for GI Endoscopy; JPAC, Joint UK Blood Transfusion Professional Advisory Committee; BTS, British Thoracic Society.
Source: Data from Nagrebetsky et al. *Br J Anaesthesia*, 2019.

have demonstrated benefit in prophylactic platelet transfusions to achieve platelet counts above a perioperative target. Table 23-3 summarizes significant platelet count thresholds for patients undergoing elective procedures, recognizing that recommendations are based on weak or ungraded levels of evidence.

Immune Thrombocytopenia (ITP). ITP is characterized by thrombocytopenia caused by increased clearance of platelets due to autoantibodies against platelet antigens. ITP can occur in association with other diseases and treatments (rheumatologic conditions, lymphoproliferative disorders, viral infections, immunodeficiency syndromes, drugs) or be idiopathic/primary. Platelet counts typically rise within 7 days following administration of glucocorticoids (prednisone 1 mg/kg daily or dexamethasone 40 mg daily). Time to response can be shortened (to usually <72 hours) with concurrent administration of intravenous immunoglobulin (IVIG). Combinations of glucocorticoids and/or IVIG can often be used preoperatively to increase platelet counts above a surgical threshold. Potential perioperative complications include hyperglycemia, hypervolemia, acute kidney injury, infection, and impaired wound healing. In cases of refractory ITP, platelet transfusion can be considered. However, duration and degree of platelet count response to platelet transfusion is often limited in the setting of ITP, and a platelet count should be repeated 1 hour after transfusion of platelets. Thrombopoietin (TPO) receptor agonists, including romiplostim, eltrombopag, avatrombopag, and lusutrombopag, can increase megakaryocyte production of platelets. Both eltrombopag and romiplostim are FDA-approved for treatment of ITP and have been shown to improve platelet counts perioperatively.

Drug-Induced Thrombocytopenia. Drugs cause thrombocytopenia via different mechanisms including induction of platelet antibodies, suppression of megakaryocytes, and activation of platelets causing consumption. At least 253 drugs have been associated with thrombocytopenia.[3] Perioperative complications are most commonly seen with glycoprotein IIb/IIIa inhibitors, amiodarone, penicillins, antipsychotics, linezolid, vancomycin, nonsteroidal anti-inflammatory drugs (NSAIDs), and trimethoprim-sulfamethoxazole. The degree of thrombocytopenia and risk of perioperative hemorrhage varies. Treatment includes discontinuation of the causative drug (if possible) and platelet transfusion as needed.

Heparin-Induced Thrombocytopenia (HIT). HIT is a prothrombotic disorder characterized by thrombocytopenia caused by activation and consumption of platelets via antibodies to the heparin-platelet factor 4 (PF4) complex. HIT most commonly occurs 5–10 days after exposure to heparins, causes a reduction in platelet count by at least 50% from baseline, and is associated with both arterial and venous thrombosis. Diagnosis is made by use of a pretest probability scoring system (the 4T test) and confirmatory labs including PF4 ELISA and serotonin-release assay. When HIT is diagnosed, all heparin products should be discontinued and alternative anticoagulation initiated with direct thrombin

inhibitors (argatroban, bivalirudin) or fondaparinux, an indirect Factor Xa inhibitor (although it is not FDA-approved for this indication). Emerging data suggest treatment with direct oral anticoagulants including factor Xa inhibitors (apixaban, rivaroxaban, edoxaban) and direct thrombin inhibitors (dabigatran) is effective in management of HIT, but these drugs have not been FDA-approved for this indication.[4]

Persons with a history of HIT can be safely exposed to heparin transiently during surgery (e.g., cardiopulmonary bypass) provided they have normal preoperative platelet count, resolution of PF4 antibodies prior to heparin reexposure, and postoperative heparin exposure is minimized.[5] PF4 antibodies peak after 14 days of final exposure to heparin, and most have resolved by 120 days following heparin cessation. Venous thromboembolism (VTE) prophylaxis with heparins (including low-molecular-weight heparin) should be avoided in persons with a prior diagnosis of HIT.

Platelet Dysfunction

Platelet function (adherence to damaged endothelium, activation/granule release, and aggregation) can be impaired in both congenital and acquired conditions. Platelet function defects tend to be associated with a mild bleeding diathesis but can be associated with surgical hemorrhage.

Medications are the most common cause of platelet dysfunction. Antiplatelet agents (aspirin, clopidogrel, prasugrel, ticagrelor, dipyridamole) and NSAIDs are typically held at least 5–7 days prior to surgical procedures. More mild antiplatelet effects can be seen with selective serotonin reuptake inhibitors (SSRIs), proton pump inhibitors (PPIs), alcohol, and antiepileptics.[6] Some herbal supplements (ginkgo, ginseng, turmeric, willow, fish oil) may be associated with bleeding and are typically stopped 1–2 weeks prior to surgery when time permits.

Renal failure has been shown to reduce platelet expression of glycoprotein-Ib, decrease platelet granule content, and increase platelet cyclic adenosine monophosphate content. It is uncertain that uremic toxins directly affect platelet function, although platelet function is impaired by both acute and chronic kidney injury. Uremic patients should undergo dialysis prior to elective surgery. Hematologic malignancies, including myeloproliferative neoplasms, myelodysplastic syndrome (MDS), multiple myeloma, and some lymphomas and leukemias, can be associated with platelet dysfunction. These disorders tend to respond well to both platelet transfusions and use of desmopressin (DDAVP) and antifibrinolytic therapy.

Congenital disorders of platelet function tend to be rare. These include Bernard-Soulier syndrome, Glanzmann's thrombasthenia, gray platelet syndrome, storage pool defects, and Wiskott-Aldrich syndrome. Recombinant factor VIIa is approved for treatment of bleeding and surgical complications in Glanzmann's thrombasthenia. Other congenital platelet defects are treated with platelet transfusion.

There is a paucity of clinical trial evidence to guide the management of bleeding due to other platelet function defects. Tranexamic acid and aminocaproic acid are inhibitors of fibrinolysis, widely used in high-risk surgery and trauma to reduce bleeding. DDAVP can stimulate hemostasis by increasing plasma levels of vWF and factor VIII, with secondary increases in platelet adhesion and activation. Platelet transfusions can be used in the setting of platelet function disorders if bleeding exceeds anticipated levels.

Coagulation Factor Defects

Adequate hemostasis requires the formation of a fibrin-based clot to stabilize a platelet plug at the site of endothelial injury. Endothelial injury and platelet activation drive thrombin generation, which acts as a regulator in fibrin formation. Deficits in clotting factors are relatively uncommon but have profound impact on perioperative care due to the severity of bleeding associated with some disorders as well as the cost of intervention. Most cases of congenital factor deficiencies are diagnosed in childhood, although mild cases and von Willebrand disease (vWD) are often diagnosed later in life.

von Willebrand Disease. vWD is the most common hereditary bleeding disorder and is caused by deficiency (types 1 and 3) or dysfunction (type 2) of vWF. vWF is responsible for platelet adherence to damaged endothelium by binding both platelet factor Ib and collagen in the subendothelial matrix. Additionally, vWF acts as a carrier protein for factor VIII, preventing rapid cleavage by normal endothelial cells. vWD has an estimated prevalence of 1–2% in the general population and can be inherited in both autosomal dominant (more common) and autosomal recessive patterns. The disease is manifested by failure of the primary phase of hemostasis, causing mucocutaneous bleeding. More severe cases can induce failure of the secondary phase of hemostasis, causing bleeding in soft tissue sites and postoperative bleeding.

Most cases of vWD are mild quantitative deficits of vWF (type 1 disease). Bleeding severity can vary, but most cases tend to be mild. Administration of IV or intranasal DDAVP releases vWF from stores in both endothelial cells and platelets, leading to a transient rise in circulating vWF. DDAVP can be used preoperatively in most patients with type 1 vWD and some subtypes of qualitative (type 2) vWD (type 2A, 2M, 2D). DDAVP can cause flushing, fluid retention, and hyponatremia, and can only be used for 2 consecutive days to avoid tachyphylaxis. Test doses should be given before use in operative settings to assure a patient sufficiently responds.

Absence of vWF (type 3 vWD) and severe type 1 and 2 vWD typically require perioperative administration of recombinant or plasma-derived vWF concentrates. Differences between vWF concentrates include differences in content of high-molecular-weight multimers, factor VIII, and need for viral inactivation. Dosing is based on vWF:ristocetin cofactor units with the goal to keep vWF activity >50% for 3–5 days and factor VIII activity >50% for 5–7 days postoperatively.[7]

Coagulation Factor Deficiencies

Hemophilia A (factor VIII deficiency) is an X-linked recessive disorder caused by mutation of the gene encoding factor VIII. It occurs in 1/5,000–1/10,000 male births and has equal prevalence among all ethnicities. The disease is classified into three forms: severe (50–60% of patients), moderately severe (25–30%), and mild (15–20%). Severity of bleeding complications is directly proportional to factor VIII activity level. Severe hemophilia A is seen with factor VIII activity <1% of normal and is characterized by spontaneous hemorrhage into joints and soft tissues. Patients with moderately severe hemophilia A have 2–5% of normal factor VIII activity and are prone to bleeding after minor trauma. In the mild form of hemophilia A, factor VIII activity ranges from 5% to 30%, and bleeding typically only occurs with significant trauma or surgery.

Hemophilia B (factor IX deficiency; Christmas disease) is another X-linked recessive disorder caused by mutation of the factor IX gene. It is less common than hemophilia A, accounting for 12% of total hemophilia cases, and is more frequently associated with de novo mutations. Bleeding complications correlate well with factor IX activity and are phenotypically identical to those seen with hemophilia A.

Hemophilia C (factor XI deficiency; Rosenthal syndrome) is a rare autosomal recessive disorder most commonly identified in Ashkenazi Jews. PTT is typically prolonged in the disorder. It is associated with a milder bleeding phenotype than deficiencies of either factor VIII or IX.

Factor XII deficiency causes prolongation of the PTT, which corrects on 1:1 mixing study. However, this effect occurs in vitro and is not associated with a bleeding diathesis.

Other inherited bleeding diatheses: Deficiencies of several other coagulation factors (II, V, VII, X, and XIII) and congenital disorders of fibrinogen also predispose patients to bleeding, but they are very rare and beyond the scope of this text.

Elective and emergent surgery can be performed safely in most cases of hemophilia. Use of recombinant or plasma-derived clotting factor concentrates allows normalization of factor VIII or IX activity during the perioperative period. For most major procedures, a target preoperative factor activity of 80–100% of normal is recommended at the time of first incision. Thereafter, factor activity is maintained above 25–50% over a period of 7–14 days.[8] Novel hemophilia therapies, including extended half-life clotting factors and emicizumab, a bispecific factor IXa–factor X antibody, promise to ease administration of therapy to patients requiring surgery.

Coagulation Factor Inhibitors. Approximately 20–30% of patients with hemophilia A and 3% with hemophilia B will develop inhibitors to coagulation factors VIII and IX. These inhibitors are antibodies against infused clotting factors that inhibit the function of the clotting factor. In addition to congenital hemophilia-associated coagulation inhibitors, spontaneous occurrence of factor VIII-inhibiting autoantibodies against factor VIII has been documented in the elderly and the peripartum period. Bleeding manifestations of hemophilia with inhibitors are severe and

often life-threatening. In the setting of a newly recognized factor inhibitor, surgery is typically deferred. If emergent surgical management is required, use of high doses of factor concentrates to overwhelm the neutralizing antibody or use of bypassing agents, such as recombinant factor VIIa or factor-VIII bypassing agent (FEIBA), to drive thrombin formation via the extrinsic pathway can be considered.

Disorders of Both Platelets and Coagulation Factors

Liver Disease. Liver disease is associated with increased perioperative morbidity and mortality, and further discussion is available in other chapters. Bleeding and thrombotic complications are both increased in the perioperative setting in patients with liver disease. Liver disease induces thrombocytopenia via multiple mechanisms including impaired TPO production, splenic sequestration of platelets in the setting of portal hypertension, and increased platelet consumption. Both procoagulant and anticoagulant proteins are predominantly synthesized in the liver, and factor activities are decreased in even mild liver disease.

Guidelines from the International Society on Thrombosis and Hemostasis (ISTH) do not recommend routine assessment of PT, PTT, platelet count, and fibrinogen before surgery, nor do they recommend prophylactic interventions to correct abnormalities of these studies.[9] Prophylactic platelet transfusions in cirrhotic patients prior to surgery are also not advised by the ISTH except for procedures with very high bleeding risks, such as neurosurgery. The TPO agonists avatrombopag and lusutrombopag are approved to raise platelet counts perioperatively in adults with chronic liver disease and thrombocytopenia.

Thrombotic Microangiopathies (TMAs). TMAs represent a series of hematologic disorders characterized by consumptive thrombocytopenia, fragmentation hemolysis, and multisystem end-organ dysfunction. Prototypes of TMA include thrombotic thrombocytopenic purpura (TTP), hemolytic uremic syndrome (HUS), HELLP syndrome, and disseminated intravascular coagulation (DIC). In the setting of an acute TMA, elective surgeries should be deferred given the risk of both thrombotic and bleeding complications. If emergent surgery is required, supportive treatment with blood transfusion support in addition to treatment of the underlying cause may be required.

Thrombophilias

Generation of thrombus is an essential component of hemostasis and involves complex regulation between the endothelium, platelets, and procoagulant and anticoagulant proteins. Surgical procedures increase the risk of thrombotic complications. Strategies to reduce the potential impact of perioperative arterial and venous thrombosis are discussed in other chapters.

While many congenital thrombophilias have now been well described, their impact on surgical outcome is disputed. Most patients with inherited thrombophilias warrant routine thromboprophylactic strategies to decrease the risk of VTE events. While many guidelines recommend prophylactic anticoagulation be considered perioperatively in those with inherited thrombophilias, these guidelines do not recommend testing for inherited thrombophilia prior to surgery. Thrombophilia testing rarely influences decision making around anticoagulation, and its routine use has been discouraged.[10]

Acquired thrombophilias are more predictive of perioperative thrombotic risk than inherited thrombophilias. Acquired risks include malignancy, chemotherapy, immobility, trauma, extended hospitalization, inflammatory disease, and infection. Scoring systems to determine appropriate thromboprophylaxis have been well described and are outlined in Chapter 6.

Factor V Leiden (FVL). Activated protein C (APC) is a potent inhibitor of the coagulation system, specifically cleaving the activated forms of factor V and VIII (FVa and FVIIIa). The FVL gene product makes factor V less susceptible to inactivation. FVL is the most common inherited thrombophilia, with a prevalence of 3–8% in Caucasian populations. Heterozygosity for FVL is moderately thrombophilic, with a lifetime sevenfold increased risk of venous thrombosis compared to the general population. Meta-analyses have demonstrated FVL heterozygosity is only weakly associated with increased risk of recurrence of venous thrombosis (odds ratio of 1.3). Because heterozygosity for FVL confers only a modest risk of recurrence, its finding alone should not

alter anticoagulation treatment decisions. Furthermore, family members of persons with FVL heterozygosity need not be routinely tested.

Prothrombin Gene Mutation. The prothrombin gene mutation is associated with threefold increased plasma levels of prothrombin. The mutation is found most commonly in those of southern European ancestry, with a prevalence throughout Europe of 0.7–4%. Heterozygosity for the prothrombin mutation is moderately thrombophilic, with a lifetime increased risk of venous thrombosis two- to threefold higher than the general population. Data suggesting that patients with prothrombin gene mutation are at increased risk of recurrent VTE are limited, with most studies failing to demonstrate an increased risk of recurrence for persons heterozygous for the gene mutation. Because heterozygosity for the prothrombin mutation confers only a modest risk of venous thrombosis, its finding alone should not alter anticoagulation treatment decisions.

Deficiencies of Anticoagulant Proteins (Protein C, Protein S, Antithrombin [AT]). APC works in conjunction with its cofactor, protein S, to inhibit factor V and thereby inhibit thrombin generation. Proteins C and S are vitamin K-dependent anticoagulant proteins responsible for the downregulation of the clotting system. Both qualitative and quantitative deficiencies in proteins C and S have been recognized since the mid-1980s as being thrombophilic. Deficiencies of proteins C and S occur in less than 1 per 1,000 persons and have variable clinical significance. Over 130 different mutations have been identified. Screening with functional and quantitative assays helps determine deficiency, although testing is not reliable if patients are using vitamin K antagonists. Treatment of protein C and S deficiency with anticoagulation requires special consideration for warfarin-induced skin necrosis. This transient hypercoagulable state is related to abrupt declines in protein C and S activity after the initiation of vitamin K antagonists. Bridging anticoagulation with a heparin product is required if warfarin is being initiated.

AT is a glycoprotein that inhibits thrombin, activated factor X, and activated factor IX. When bound to heparin, the AT-mediated inhibition of thrombin is increased 4,000-fold. AT deficiency occurs in 1 in every 2,500 persons and more than 120 different mutations have been described. Relative risk of VTE in AT deficiency is increased by 20 times, and the lifetime risk of VTE approaches 100% by the time the affected individual reaches 70 years of age. AT concentrates are commercially available and can be given perioperatively to decrease thrombotic risk. AT deficiency can cause heparin resistance, and close monitoring of factor Xa or PTT levels while using heparin or low-molecular-weight heparin is required in AT deficiency to ensure therapeutic anticoagulation.

Antiphospholipid Antibody (APLA) Syndrome. APLAs are acquired autoantibodies targeted against phospholipids and phospholipid-binding proteins such as beta-2 glycoprotein-I. These autoantibodies trigger the coagulation system and have been associated with increased risk of venous and arterial thrombosis. Diagnosis of APLA syndrome requires both evidence of a thrombotic event (venous or arterial thrombosis or recurrent late gestational loss) and persistent laboratory evidence of APLA over a 12-week period. APLAs are highly thrombophilic, and due to the high rate of recurrent thrombosis, patients with APLA syndrome should receive full dose anticoagulation pre- and postoperatively. Randomized controlled trials in APLA syndrome suggest warfarin is superior to DOACs and other anticoagulation. Patients with APLA syndrome should receive heparin bridging for most procedures.

> ### Clinical pearls
>
> - A complete history and physical examination remain the best screening tools to assess thrombotic and bleeding disorders preoperatively. Routine screening for bleeding disorders with lab testing is not recommended.
>
> - Thrombocytopenia is among the most common defects of coagulation. Clinical history and labs to determine the etiology of thrombocytopenia are warranted preoperatively.
>
> - Treatment of defects in coagulation proteins including vWD and hemophilia is effective for achieving surgical hemostasis, but coordination with hematology should be performed. Therapies differ among the different subtypes of vWD and hemophilia.
>
> - Thrombotic disorders are associated with increased risk of perioperative venous thrombosis.

REFERENCES

1. Chee YL, Crawford JS, Watson HG, et al. Guidelines on the assessment of bleeding risk prior to surgery or invasive procedure. *British J Haematol.* 2008;140(5):496. PMID: 18275427
2. Nagrebetsky A, Al-Samkari H, Davis NM, et al. Perioperative thrombocytopenia: evidence evaluation, and emerging therapies. *British J Anaesth.* 2019;122(1):19-31. PMID: 30579402
3. Reese JA, Li X, Hauben M, et al. Identifying drugs that cause acute thrombocytopenia: an analysis using 3 distinct methods. *Blood.* 2010;116(112):2127-2133. PMID: 20530792
4. Warkentin TE, Pai M, Linkins LA. Direct oral anticoagulants for treatment of HIT: update of the Hamilton experience and literature review. *Blood.* 2017;130(9):1104. PMID: 28646118
5. Tucker MJ, Sabnani I, Baran MA, et al. Cardiac transplantation and/or mechanical circulatory support device placement using heparin anti-coagulation in the presence of acute heparin-induced thrombocytopenia. *J Heart Lung Transplant.* 2010;29(1):53-60. PMID: 19819167
6. Brennan Y, Levade M, Ward CM. Acquired platelet function disorders. *Thromb Res.* 2020;196:561-568. PMID: 31229273
7. Laffan MA, Lester W, O'Donnell JS, et al. The diagnosis and management of von Willebrand disease: a United Kingdom Haemophilia Centre Doctors Organization guideline approved by the British Committee for Standards in Haematology. *Br J Haematol.* 2014;167(4):453-465. PMID: 25113304
8. Srivastava A, Brewer AK, Mauser-Bunschoten EP, et al. Guidelines for the management of hemophilia. *Haemophilia.* 2013;19(1):e1-e47. PMID: 22776238
9. Roberts LN, Lisman T, Stanworth S, et al. Periprocedural management of abnormal coagulation parameters and thrombocytopenia in patients with cirrhosis: guidance from the SSC of the ISTH. *J Thromb Haemost.* 2022;20(1):39-47. PMID: 34661370
10. Middledorp S, Vlieg AVH. Does thrombophilia testing help in the clinical management of patients? *British J Haematology.* 2008;143(3):321-335. PMID: 18710381

## 24

Immunocompromised Patients

J. Njeri Wainaina, MD, FACP, FHM, FIDSA, Avital Y. O'Glasser, MD, FACP, SFHM, DFPM, and Nidhi Rohatgi, MD, MS, SFHM

COMMON CLINICAL QUESTIONS

1. How do I know if my patient who recently had a COVID-19 infection is medically appropriate to proceed with surgery?
2. Are there any special considerations in preoperative evaluation of patients with a history of solid organ transplant planned for nontransplant surgery?
3. What should be considered in the perioperative management of patients with HIV infection?

INTRODUCTION

This chapter includes perioperative considerations for patients with a history of COVID-19, nontransplant surgery in patients with a history of solid organ transplantation, and patients with human immunodeficiency virus (HIV) infection.

COVID-19

The emergence of SARS-CoV-2, and the onset of the COVID-19 pandemic in March 2020, brought many new clinical and logistical challenges to the perioperative space. Especially with the sequential variants, perioperative management in the setting of COVID-19 has involved a very rapidly shifting clinical landscape since the pandemic was declared in March 2020. This includes clinical questions regarding patient risk, recovery time, post-COVID clinical evaluations, and preoperative testing for symptomatic and asymptomatic patients—all of which have had rapidly shifting clinical answers, often with differences in practice between institutions.[1,2] As of the last major published update by The Society for Healthcare Epidemiology of America (SHEA) in December 2022,[3] which was published since the last American Society of Anesthesiologists (ASA) and Anesthesia Patient Safety Foundation (APSF) statement[4] on the matter, routine preprocedure COVID-19 screening is no longer indicated.

Research by multiple groups identified a steep increase in morbidity and mortality associated with perioperative COVID-19 early in the pandemic when the wild type and alpha variant were predominant and prior to the introduction of vaccines and treatments. Unique to COVID-19 was the elevated risk of poor outcomes in asymptomatic patients as identified by the COVIDSurg group in early 2021. In addition to respiratory complications, increased perioperative morbidity and mortality was largely due to respiratory, thromboembolic, and cardiac complications driven by the prothrombotic and pro-inflammatory state induced by COVID-19.[1,5] Interval outcome data, reflecting newer variants and a higher percentage of the population with some type of immunity (via vaccinations and/or history of infection), continues to trend in reassuring directions, so perioperative risk and surgical delay time may be approaching levels similar to those applied for any preoperative patient recovering from a respiratory tract infection caused by any viral or bacterial pathogen (e.g., 2–4 weeks).[6] So, although earlier data found a higher incidence of pulmonary complications and death associated with surgery performed within 7 weeks of COVID-19 infection and worse outcomes in those patients with more severe symptoms, more recent guidance from the ASA/APSF[4] as well as that from the Association of Anaesthetists, Centre for Perioperative Care, Federation of Surgical Specialty Associations, Royal College of Anaesthetists, and Royal College of Surgeons of England[7] recommend that elective surgery should not occur within 2 weeks of SARS-Cov-2 infection but can be performed between 2 and 7 weeks after assessment of individual risk.

Akin to the preoperative assessment of any patient with a recent URI, when assessing a patient with recent COVID-19 in the preoperative setting, it is appropriate to review illness-specific history (including presence, severity, and duration of associated symptoms), recovery trajectory, and comorbid illnesses like chronic pulmonary disease (Tables 24-1 and 24-2). Patients with ongoing symptoms related to COVID-19 should be assessed for post-COVID complications such as long COVID or other COVID-induced complications like cardiac manifestations. There are very limited data regarding best practice for the preoperative assessment and perioperative management of patients with long COVID.[8] Even though COVID-19 overall has decreased in clinical severity, it is still prudent to perform patient-centered evaluations for patients who did experience more significant illness, ranging from prolonged duration to inpatient or ICU stays, as well as potential post-COVID infection symptoms that might signal ongoing increased perioperative risk. This includes, but may not be limited to, residual pulmonary disease, cardiac complications, VTE, "brain fog" or cognitive changes, ongoing fatigue, or deconditioning.[1] For patients with symptoms concerning for long COVID, reviewing disease specific history and long COVID "phenotype" (e.g., cardiac symptoms, myalgic encephalomyelitis/chronic fatigue syndrome-type symptoms, or postural hypotension syndrome-type symptoms) including confirming past testing a

TABLE 24-1. COVID-19 Focused Preoperative Evaluation

QUESTION	EXAMPLE OF POTENTIAL ASSOCIATED INFORMATION
Date of positive test and/or symptom onset	• PCR or antigen test (office or home-based) • Symptomatic vs. asymptomatic infection • Negative test but high probability of symptomatic illness (i.e., false negative) • Duration of test positivity
Duration of symptoms	• Asymptomatic • Less than 1 week • 1-2 weeks • Ongoing symptoms beyond 2 weeks
Treatment	• Any prescription antiviral use • Any non-FDA-approved treatments
Symptoms with acute illness	• Upper respiratory • Lower respiratory • Gastrointestinal • Myalgias • "Brain fog" • Other
Residual or subsequent symptoms	• Pulmonary symptoms (e.g., cough, dyspnea) • Cardiac symptoms (e.g., palpitations) • Syncope/pre-syncope, orthostasis • Asymmetric lower extremity edema • Reduced exercise tolerance • Cognitive changes • Concern for long COVID • Other
Patient-specific factors	• Age • Comorbid cardiopulmonary conditions • Comorbid immunosuppression including pharmacologic • Vaccination status

TABLE 24-2. COVID-19 and Perioperative Complications

PROTECTIVE FACTORS	
Vaccination	
Recovery with complete resolution of symptoms	
Mild to moderate well-controlled or no chronic comorbidities	
DISADVANTAGEOUS FACTORS	
Severe or critical infection	Defined as requiring hospitalization or intensive care for COVID-19
Complicated infection	Chronic respiratory failure
	Cardiomyopathy
	Arrhythmia
	Acute kidney injury/chronic kidney disease
	Venous thromboembolism
Long COVID syndrome	Chronic fatigue
	Postural orthostatic tachycardia syndrome (POTS)
	Cognitive impairment
Age > 65 years	

patient has completed (e.g., transthoracic echocardiogram, cardiac event monitor, pulmonary imaging, laboratory assessment) is prudent.[1]

SOLID ORGAN TRANSPLANT RECIPIENTS

As rates and success of solid organ transplantation are increasing, many more patients with a prior solid organ transplant may present for nontransplant surgeries. Although a complete discussion on perioperative considerations for this complex population is beyond scope, a few key points are discussed.

PREOPERATIVE EVALUATION

Preoperative risk assessment of a patient with a history of solid organ transplant planned for nontransplant surgery is fairly similar to that of patients with no transplant, except for a few special considerations. Patients with a prior solid organ transplant have had cardiac testing (e.g., electrocardiogram, echocardiogram, stress test) prior to receiving the transplant; results of these tests, especially if performed recently, can be reviewed in preparation for the nontransplant surgery. During preoperative evaluation of a patient with a prior solid organ transplant, a comprehensive history related to the transplant should be obtained (e.g., when was the transplant surgery performed, any history of transplant rejection or failure of the transplanted organ, any post-transplant complications including cardiac, immunosuppressive therapy regimen, any adverse effects with immunosuppressive therapy including chronic steroid use, target trough levels for the immunosuppressants, any antimicrobial prophylaxis).[9] Patients who have received a transplant are often very well informed and can provide a good history. In addition, the patient's transplant team should be involved during preoperative evaluation for nontransplant surgery to provide recommendations on the appropriate timing of elective nontransplant surgery and any special precautions for that patient or procedure. Appropriate laboratory data should be obtained to assess the graft function and to titrate the doses of any medications. Anemia should be corrected in the preoperative setting prior to elective surgery. Patients who are seronegative for cytomegalovirus (CMV) and received seronegative organ transplant should receive blood from CMV seronegative donor or leukocyte-reduced blood.[10] The blood bank should be prepared to provide appropriately matched and processed blood for any major surgery in a transplanted patient. Every effort should be made to avoid interruption or missed doses of patient's immunosuppressive therapy unless specifically recommended by patient's transplant team—if the immunosuppressive therapy is not on the hospital formulary, the patient should be advised to bring their home supply of medications. If the patient is anticipated to not have enteral access postoperatively, alternative options should be discussed with the patient's transplant team, including the potential for any drug-drug interactions.

POSTOPERATIVE MANAGEMENT

The patient's transplant team or local institutional expert should be involved in the postoperative care after nontransplant surgery to monitor graft function, manage immunosuppressive therapy, and provide guidance on any special considerations for that particular patient in the context of their history of solid organ transplant. Doses of immunosuppressive therapy may require titration in the postoperative period due to drug-drug interactions (including through cytochrome P450 mechanisms) or fluctuations in hepatic or renal function. Relevant laboratory data such as trough levels of immunosuppressive therapy or chemistry panel should be obtained for dose titration and monitoring. Every effort should be made to avoid an infectious complication that could be catastrophic in this population, including avoiding lines and drains as much as possible. The surgical site should be monitored carefully as wound healing may be impaired with certain immunosuppressants.

HUMAN IMMUNODEFICIENCY VIRUS

The advent and evolution of effective antiretroviral therapy (ART) has led to a stark drop in mortality attributable to HIV infection. The downstream effect of better survival has been longer life spans such that persons living with HIV/AIDS (PLWHA) are increasingly likely to need surgical interventions similar to the general population.

The risk of HIV transmission from patients to healthcare providers during a surgical procedure is very low as long as universal precautions are maintained by all members of the surgical team. Operative treatments should not be denied solely because of HIV infection. No benefit has been found for routine preoperative screening for HIV infection.[11]

PREOPERATIVE EVALUATION

In the United States, 50% of patients diagnosed with HIV infection are not retained in care[12] and so have suboptimal disease control, which may be accompanied by poorly controlled acute or chronic comorbidities. It is thus necessary to determine the level and stability of virological suppression and immunological recovery prior to surgery. This can be accomplished by reviewing records for recent HIV viral load, CD4 count, and adherence to follow-up. Where this is not easily available electronically, the patient's HIV clinician should be contacted directly for current status and HIV-specific perioperative recommendations.

Clinicians should also be aware that noninfectious comorbidities that impact anesthetic and surgical risk, including diabetes mellitus, adrenal insufficiency, and cardiovascular, pulmonary, and renal disease,[13] occur at a higher rate and younger age than in groups without HIV. Additionally, substance abuse, mental health disorders, and socioeconomic instability, which can contribute to poor postoperative outcomes, are more prevalent in PLWHA.

Preoperative risk assessment, mitigation, and optimization should follow general principles with the addition of ensuring that HIV is maximally treated. Most commonly used ART regimens do not require preoperative toxicity testing. The preoperative visit also allows for patient education, provision of anticipatory guidance regarding pain management and acute withdrawal risk, and advance planning for support systems after discharge. Multiple studies have shown that when medically optimized prior to surgery, patients with and without HIV infection have no difference in postoperative outcomes.[13-15]

Table 24-3 illustrates a checklist of important considerations when evaluating PLWHA before surgery.

MEDICATION MANAGEMENT

During preoperative medication reconciliation, the patient's current ART regimen and adjunctive prophylactic medications should be confirmed, and all efforts should be made to avoid interruption of ART around surgery. For most patients, ART will be two to four agents combined into a single tablet. Many of these are not on hospital formularies, but they may be available as individual components. If staying overnight after surgery, patients should be advised to bring their own supply to the hospital to avoid missed doses.

For procedures where it is anticipated that there will be no oral intake for a prolonged period postoperatively, consultation with the patient's HIV provider and the hospital pharmacy is recommended prior to surgery. This facilitates medication adjustments to those with liquid formulations or that can be crushed for delivery via gastric tubes along with more

TABLE 24-3. Checklist for Preoperative Evaluation of Patients with HIV
HIV CARE
• Name and contact of provider
• Visit frequency and last visit
• Social support need and current structure
• Antiretroviral regimen
• Availability and formulation(s) at site of surgery
• Modifications if necessary
• Level of control
• Last viral load, when and trend
• Last CD4, when and trend
• Prophylactic antimicrobials

COMORBIDITIES PRESENT AND LEVEL OF CONTROL	
Cardiovascular	Neurological
Pulmonary	Endocrine: diabetes; adrenal insufficiency risk
Hematology	Psychiatric
Renal	Substance use: tobacco, alcohol, opioids, other

SOCIAL
• Housing stability
• Transport availability

sophisticated measures such as matching pharmacokinetics to avoid inadvertent single drug therapy.[16]

Clinicians should keep in mind that drug interactions are common with antiretroviral medications, particularly ritonavir and cobicistat. These are potent inhibitors of CYP cytochromes that are used to boost the effect of other components of the ART cocktail. Consequently, prolonged action of some drug classes such as opioids may occur. For the newly diagnosed or uncontrolled patient, HIV infection is never a contraindication for emergency surgery. Barring other medical instability, time-sensitive surgery should not be delayed to start or optimize treatment of HIV. On the other hand, the need for elective surgery can be leveraged to motivate patients to connect to and engage in HIV treatment. Resources to aid with this can be found at local HIV clinics or accessed through infectious disease specialists.

POSTOPERATIVE MANAGEMENT

Patients with controlled HIV infection on ART have postoperative outcomes that are similar to the general population. Uncontrolled disease, including AIDS, is associated with a greater likelihood of mortality, sepsis, and wound complications including surgical site infections. Factors predictive of poor outcomes include trauma as the indication for surgery, hypoalbuminemia which may be a flag for malnutrition, increasing age, and CD4 cell count. Compared to surgery to correct dysfunction, surgery for acute trauma can increase the risk of postoperative sepsis in HIV patients up to tenfold, and the severity of trauma correlates directly with associated morbidity. In the same population, the risk of postoperative sepsis after surgery to manage tumors and infection has been reported to be 1.5–2 times higher.[17] In the era of widely available simple ART regimens and improved engagement in care, HIV RNA levels or viral load has not been found to have a consistent impact on perioperative morbidity or mortality, but CD4 cell count seems to be inversely related to mortality.[18]

Clinical pearls

- COVID-19 can be a protean illness with multiple organ–system–related effects and complications. Preoperative assessment of a post-COVID-19 patient should include illness-specific review in addition to considering the impact of underlying comorbid conditions.

- A solid organ transplant team should be involved in the perioperative management of patients with a history of solid organ transplantation undergoing nontransplant surgery to monitor graft function and titrate doses of immunosuppressive therapy based on enteral access, drug-drug interactions, and fluctuations in hepatic or renal function.

- The approach to preoperative risk assessment and stratification in patients living with HIV/AIDS is no different to that in patients without HIV. However, attention should be paid to assessing the level of virological control, medication reconciliation to minimize ART interruption, and care coordination to avoid HIV care continuum discontinuity.

- Postoperative complications in patients with HIV are related to immunological recovery as measured by CD4 cell count, surgical procedure, individual patient comorbidities, and lifestyle risk factors.

REFERENCES

1. O'Glasser AY. COVID-19 in the perioperative setting: 2023 updates. *Perioper Care Oper Room Manag.* 2023;33:100353.

2. Liu JK, Porras PA, Hari DM, Chen KT. Routine preoperative Covid testing in elective surgeries: is it worth it? *Am J Surg.* 2022;224(6):1380-1384. PMID: 36424202

3. Talbot TR, Hayden MK, Yokoe DS, et al. SHEA Board of Trustees. Asymptomatic screening for severe acute respiratory coronavirus virus 2 (SARS-CoV-2) as an infection prevention measure in healthcare facilities: challenges and considerations. *Infect Control Hosp Epidemiol.* 2023;44(1):2-7. PMID: 36539917

4. ASA and APSF Statement on Perioperative Testing for the COVID-19 Virus. Updated June 15, 2022. Accessed June 2, 2024. https://www.asahq.org/about-asa/newsroom/news-releases/2022/06/asa-apsf-statement-on-perioperative-testing-for-covid.

5. Rohatgi N, Smilowitz NR, Reejhsinghani R. Perioperative cardiovascular considerations prior to elective noncardiac surgery in patients with a history of COVID-19. *JAMA Surg.* 2022;157(3):187-188. PMID: 35019990

6. Lam F, Liao CC, Chen TL, et al. Outcomes after surgery in patients with and without recent influenza: a nationwide population-based study. *Front Med (Lausanne).* 2023;10:1117885. PMID: 37358993

7. El-Boghdadly K, Cook TM, Goodacre T, et al. Timing of elective surgery and risk assessment after SARS-CoV-2 infection: an update: a multidisciplinary consensus statement on behalf of the Association of Anaesthetists, Centre for Perioperative Care, Federation of Surgical Specialty Associations, Royal College of Anaesthetists, Royal College of Surgeons of England. *Anaesthesia.* 2022;77:580-587. PMID: 35194788

8. Boles S, Ashok SR. Pre-assessment and management of long COVID patients requiring elective surgery: challenges and guidance. *Perioper Med.* 2023;12(1):20. PMID: 37277879

9. Holt CD. Overview of immunosuppressive therapy in solid organ transplantation. *Anesthesiol Clin.* 2017;35(3):365-380. PMID: 28784214

10. Herborn J, Parulkar S. Anesthetic considerations in transplant recipients for nontransplant surgery. *Anesthesiol Clin.* 2017;35(3):539-553. PMID: 28784225

11. Weber P, Eberle J, Bogner JR, et al. Is there a benefit to a routine preoperative screening of infectivity for HIV, hepatitis B and C virus before elective orthopaedic operations? *Infection.* 2013;41:479-483. PMID: 23225209

12. HIV Care Continuum Updated October 28, 2022. Available at https://www.hiv.gov/federal-response/policies-issues/hiv-aids-care-continuum/.

13. Guaraldi G, Orlando G, Zona S, et al. Premature age-related comorbidities among HIV-infected persons compared with the general population. *Clin Infect Dis.* 2011;53:1120-1126. PMID: 21998278

14. Issa K, Pierce TP, Harwin SF, et al. No decrease in knee survivorship or outcomes scores for patients with HIV infection who undergo TKA. *Clin Orthop Relat Res.* 2017;475:465-471. PMID: 27743304

15. Boccara F, Cohen A, Di Angelantonio E, et al. Coronary artery bypass graft in HIV-infected patients: a multicenter case control study. *Current HIV Research.* 2008;6:59. PMID: 18288976

16. Cimino C, Binkley A, Swisher R, Short WR. Antiretroviral considerations in HIV-infected patients undergoing bariatric surgery. *J Clin Pharm Ther.* 2018;43:757-767. PMID: 30110123

17. Tienan F, Xiuling F, Chenghua J, et al. Sepsis risk factors associated with HIV-1 patients undergoing surgery. *Emerg Microbes Infect.* 2015;4:e59. PMID: 26954996

18. King JT Jr, Perkal MF, Rosenthal RA, et al. Thirty-day postoperative mortality among individuals with HIV infection receiving antiretroviral therapy and procedure-matched, uninfected comparators. *JAMA Surg.* 2015;150:343. PMID: 25714794

## 25

Renal Disease

Barbara Slawski, MD, MS, SFHM

COMMON CLINICAL QUESTIONS

1. How common is chronic kidney disease (CKD) in the surgical population?
2. How does CKD affect perioperative risk for adverse outcomes?
3. What preoperative assessments and interventions can ameliorate risk?

INTRODUCTION

Chronic Kidney Disease in the Surgical Population

Chronic kidney disease (CKD) is defined as abnormalities of kidney structure or function, present for ≥3 months. Approximately 2–17% of the global population has CKD, but this may be an underestimation because CKD is usually asymptomatic.[1]

The 2024 Kidney Disease Improving Global Outcomes (KDIGO) criteria are now the commonly accepted criteria for defining CKD, specifying six stages based on increasing severity of estimated glomerular filtration rate (eGFR) (Table 25-1).[2] Additional data regarding the presence and severity of albuminuria can provide prognostic information about the likelihood of CKD progression in the general medical population.[2] In recent studies examining the effect of CKD on perioperative outcomes, the reported prevalence of stage 3 and higher CKD in cardiac surgery patients was over 25%,[3] and in noncardiac surgery patients (including vascular surgery), it was >20%.[4,5]

CKD and Perioperative Outcomes

CKD is one of the most significant risk factors for postoperative acute kidney injury (AKI) and is associated with several adverse outcomes. Risks of kidney injury in cardiac and noncardiac surgery patients are different not only because of surgical risk factors such as cardiopulmonary bypass, but also due to differences in underlying patient demographics. In addition to the risk for AKI on CKD, the presence of CKD by itself is associated with adverse perioperative outcomes. In cardiac surgery patients, CKD is correlated with postoperative mortality, with one recent study demonstrating an adjusted odds ratio (OR) for mortality of 3.4 in CABG patients with CKD.[3]

Noncardiac surgery patients with preoperative CKD also have higher rates of postoperative mortality than those with normal renal function, with the OR for mortality also increasing by CKD stage.[4,5] For example, compared with patients with an eGFR > 90 mL/min/1.73 m^2, the ORs for mortality are 2.8 in patients with eGFRs of >30–<45 and 5.8 for patients with eGFR < 15. Besides mortality, CKD is also associated with other adverse perioperative outcomes. Preoperative CKD in cardiac surgery is associated with infection, AKI, myocardial infarction, stroke, gastrointestinal bleeding, prolonged ventilation,

TABLE 25-1. Criteria for Defining Chronic Kidney Disease

STAGE	eGFR RANGE (ml/min/1.73 m²)
G1	>90
G2	60–89
G3a	45–59
G3b	30–44
G4	15–29
G5	<15

sepsis, the need for renal replacement therapy, prolonged length of stay, return to the operating room, and mortality.[3]

Long-term dialysis patients have even higher rates of postoperative complications, including death, pneumonia, unplanned intubation and ventilator dependence, reoperation within 30 days, and vascular complications.[6]

PREOPERATIVE EVALUATION

Indications for Preoperative Tests of Renal Function

Preoperative kidney function testing should be targeted to identify patients with risk factors for CKD while decreasing wasteful testing in patients at lower risk. Preoperative creatinine levels are indicated for patients with known history of CKD or risk factors for it, age > 50 undergoing intermediate or high-risk surgery, and those on medications that may affect kidney function.

Preoperative Assessment and Management (Figure 25-1)

Patients with CKD often have multiple comorbidities that are associated with adverse perioperative outcomes. Considerations in surgical patients with CKD include[7]:

- Chronicity, severity, and etiology of CKD—If unidentified, untreated, or ≥stage 4, patients may benefit from a preoperative nephrology evaluation.

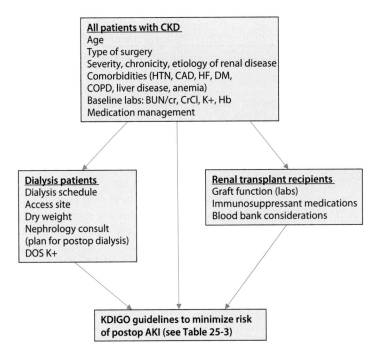

FIGURE 25-1. Algorithm for preoperative evaluation of the patient with renal disease.

- Cardiovascular disease risk is elevated in the CKD population. See Chapter 11 for additional information on preoperative cardiovascular testing.

- Anemia is common—Additional assessment and intervention may be required before cases with large, anticipated blood loss. KDIGO Hb target is 10–11.5 g/dL for HD patients, but PRBC use can lead to sensitization to HLA antigens, which can affect the patient's ability to receive a future kidney transplant. See Chapter 22 on anemia.

- Hypertension is frequently seen in this population. Cautious blood pressure (BP) management is important, both to manage significant elevations in BP and avoid hypotension. Patients with CKD often have additional medical comorbidities that put them at risk of developing acute tubular necrosis (ATN).

- Medications—Renally cleared medications should be dose-adjusted, and contraindications need to be considered. For example, opioids and several anticoagulants used perioperatively are renally cleared. Nephrotoxic medications should be identified and avoided.

- Glycemic control—Many patients with CKD also have diabetes mellitus. Impaired glycemic control is associated with development of AKI in the perioperative period and should be optimized if possible.

- Central lines in the subclavian vein or PICC lines in the cephalic, brachial, or basilic vein should be avoided if possible because CKD patients may need upper extremity AV access for dialysis in the future.

Special Considerations for End-Stage Renal Disease (ESRD) Patients on Dialysis

- Dialysis timing—Dialysis patients undergoing procedures should be euvolemic and have near-normal electrolytes. It is often most feasible to schedule surgery on a nondialysis day, preferably the day after dialysis, because of the timeframes required for both hemodialysis and the surgical procedure. In noncardiac surgery patients with end-stage kidney disease, *intervals longer than 1 day between hemodialysis and surgery were associated with slightly higher risk of postoperative mortality.*[8] Peritoneal dialysis patients who are having abdominal surgeries may need to transition to hemodialysis for a short duration of time. For nonabdominal surgeries, peritoneal dialysis can be continued. It is

important to consult the nephrology team early to coordinate dialysis needs of the patients.

- Access—Identify the type of hemodialysis access and its patency. In patients with advanced CKD who are not on dialysis, a proactive plan for potential perioperative AKI or need for renal replacement therapy should be considered.

- Heparin use—If hemodialysis will take place on the day of surgery, avoid the use of heparin during dialysis.

- Dry weight—Document the patient's dry weight and ascertain if they are euvolemic. Since many ESRD patients are anuric, avoid overhydration.

- Potassium—Consider checking a potassium level on the day of surgery.

- Postoperative dialysis—Provide anticipatory guidance to the care teams regarding a postoperative dialysis plan.

Renal Transplant

Patients with renal transplants have unique risks for perioperative complications. Important perioperative considerations in the renal transplant population include the following[9]:

- Graft function—Review recent routine transplant labs and assess risk for postoperative AKI and existing electrolyte abnormalities.

- Immunosuppression—These medications have the potential for infectious complications and impaired wound healing, and the regimen should not be changed without consulting the kidney transplant physician.

- Blood bank considerations—Transfused packed red blood cells should be leukocyte reduced.

- For cytomegalovirus (CMV) seronegative patients, CMV-negative blood products should be available.

- Comorbid diseases are common in renal transplant patients and need to be identified and assessed preoperatively. Kidney transplant recipients are at risk for normotensive ATN.

  Clinicians may also be asked to evaluate patients with CKD who are planning a future renal transplant. Preoperative evaluation for the transplant candidate is extensive and may include items performed by the transplant team or the preoperative clinician[10]:

- The cause of ESKD should be elucidated, if possible. Some underlying etiologies place the patient at risk for recurrence after transplant.

- Cardiac evaluation—History, physical, and ECG are recommended for all patients. Although guidelines recommend that asymptomatic patients at high cardiac risk or with poor functional capacity undergo noninvasive testing,[10] stress testing in the 18 months prior to kidney transplantation is not associated with a reduction in mortality of MI within 30 days of surgery.[11] Guidelines also recommend excluding patients with uncorrectable, symptomatic NHYA III/VI disease from renal transplant.[10]

- Psychosocial and adherence to treatment requires assessment.

- Pulmonary—Assess for lung disease. Patients with severe, irreversible restrictive or obstructive disease are at increased risk for premature post-transplant mortality and should be excluded from transplantation. Tobacco use should be avoided, and patients with ≥30 pack years may have CT to screen for occult malignancy.

- Endocrine—Test for abnormal glucose metabolism and hyperparathyroidism.

- Active infectious diseases are an indication for surgical delay due to increased risk with subsequent immunosuppression. Vaccinations should be up to date.

- Routine cancer screening should be complete because most active cancers are contraindications to transplantation.

- Vascular screening for peripheral arterial disease (PAD) is suggested for patients at high risk; however, routine carotid evaluations are not indicated.

- Gastrointestinal evaluation includes assessment for liver disease with laboratory testing and referral for patients with suspected disease.

- HLA testing is routinely performed.

Risk Factors for Developing Postoperative AKI

Risk factors for AKI can be identified preoperatively. In addition to potential preventive measures, counseling patients and other care team members regarding the potential for AKI and associated outcomes is key. Postoperative AKI is associated with high rates of inhospital, 90-day, and 1-year mortality in both cardiac and noncardiac surgery patients. In addition, both cardiac and noncardiac surgery patients had significantly higher risks of hospital readmissions and 1-year progression to ESRD.[12] In surgical patients, the kidney can be injured by multiple mechanisms including ischemic injury due to hemodynamic changes, nephrotoxic medications, mechanical obstruction, and nephrotoxic effects of inflammatory mediators. Specific preoperative risk factors associated with postoperative AKI in patients undergoing both cardiac and noncardiac major surgeries are listed in Table 25-2.[12,13]

TABLE 25-2. Risk Factors for Postoperative Acute Kidney Injury

SURGICAL	PREOPERATIVE PATIENT-RELATED	INTRAOPERATIVE
Emergent	eGFR < 90 mL/min	Vasopressor infusion
High risk	Diabetes mellitus	Vasopressor dose
Open (vs. laparoscopic)	Advancing age	Hypotension
Coronary artery bypass (on pump)	Male gender	Diuretic use
Long cardiopulmonary bypass time	Hypertension	
	Congestive heart failure	
	Vascular disease/AAA	
	ACE-I/ARB use	
	Diuretic use	
	Lung disease/COPD requiring bronchodilators	
	Liver disease	
	Elevated body mass index	

AKI Risk Assessment Tools

The strongest predictor of postoperative AKI is preoperative CKD. Multiple risk-prediction models are available to assess the risk of perioperative AKI, with newer ones developed using machine learning. These models can identify risk factors and potentially the risk of AKI; however, because many also include data points that are not easily available to practicing clinicians, their clinical utility is not clear. A recent study compared nine different risk models in their ability to predict AKI based on the KDIGO definition. Only three models[14-16] had fair discrimination (AUROC 0.71–0.75) and shared common risk predictors including age, sex, eGFR, ASA physical status, and diabetes mellitus.[17] There is no evidence that a single model can be currently recommended.[18]

PERIOPERATIVE MANAGEMENT/RISK REDUCTION

Prevention of Postoperative Complications

The KDIGO guidelines recommend several measures (Table 25-3) in patients who are at risk for or experience AKI.[19]

- Maintenance of volume status
  - Hyper and hypovolemia—Several studies have examined both liberal and restrictive perioperative fluid administration strategies. Liberal strategies have been linked to longer hospital length of stay and complications. Volume overload is associated with organ edema that can lead to AKI. Restrictive strategies may also lead to AKI. Standard strategies for fluid replacement and ideal urine output have yet to be determined.[7]

- IV fluid selection—Large volume infusions of normal saline are associated with renal vasoconstriction and hyperchloremic acidosis that increase the risk of AKI. In addition, hydroxyethyl starch has also been associated with perioperative AKI. Balanced crystalloids are suggested for IVF replacement to maintain hemodynamic stability.[7]

- Hemodynamic control/maintenance of perfusion pressure—Intraoperative hypotension and hypertension have been linked to postoperative AKI. Despite multiple studies, a general recommendation for a directed intraoperative mean arterial pressure is not available and likely needs an individual approach.

- Discontinuation and avoidance of nephrotoxins is recommended.

- Avoid CT radiocontrast agents and consider non-contrast CT or ultrasound.

- Maintain normoglycemia.

- Monitor serum creatinine and urine output—see Chapter 41.

Multiple interventions have been studied with an intent to prevent perioperative AKI or decrease the impact of AKI on perioperative outcomes including aspirin, statins, N-acetylcysteine, human atrial natriuretic peptide, fenoldopam, dexmedetomidine, levosimendan, and remote ischemic preconditioning. There is not enough evidence at this point to recommend their use. Remote ischemic preconditioning does not reduce AKI rates but does demonstrate some improvements in other surrogate markers of renal function.[19]

SUMMARY

Preoperative CKD is a strong predictor of adverse perioperative outcomes. CKD patients planning surgery require additional assessment and management to reduce the risk of postoperative complications, including AKI, cardiovascular complications, infections, pulmonary complications, and death. Preoperative assessment includes evaluation of risk for AKI, management of associated comorbidities, and evaluation of the etiology of CKD if indicated.

TABLE 25-3. Risk Reduction Strategies—KDIGO Guidelines
Maintain volume status
Maintain perfusion pressure—BP control
Avoid/discontinue nephrotoxins (meds, IV contrast)
Maintain normoglycemia
Monitor creatinine and urine output

REFERENCES

1. Murton M, Goff-Leggett D, Bobrowska A, et al. Burden of chronic kidney disease by KDIGO categories of glomerular filtration rate and albuminuria: a systematic review. *Adv Ther*. 2021;38(1):180-200. PMID: 33231861

2. Kidney Disease: Improving Global Outcomes (KDIGO) CKD Work Group. KDIGO 2024 clinical practice guideline for the evaluation and management of chronic kidney disease. *Kidney Int*. 2024;105(4S):S117-S314. PMID: 38490803

3. Li X, Zhang S, Xiao F. Influence of chronic kidney disease on early clinical outcomes after off-pump coronary artery bypass grafting. *J Cardiothorac Surg*. 2020;15:199. PMID: 32727495

4. Mases A, Sabaté S, Guilera N, et al. Preoperative estimated glomerular filtration rate and the risk of major adverse cardiovascular and cerebrovascular events in non-cardiac surgery. *Br J Anaesth*. 2014;113(4):644-651. PMID: 24929634

5. Mathew A, Devereaux PJ, O'Hare A, et al. Chronic kidney disease and postoperative mortality: a systematic review and meta-analysis. *Kidney Int*. 2008;73(9):1069-1081. PMID: 18288098

6. Gajdos C, Hawn MT, Kile D, et al. Risk of major nonemergent inpatient general surgical procedures in patients on long-term dialysis. *JAMA Surg*. 2013;148(2):137-143. PMID: 23560284

7. Zarbock A, Koyner JL, Hoste EA, Kellum JA. Update of perioperative acute kidney injury. *Anesth Analg*. 2018;127(5)1236-1245. PMID: 30138176

8. Fielding-Singh V, Vanneman MW, Grogan T, et al. Association between preoperative hemodialysis timing and postoperative mortality in patients with end-stage kidney disease. *JAMA*. 2022;328(18):1837-1848. PMID: 36326747

9. Herborn J, Parulkar S. Anesthetic considerations in transplant recipients for nontransplant surgery. *Anesthesiol Clin*. 2017;25:539-553. PMID: 28784225

10. Chadban S, Ahn C, Axelrod D, et al. Summary of the Kidney Disease: Improving Global Outcomes (KDIGO) clinical practice guideline on the evaluation and management of candidates for kidney transplantation. *Transplantation*. 2020;104:708-714. PMID: 32224812

11. Dunn T, Saeed MJ, Shpigel A, et al. The association of preoperative cardiac stress testing with 30-day death and myocardial infarction among patients undergoing kidney transplantation. *PLoS ONE*. 2019;14(2):e0211161. PMID: 30707723

12. Grams ME, Sang Y, Coresh J, et al. Acute kidney injury after major surgery: a retrospective analysis of Veterans Health Administration data. *Am J Kidney Dis*. 2016;67(6):872-880. PMID: 26337133

13. Kheterpal S, Tremper KK, Englesbe MJ, et al. Predictors of postoperative acute renal failure after noncardiac surgery in patients with previously normal renal function. *Anesthesiology*. 2007;107(6):892-902. PMID: 18043057

14. Bell S, Dekker FW, Vadiveloo T, et al. Risk of postoperative acute kidney injury in patients undergoing orthopaedic surgery—development and validation of a risk score and effect of acute kidney injury on survival: observational cohort study. *BMJ*. 2015;351:h5639. PMID: 26561522

15. STARSurg Collaborative. Prognostic model to predict postoperative acute kidney injury in patients undergoing major gastrointestinal surgery based on a national prospective observational cohort study. *BJS Open*. 2018;2(6):400-410. PMID: 30513129

16. Park S, Cho H, Park S, et al. Simple postoperative AKI risk (SPARK) classification before noncardiac surgery: a prediction index development study with external validation. *J Am Soc Nephrol*. 2019;30(1):170-181. PMID: 30563915

17. Zhuo XY, Lei SH, Sun L, et al. Preoperative risk prediction models for acute kidney injury after noncardiac surgery: an independent external validation cohort study. *Br J Anaesth*. 2024;24:S0007-0912(24)00097-7. PMID: 38527923

18. Tinica G, Brinza C, Covic A, et al. Determinants of acute kidney injury after cardiac surgery: a systematic review. *Rev Cardiovasc Med*. 2020;21(4):601-610. PMID: 3338805

19. Kidney Disease: Improving Global Outcomes Acute Kidney Injury Work Group. KDIGO clinical practice guideline for acute kidney injury. *Kidney Int Suppl*. 2012;2:1-138. PMID: 22890468

26

Liver Disease

Avital Y. O'Glasser, MD, FACP, SFHM, DFPM and Kay M. Johnson, MD, MPH

COMMON CLINICAL QUESTIONS

1. How do liver disease and cirrhosis impact perioperative risk?
2. What tools/risk calculators can be used to quantify cirrhosis-related perioperative risk?
3. What can be done to mitigate the risk of cirrhosis-related postoperative complications?

INTRODUCTION

Liver disease may range from acute hepatic injury/hepatitis to chronic liver disease, which encompasses a spectrum from asymptomatic inflammation, to progressive hepatic fibrosis leading to cirrhosis, hepatic dysfunction, and eventually to end-stage liver disease and liver failure. Multiple etiologies exist, including viral, metabolic, autoimmune, or toxin/medication, including alcohol-related liver disease. One and a half million people worldwide have chronic liver disease, with metabolic dysfunction-associated steatotic liver diseases (MASLD, formerly known as nonalcoholic fatty liver disease) now the most common etiology (60%); hepatitis B vaccination and effective hepatitis C treatment have contributed to shifting epidemiology.[1] With improved survival, more patients with chronic liver disease may present for surgical care and with more comorbidities.

Liver disease, especially cirrhosis and end-stage liver disease, is clearly associated with increased risk of perioperative morbidity and mortality. Impaired homeostasis and extrahepatic complications can have significant adverse effects and contribute to perioperative risk.

Liver Disease, Homeostasis, and Perioperative Risk

Acute or chronic liver failure impairs many vital metabolic and synthetic functions that have clear implications in the perioperative period (Table 26-1). Additionally, perioperative factors including intraoperative hypotension or changes to hepatic perfusion may acutely worsen baseline liver function. Anesthetic agents, centrally acting medications including opioids, and impaired bowel function may increase the risk of hepatic encephalopathy. Portal hypertension contributes to the risk of perioperative complications. Esophageal and, to a lesser extent, gastric varices contribute to the risk of anemia and acute blood loss. Splenomegaly contributes to thrombocytopenia through platelet sequestration. Poor ascites control postoperatively increases the risk of postoperative acute kidney injury or further complications after intra-abdominal surgeries, given the risk of volume loss and poor wound healing due to seepage and compromised incision integrity or loss through drains.

TABLE 26-1. Correlation of Altered Homeostasis, Derangements in Cirrhosis, and Potential Perioperative Complications[2,5]

ROLE IN NORMAL HOMEOSTASIS	EFFECT IN CHRONIC LIVER DISEASE	POTENTIAL PERIOPERATIVE COMPLICATIONS
Coagulation factor synthesis	Decreased clotting factors synthesis Impaired fibrinolysis	Bleeding Thrombosis
Protein synthesis	Hypoalbuminemia Low oncotic pressure Low complement levels Malnutrition Sarcopenia syndrome	Impaired wound healing Edema and third spacing Infections Delayed physical recovery Deconditioning
Glucose homeostasis	Impaired gluconeogenesis and glycogenolysis	Hypoglycemia
Bilirubin excretion	Fat-soluble vitamin deficiency	Impaired coagulation Malnutrition
Drug metabolism and elimination	Delayed metabolism of anesthetic agents and analgesics Drug-drug interactions	Sedation Hepatic encephalopathy
Metabolic waste metabolism	Nitrogenous waste metabolism	Hepatic encephalopathy and delirium

Extrahepatic Complications of Liver Disease and Perioperative Risk

Patients with liver disease can develop extrahepatic complications and end-organ damage due to the multisystem effects of the vasodilatory and neurohormonal dysregulation seen in chronic liver disease and cirrhosis. These, too, contribute to perioperative risk in addition to synthetic dysfunction and portal hypertension (Table 26-2).

PREOPERATIVE EVALUATION/RISK FACTORS

Patient-Related Risk Factors (Table 26-3)

A comprehensive history and physical exam is a crucial element of a preoperative assessment. If liver disease is present, the clinician should assess the level of hepatic inflammation (i.e., transaminase elevation) and if chronic, whether it has progressed to cirrhosis,

and, if so, whether there is a history of decompensation (e.g., ascites, hepatic encephalopathy, spontaneous bacterial peritonitis, variceal bleeding, hepatorenal syndrome or jaundice), or hepatocellular carcinoma. Past medical history and social history may reveal risk factors for undiagnosed liver disease (e.g., intravenous drug use, alcohol misuse, metabolic syndrome, birth in HBV endemic countries, sexual history, history of blood transfusions).

The physical exam may prompt concern for undiagnosed cirrhosis, revealing ascites, hepatomegaly, splenomegaly, lower extremity edema, or other manifestations (jaundice, scleral icterus, spider telangiectasias, palmar erythema, gynecomastia, caput medusa). In a patient with known cirrhosis, the examination should assess the presence or control of ascites, lower extremity edema, and asterixis.

Several blood tests are required for various risk calculators (discussed below) used to quantify severity of liver disease. In patients with established liver disease

TABLE 26-2. Extrahepatic Manifestations of Cirrhosis and Their Associated Complications[3]

ORGAN SYSTEM	EFFECT SEEN IN CHRONIC LIVER DISEASE	POTENTIAL PERIOPERATIVE COMPLICATION
Cardiovascular	Increased cardiac index Vasodilation Decreased effective circulating volume	Hemodynamic instability
Immune function	Decreased complement levels	Infection risk
Renal	Impaired renal perfusion Decreased effective circulating volume	Acute kidney injury Hepatorenal syndrome Hyponatremia
Marrow function and hematologic parameters	Anemia Thrombocytopenia Coagulopathy	Bleeding Risks associated with transfusions
Pulmonary	Hepatic hydrothorax Hepatopulmonary syndrome Portopulmonary syndrome Impaired respiration	Acute respiratory failure Atelectasis Hypoxia Right heart failure

TABLE 26-3. Patient- and Surgery-Specific Risk Factors for Perioperative Complications with Cirrhosis[2,3,6,7]

CIRRHOSIS-SPECIFIC RISK FACTORS	OTHER PATIENT-SPECIFIC RISK FACTORS	SURGERY-SPECIFIC RISK FACTORS
More advanced cirrhosis • MELD > 10 • CTP B or C History of portal HTN and/or decompensated cirrhosis • Ascites • Encephalopathy • Variceal bleeding • Hepatorenal syndrome Impaired synthetic function • Hypoalbuminemia • Coagulopathy	Age Malnutrition Active alcohol use Tobacco use ASA class Functional status Comorbid conditions • Cardiovascular disease • Diabetes • COPD • Hypoxia • Cancer • Sepsis • Frailty	Type of surgery • Hepatic resection • Hepatobiliary • Major intra-abdominal • Cardiac Emergency surgery Longer surgery Intraoperative blood loss Intraoperative transfusions Facility expertise Anesthetic technique and agents

or risk factors for such, it is reasonable to check liver function tests (LFTs), renal function, complete blood count (CBC), and INR. LFTs, especially ALT and AST, can fluctuate for stable patients, but new elevations significantly outside a patient's established baseline should prompt further attention. A high INR can be a marker for severe liver disease. However, abnormal INR correlates poorly with bleeding risk,[2] as patients with liver disease can be prothrombotic. A CBC should be checked to evaluate for cytopenias, especially thrombocytopenia, which often indicates the presence of portal hypertension. It is reasonable to have a lower threshold to obtain a Type and Screen given bleeding risk from impaired coagulation and thrombocytopenia.

Perioperative evaluation of patients with liver disease must also include assessment of other comorbid conditions such as diabetes, cardiovascular disease, chronic kidney disease, and frailty.

Risk Calculators (Table 26-4)

Patients with mild chronic liver disease or early stages of cirrhosis generally have a lower and likely acceptable risk of perioperative complications. Conversely, patients with advanced or decompensated liver disease have extremely high postoperative morbidity and mortality levels. This is shown by multiple studies examining the predictive ability of the CTP class and MELD score in the perioperative setting, with patients overall having two- to tenfold increased risk.[3]

Child-Turcotte-Pugh (CTP): In general, CTP class correlates well with perioperative mortality, where most procedures are safe in patients with CTP A but prohibitively dangerous for patients with CTP C. However, using CTP alone to estimate postop mortality is no longer recommended because sources using CTP class frequently quote estimates that are from very old studies or that do not take into account the type or urgency of surgery.[4,5] For instance, even within abdominal surgeries, there is a wide range of perioperative mortality, depending on the specific procedure and urgency.[2,6]

Model of End-Stage Liver Disease (MELD): The MELD was originally developed to predict prognosis after transjugular intrahepatic portosystemic shunt (TIPS) placement and then validated to predict mortality in liver disease and used for liver transplantation allocation. Postoperative mortality is predicted by MELD score in a progressive fashion, with 30-day mortality 5.7% for MELD < 8 to more than 50% for MELD > 20.[7] The recent narrative review confirmed that patients with MELD < 10 had minimally increased risk of mortality; it is recommended to avoid elective surgery in patients with MELD > 15, especially higher risk surgeries such as abdominal or cardiothoracic cases.[3]

Since the original MELD score was created, updated models that incorporate serum sodium levels have been developed and introduced. The *MELD-Na* adds serum sodium to the MELD score. The integrated MELD (*iMELD*) adds age and sodium and was shown to be somewhat better than CTP and similar to the original MELD in predicting perioperative mortality.[8] The model for end-stage liver disease to sodium (*MESO index*) is a *function* of the MELD score *divided by* serum sodium levels. As of 2023, an even newer *MELD 3.0* is being used to triage liver transplant recipients. These newer models improve prognostic accuracy for patients awaiting liver transplantation,[9] but there are currently limited data regarding perioperative risk prognostication or cut-off values outside the transplant setting beyond data that MELD-Na might underestimate perioperative morbidity and mortality for general surgery patients.[10,11]

Other Calculators

Mayo Postoperative Mortality Risk Calculator in Patients with Cirrhosis added ASA class and age to the MELD score.[7] In this 2007 study, age and ASA score were significantly associated with the risk of mortality. However, the Mayo score also does not take into account the type of surgery or whether it is emergent. A 2021 study showed that the Mayo calculator overestimates risk and that its calibration worsened over time since its publication.[4]

VOCAL-Penn Score: Currently, the most useful perioperative risk estimation model for patients with cirrhosis is the Veterans Outcomes and Costs Associated with Liver Disease study group's VOCAL-Penn score.[4] The model is based on a national cohort of 3,785 U.S. veterans diagnosed with cirrhosis between 2008 and 2016 who received a surgical procedure at a VA medical center in one of six categories: (1) open abdominal, (2) laparoscopic abdominal, (3) abdominal wall, (4) vascular, (5) cardiac/chest, and (6) major orthopedic. The authors excluded minor surgeries and hepatic surgeries. The model estimates 30-, 90-, and 180-day postoperative mortality and 90-day decompensation using the following variables: age, ASA class (2–4), emergency status, surgery anatomic category BMI, whether NAFLD was the etiology of cirrhosis, and lab variables quantifying severity of cirrhosis: hypoalbuminemia, thrombocytopenia, and

TABLE 26-4. Available Perioperative Risk Calculators for Patients with Cirrhosis

CALCULATOR	VARIABLES				AVAILABLE AT:
Child-Turcotte Pugh (CTP)	FACTOR	1 POINT	2 POINTS	3 POINTS	https://www.mdcalc.com/child-pugh-score-cirrhosis-mortality
	Ascites	None	Medically controlled	Poorly controlled	
	Encephalopathy	None	Grades I–II	Grades III–IV	
	Total bili, mg/dL	<2	2–3	> 3	
	Albumin, g/dL	>3.5	2.5–3.5	<2.5	
	INR	<1.7	1.7–2.2	>2.2	
	CTP classes: A: 5–6 points B: 7–9 points C: 10–15 points				
MELD[7]	INR, creatinine, bilirubin				https://www.mdcalc.com/calc/10437/model-end-stage-liver-disease-meld
MELD-Na[9,11]	INR, creatinine, bilirubin Sodium Dialysis (at least twice in the past week)				https://www.mdcalc.com/calc/10437/model-end-stage-liver-disease-meld
iMELD[4,9]	INR, creatinine, bilirubin Age				http://www.livercancer.eu/calculators.html
MELD 3.0	INR, creatinine, bilirubin Sodium Albumin Sex				https://www.mdcalc.com/calc/10437/model-end-stage-liver-disease-meld
MESO[9]	MELD Sodium				MELD/SNa × 10
Mayo Risk Score[7]	INR, creatinine, bilirubin Age ASA class Etiology of liver disease				https://www.mayoclinic.org/medical-professionals/transplant-medicine/calculators/post-operative-mortality-risk-in-patients-with-cirrhosis/itt-20434721
VOCAL-Penn[4]	Age Albumin Bilirubin Platelets BMI > 30 ASA class Surgery type (including emergency)				https://www.vocalpennscore.com/

hyperbilirubinemia. VOCAL-Penn's 30-day mortality discrimination and calibration were better than prior tools, including MELD and Mayo calculator.

A limitation of the VOCAL-Penn study is that many common surgeries were not included, and the categories of surgery were still quite broad, encompassing a wide range of perioperative risks. The major limitation of all retrospective surgical outcome studies mentioned in this chapter is that the cohorts represent a preselected population. All patients in the studies, by definition, were felt to be surgical candidates, so the models likely underestimate risk when applied to all patients with cirrhosis who may seek surgery, and clinical judgment is necessary. This is also why the vast majority of patients included in VOCAL-Penn were CTP A, while only 11.2% were CTP class B and 0.5% were CTP class C. Because patients with cirrhosis also have other perioperative risks, a standard preoperative assessment should be performed first before applying the VOCAL-Penn score.

Surgery-Related Risk Factors (Tables 26-3 and 26-5)

Surgery-specific risk factors add to patient-specific risk factors. In general, more invasive, higher-risk surgeries with prolonged time under anesthesia carry higher risk of perioperative complications in patients with liver disease, with risk additionally stratified by CTP class or MELD score (Table 26-5). Emergency or urgent surgery also carries an increased risk of complications.[6]

Intra-abdominal surgeries carry a high risk of complications due to intraoperative factors, such as traction on the splanchnic vasculature leading to decreased hepatic perfusion, along with challenges with ascites management and incisional integrity.[12]

Hernia repairs create unique challenges for patients with liver disease, with the need to balance the risk of perioperative complications and ascites management versus the risk of more significant complications should emergency surgery for strangulated or incarcerated bowel become necessary. A study of 1,475 patients with cirrhosis receiving umbilical hernia repair at VA medical centers 2001–2014 found that 30-day mortality was 12.2% after emergent repair compared to 1.2% after nonemergent repair (0.7% in those without ascites in the prior month). For non-emergent repair in patients with recent ascites, mortality was still low if MELD was <15.[13]

TABLE 26-5. Surgery-Specific Mortality Estimates for Highest-Risk Procedures for Patients with Chronic Liver Disease, Stratified by Severity of Underlying Liver Disease[2,3,11]

TYPE OF SURGERY	CTP/MELD	POSTOPERATIVE MORTALITY
Hepatobiliary	A	0–3%
	B	0–55%
	C	21–100%
	MELD <10 >20	0–15% 60–70%
Non-hepatobiliary intra-abdominal	A	0–24%
	B	7–50%
	C	20–100%
	MELD <10 >20	3–15% 30–70%
Cardiac	A	0–20%
	B	15–50%
	C	20–100%
	MELD <15 >15	0–20% 20–60%

Very high-risk surgeries for patients with liver disease include liver resection and cardiothoracic surgery. Liver resection is often indicated for hepatic malignancy related to underlying liver disease but results in further reduction in liver mass. Cardiac surgery is appropriate in CTP A and select CTP B patients, though it carries a 67% risk of inhospital mortality for patients with CTP C disease.[14]

Unique Patient Circumstances

Liver Transplant Evaluation. Considerations for transplant involve unique and robust evaluation pathways because of the high-risk nature of the procedure combined with rare resource allocation (the small number of donor organs) and long-term risk considerations (including immunosuppression).[15] Transplant centers thoroughly evaluate potential liver transplant candidates through objective testing and committee selection, with consideration of life-limiting comorbid conditions that may limit transplant survival (e.g., cardiovascular disease, diabetes, malignancies, and frailty). The onus on objective testing, including imaging, labs, and testing for ischemic heart disease, is higher than it is for nontransplant perioperative risk assessments. For example, preoperative cardiac evaluation prior to liver transplant typically involves obtaining a TTE and a stress test, whereas these tests would not necessarily be indicated before nontransplant surgery.[16]

Listed for Liver Transplant. Patients on the liver transplant list or being evaluated for listing typically have more severe disease, which would increase risk of complications including mortality. Elective surgery should be deferred in patients with advanced disease and on the transplant waiting list, as evidenced by high mortality rates for patients with higher MELD scores. However, surgery might become necessary in nonelective situations or to maintain transplant candidacy (e.g., dental rehabilitation, diagnostic procedures to exclude malignancy or address infections). Risk-benefit discussions and planning must be performed in close coordination with the transplant team.

Acute Hepatitis and Acute Liver Failure. Acute hepatitis may be caused by acute alcoholic hepatitis, acute viral hepatitis, or other etiologies such as medications, Wilson's disease, or autoimmune hepatitis. Patients may or may not have underlying cirrhosis. Surgery should be avoided while the patient recovers from the acute injury given further increased risk of morbidity and mortality. Except for liver transplant, surgery should not be performed in patients with acute hepatitis or fulminant hepatic failure.[12]

Incidental Abnormal LFTs. Routine LFTs preoperatively are not recommended for patients without signs/symptoms or concerning risk factors for chronic or acute liver disease (e.g., alcohol use disorder). However, the preoperative clinician might encounter abnormal LFTs on prelim labs or in the medical record for previous reasons. There are limited data to guide thresholds for further evaluation before surgery, though ALT/AST more than three times the upper limit normal or any bilirubin elevation are proposed as reasons for surgical delay and further investigation. Based on history and physical exam, origins of ALT/AST elevations from muscle, alkaline phosphatase elevations from bone, and bilirubin elevations from hemolysis or benign etiologies (e.g., Gilbert syndrome) should also be considered.

PERIOPERATIVE MANAGEMENT/ RISK REDUCTION

Medical Optimization

Patients with chronic liver disease should be optimized in terms of manifestations of cirrhosis and risk (Figure 26-1), for example, using a structured approach.[2,5,12] Ascites or other manifestations of third spacing, such as hepatic hydrothorax, should be optimized, with therapeutic paracentesis, thoracentesis, or TIPS considered preoperatively. Treatment of active hepatitis C or alcohol use disorder can improve hepatic function. Alcohol cessation is prudent especially for patients with alcohol-related hepatitis, as is nutritional optimization.

Multidisciplinary coordination should be ensured, with clear coordination between surgeons, anesthesiologists, and hepatologists along with other potential members of the perioperative team including internists, hospitalists, or critical care physicians. Surgery should be performed at a center with experience in the perioperative care of patients with cirrhosis. Clinical teams should have a low threshold to schedule surgeries as inpatient or overnight observation cases rather than plan for same-day discharge or have surgeries occur at ambulatory surgery centers.

Preoperative Medication Management

Consider holding loop diuretics and spironolactone in patients NPO for surgery to avoid the risk of intravascular volume depletion and acute kidney injury. Rifaximin may be better tolerated than lactulose when NPO. Patients on steroids for autoimmune liver disease should take them on their surgery day. Nonselective beta-blockers prescribed for esophageal varices should be continued. Any immunosuppressants prescribed for liver transplant recipients should be continued as should agents prescribed for autoimmune liver disease.

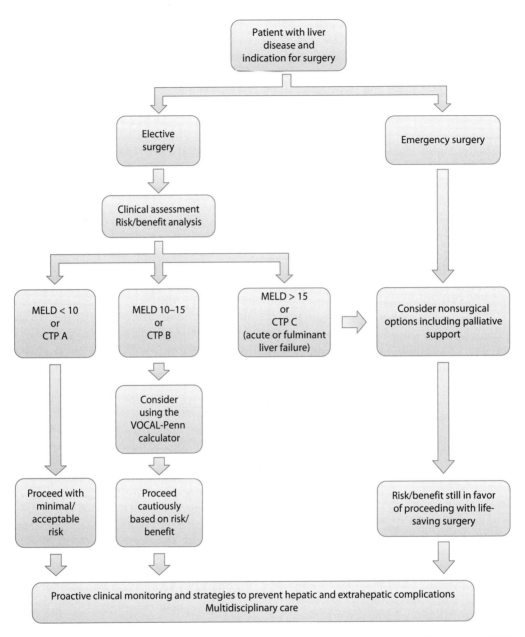

FIGURE 26-1. Risk evaluation pathway for patients with liver disease presenting for potential surgery. (Note that the MELD cut-offs may vary across the literature depending on author.)

Management of Coagulopathy

Platelet levels > 50,000/mm³ are adequate for stable clot formation[2,3,12]; platelet transfusions are likely only warranted for platelet levels < 50,000/mm³: and do not have long-lasting effects. The TPO agonists avatrombopag and lusutrombopag are approved to raise platelet counts perioperatively in adults with chronic liver disease and thrombocytopenia. INR levels do not correlate well with clotting function in patients with cirrhosis. Fresh frozen plasma (FFP) has a short half-life and also risks volume overload, so FFP transfusions are not recommended to reach a specific INR goal perioperatively.[2] Vitamin K can be administered to address coagulopathy due to nutritional or bile salt deficiency[12]; it will not correct INR elevations due to impaired hepatic synthetic function. There is no clear value in prophylactic use of other blood products or clotting factors such as factor VIIa or cryoprecipitate although they may be useful to treat bleeding.[3,17,18]

Postoperative Management

Patients should be monitored closely for early signs and symptoms of postoperative complications. Lab monitoring for hepatocellular or cholestatic injury (AST/ALT/alkaline phosphatase) and acutely worsened synthetic function (INR), as well as renal function and electrolytes, should be checked at least daily.

Volume status management can be very challenging postoperatively, with patients at risk of complications from both hypervolemia and hypovolemia. Volume overload can worsen portal hypertension, leading to an increased risk of variceal bleeding. Ascites management can also lower the risk of complications, including pulmonary complications from impaired diaphragmatic effort. However, decisions to stop intravenous fluids versus resume diuretics should be weighed carefully as hypovolemia and intravascular volume depletion can lead to acute kidney injury and precipitate hepatorenal syndrome. Colloids such as 5% albumin may be preferred over crystalloids as they can augment oncotic pressure.[12] Sodium or fluid restriction should be individualized. Monitor volume of ascites fluid loss after abdominal surgery (e.g., through postsurgical drains or using ultrasound) to closely track volume status. Ascites control is also important for facilitating healing and incision integrity after abdominal surgeries to avoid pressure on the wound and wound dehiscence; therapeutic paracentesis might be necessary.

Centrally acting medications should be judiciously prescribed to avoid exacerbating encephalopathy given poor hepatic metabolism and elimination. Benzodiazepines should be avoided in patients with liver disease (the exception being treatment for alcohol withdrawal). Narcotics should be cautiously prescribed and minimized, for example, at lower than typical starting doses and with longer dosing intervals.

Acetaminophen is safe to administer to patients with liver disease at reduced doses of 2 g maximum per day. Opioid-acetaminophen combinations should be avoided to prevent the risk of accidental overdosing of acetaminophen. NSAIDs should be avoided given the resultant impairment in renal blood flow and the risk of acute kidney injury.

In addition to analgesic choices, hepatic encephalopathy should be prevented by avoiding postoperative constipation and actively monitoring the number of stools per day. A low threshold for administration of lactulose and/or rifaximin may be needed, with rifaximin preferred as lactulose is a secretory laxative and can cause bowel distension or worsen hypovolemia by inducing diarrhea.[2,12] Lactulose enemas can be given for patients unable to take lactulose orally or through feeding tubes such as in the case of ileus or impaired bowel function.

If hepatic encephalopathy occurs, one should consider and investigate additional causes including surgical site infections, pneumonia, urinary tract infections, gastrointestinal bleeding, or acute or chronic liver failure. There should also be a low threshold to perform diagnostic paracentesis to assess for spontaneous bacterial peritonitis.

Patients with hepatic synthetic dysfunction are at increased risk of hypoglycemia due to impaired glucose metabolism and NPO states, and glucose should be monitored.

Venous thromboembolic (VTE) prophylaxis can be challenging for patients with liver disease and baseline coagulopathy or thrombocytopenia. Elevated INR levels, which poorly predict bleeding risk, do not correspond with decreased risk of VTE.[19] The risk-benefit of pharmacologic VTE prophylaxis should be carefully weighed, and nonpharmacologic strategies such as frequent ambulation and compression stockings are also valuable methods to reduce other postoperative complications.[12]

Encourage lung expansion maneuvers such as incentive spirometry and proactive ambulation or physical therapy assessments. Additionally, patients with liver disease should receive appropriate nutritional support, including a high-protein diet, which is no longer thought to increase risk of encephalopathy. Postoperative fevers or concerning exam findings (wound appearance, pulmonary exam) should prompt a low threshold for infectious evaluations.

SUMMARY

Cirrhosis increases the risk of perioperative morbidity and mortality. A comprehensive assessment as well as the use of risk calculators can inform perioperative optimization and risk-benefit discussions. While patients with mild, stable chronic liver disease may tolerate surgery well with nominally or acceptably increased risk of complications, patients with cirrhosis may need optimization or discussions about nonsurgical management, goals of care, and overall prognosis. Proactive postoperative monitoring for anticipated intra- and extrahepatic complications, as well as multidisciplinary collaboration with surgeons and specialists, can empower risk mitigation strategies.

Clinical pearls

- Avoid surgery in patients with acute hepatitis.
- Patients in CTP class A or MELD < 10 without evidence of portal hypertension can generally proceed to surgery; CTP B may be able to proceed to surgery after further assessing cirrhosis severity, comorbidities, and procedure-specific risk; CTP C or MELD > 15 should be counseled about nonsurgical options and avoid/delay surgery until after liver transplant unless it is urgent or potentially lifesaving.
- The VOCAL-Penn score may be the most useful model to estimate perioperative risk.
- Surgery-specific risks in the setting of chronic liver disease include high-risk surgeries (hepatobiliary, cardiac, pulmonary, and intra-abdominal) and emergency surgeries.
- Patients with chronic liver disease should be monitored closely for postoperative complications such as decompensated liver function, acute kidney injury, hepatic encephalopathy, and infections.

REFERENCES

1. Moon AM, Singal AG, Tapper EB. Contemporary epidemiology of chronic liver disease and cirrhosis. *Clin Gastroenterol Hepatol.* 2020;18(12):2650-2666. PMID: 31401364
2. Northup PG, Friedman LS, Kamath PS. AGA clinical practice update on surgical risk assessment and perioperative management in cirrhosis: expert review. *Clin Gastroenterol Hepatol.* 2019;17(4):595-606. PMID: 30273751
3. Newman KL, Johnson KM, Cornia PB, et al. Perioperative evaluation and management of patients with cirrhosis: risk assessment, surgical outcomes, and future directions. *Clin Gastroenterol Hepatol.* 2020;18(11):2398-2414.e3. PMID: 31376494
4. Mahmud N, Fricker Z, Hubbard RA, et al. Risk prediction models for post-operative mortality in patients with cirrhosis. *Hepatology.* 2021;73(1):204-218. PMID: 32939786
5. Grossniklaus EJ, Redinger JW, Johnson KM. Cirrhosis and the surgical patient. *Perioperative Care and Operating Room Management.* Available online before print: https://doi.org/10.1016/j.pcorm.2023.100348.
6. Johnson KM, Newman KL, Green PK, et al. Incidence and risk factors of postoperative mortality and morbidity after elective versus emergent abdominal surgery in a national sample of 8193 patients with cirrhosis. *Ann Surg.* 2021;274(4):e345-e354. PMID: 31714310
7. Teh SH, Nagorney DM, Stevens SR, et al. Risk factors for mortality after surgery in patients with cirrhosis. *Gastroenterology.* 2007;132(4):1261-1269. PMID: 17408652
8. Costa BP, Sousa FC, Serodio M, Carvalho C. Value of MELD and MELD-based indices in surgical risk evaluation of cirrhotic patients: retrospective analysis of 190 cases. *World J Surg.* 2009;33(8):1711-1719. PMID: 19513784
9. Huo TI, Lin HC, Huo SC, et al. Comparison of four model for end-stage liver disease-based prognostic systems for cirrhosis. *Liver Transpl.* 2008;14(6):837-844. PMID: 18508377
10. Godfrey EL, Kueht ML, Rana A, Awad S. MELD-Na (the new MELD) and peri-operative outcomes in emergency surgery. *Am J Surg.* 2018;216(3):407-413. PMID: 29871737
11. Maassel NL, Fleming MM, Luo J, et al. Model for end-stage liver disease sodium as a predictor of surgical risk in cirrhotic patients with ascites. *J Surg Res.* 2020;250:45-52. PMID: 32018142
12. Im GY, Lubezky N, Facciuto ME, Schiano TD. Surgery in patients with portal hypertension: a preoperative checklist and strategies for attenuating risk. *Clin Liver Dis.* 2014;18(2):477-505. PMID: 24679507
13. Johnson KM, Newman KL, Berry K, et al. Risk factors for adverse outcomes in emergency versus nonemergency open umbilical hernia repair and opportunities for elective repair in a national cohort of patients with cirrhosis. *Surgery.* 2022;172(1):184-192. PMID: 35058058

14. Filsoufi F, Salzberg SP, Rahmanian PB, et al. Early and late outcomes of cardiac surgery in patients with liver cirrhosis. *Liver Transplantation.* 2007;13:990-995. PMID: 17427174

15. Kriss M, Biggins SW. Evaluation and selection of the liver transplant candidate: updates on a dynamic and evolving process. *Curr Opin Organ Transplant.* 2021;26(1):52-61. PMID: 33278150

16. Cheng XS, VanWagner LB, Costa SP, et al., American Heart Association Council on the Kidney in Cardiovascular Disease and Council on Cardiovascular Radiology and Intervention. Emerging evidence on coronary heart disease screening in kidney and liver transplantation candidates: a scientific statement from the American Heart Association: endorsed by the American Society of Transplantation. *Circulation.* 2022;146(21):e299-e324. PMID: 36252095

17. Northup PG, Garcia-Pagan JC, Garcia-Tsao G, et al. Vascular liver disorders, portal vein thrombosis, and procedural bleeding in patients with liver disease: 2020 practice guidance by the American Association for the Study of Liver Diseases. *Hepatology.* 2021;73(1):366-413. PMID: 33219529

18. Roberts LN, Lisman T, Stanworth S, et al. Periprocedural management of abnormal coagulation parameters and thrombocytopenia in patients with cirrhosis: guidance from the SSC of the ISTH. *J Thromb Haemost.* 2022;20(1):39-47. PMID: 34661370

19. Dabbagh O, Oza A, Prakash S, et al. Coagulopathy does not protect against venous thromboembolism in hospitalized patients with chronic liver disease. *Chest.* 2010;137(5):1145-1149. PMID: 20040609

## 27

Cerebrovascular Disease

Nidhi Rohatgi, MD, MS, SFHM

COMMON CLINICAL QUESTIONS

1. What are the strategies to mitigate the risk of perioperative stroke in patients undergoing noncardiac, nonneurologic surgery?
2. What is the appropriate timing for elective surgery in patients with a recent ischemic stroke?

INTRODUCTION

Perioperative stroke is a devastating complication associated with 30-day mortality ranging from 16% to 26% for ischemic stroke after noncardiac or non-neurological surgery and up to 32% for perioperative hemorrhagic stroke.[1] Approximately 50% of perioperative strokes occur within postoperative days 1–3, with a significant proportion of these occurring intra-operatively. Most perioperative strokes are ischemic, primarily embolic after cardiac and carotid surgeries, and embolic or thrombotic after noncardiac surgeries. Hemorrhagic strokes comprise less than 5% of all perioperative strokes.[1]

Incidence of Perioperative Stroke

The average incidence of perioperative stroke is 0.3%[1] but varies with the type of surgery, history of prior stroke, and the patient's comorbidities. It is highest with cardiac, carotid, and neurologic surgeries[1,2]— 1.3% to 20% after cardiac surgeries,[1] 6.7% and 2.7% after carotid artery stenting (CAS), and 4.3% and 1.4% for carotid endarterectomy (CEA) for patients with symptomatic and asymptomatic carotid stenosis, respectively,[3] and 1.25% after neurological surgeries.[1]

The incidence of *overt* perioperative stroke after noncardiac, noncarotid, nonneurologic surgery in multiple studies has been reported to be less than 1% overall—less than 0.5% in patients without a history of prior stroke and 1–2% in patients with a history of prior stroke. The incidence of *covert stroke* after elective noncardiac surgeries in patients ≥65 years old has been reported to be 7%.[4]

Pathophysiology

Mechanisms and pathophysiology of perioperative stroke vary with the type of surgery and risk factors.[1] Large vessel and cardioembolic etiologies are the most common. Inflammation and hypercoagulability in the perioperative period predispose to thrombogenesis and plaque rupture, especially in patients with multiple preexisting risk factors. Cardioembolic ischemic stroke may occur in the perioperative setting in patients with prior or new-onset atrial fibrillation (compounded by interruption of antithrombotics in the perioperative period) or in patients with direct manipulation of the heart or aortic arch during cardiac surgeries. Another potential mechanism by which perioperative ischemic stroke may occur is cerebral hypoperfusion in the setting of anemia, hypotension, and hypocarbia. Reperfusion injury after CEA may predispose to hemorrhagic stroke or after neurological procedures, direct injury to intracranial vessels may predispose to perioperative stroke.

PREOPERATIVE EVALUATION

For patients at high risk of perioperative stroke, a risk-benefit discussion should occur prior to proceeding with elective surgery along with risk factor modification and discussion on the appropriate timing of the elective surgery.

Risk Factors

Any modifiable cardiovascular risk factors should be optimized prior to elective surgeries (Table 27-1).[2,5] The risk factors for perioperative stroke are similar to those in nonsurgical patients. As noted above, after the type of surgery, a history of prior stroke or transient ischemic attack (TIA) is the most important risk factor.

In the PeriOperative ISchemic Evaluation (POISE) trial of 8,351 patients undergoing noncardiac surgery, prophylactic use of metoprolol started shortly before surgery was associated with twice the risk of stroke (1% vs. 0.5%) compared to those who did not receive metoprolol.[6] In this study, independent predictors of stroke with the highest population attributable risk in decreasing order were history of stroke or TIA, clinically significant hypotension, significant bleeding, use of clopidogrel or ticlopidine in the 24 hours before surgery, and new clinically significant atrial fibrillation.[6]

The association between the severity or duration of hypotension and perioperative stroke is not clearly established. There are multiple definitions of hypotension in the perioperative setting; systolic blood pressure < 80 mmHg or mean arterial pressure < 60 mmHg or a drop in systolic blood pressure by >20% below baseline are the more common definitions.[2] The 2020 guidelines from the Society for Neuroscience in Anesthesiology and Critical Care (SNACC) concluded that the effect of relative hypotension on the stroke risk cannot be excluded based on the current evidence.[5] The recent POISE-3 trial reported no difference in the incidence of stroke (and other vascular outcomes) after noncardiac surgery between patients in the hypotension avoidance group (intraoperative goal mean arterial pressure ≥ 80 mmHg) and the hypertension avoidance group (intraoperative goal mean arterial pressure ≥ 60 mmHg).[7] Finally, although the evidence is quite limited, patient positioning during surgery may alter cerebral perfusion and increase the risk of perioperative stroke (e.g., sitting or beach chair position during shoulder or cervical spine surgeries, Trendelenburg position that may increase intracranial pressure, or prone position that may affect cerebral venous drainage).[1,2,5]

No clear association between stroke and the choice of the anesthetic agent or regional versus general anesthesia has been reported.[1,2] An association between patent foramen ovale (PFO) and perioperative stroke has been reported. A study comprising 639,985 patients

TABLE 27-1. Risk Factors Associated with Perioperative Stroke

PATIENT-RELATED FACTORS	PROCEDURE-RELATED FACTORS
• Previous stroke or transient ischemic attack • Atrial fibrillation • Acute renal failure or chronic kidney disease • Cardiac disease (heart failure, myocardial infarction, unstable angina, valvular disease) • Perioperative interruption of antithrombotics • New beta-blocker within 24 hours of surgery • Atrial septal defect/patent foramen ovale • Carotid stenosis • Other factors: age, hypertension, diabetes, hyperlipidemia • Female sex	• Type of surgery (cardiac>carotid>vascular>other noncardiac) • Emergency surgery • Hypotension • Acute anemia (limited evidence) • Hypercoagulable state • Intraoperative metoprolol

in the National Inpatient Sample reported the incidence of perioperative stroke after major noncardiac surgery to be 6.3 times higher in patients with an atrial septal defect compared to those without an atrial septal defect.[8]

Perioperative Risk Calculators

Risk calculators for prediction of perioperative stroke have been developed. In one study, myocardial infarction or cardiac arrest (MICA) risk score and American College of Surgeons Surgical Risk Calculator (ACS-SRC) provided excellent risk discrimination for perioperative stroke in most patients undergoing noncardiac surgery (*c*-statistic 0.833 and 0.836, respectively), compared to the Revised Cardiac Risk Index, $CHADS_2$, CHA_2DS_2-VASc, or Mashour risk score.[9] MICA was the most accurate for predicting perioperative stroke after nonvascular surgeries, and ACS-SRC was the best for vascular surgeries.[9] A newer risk calculator developed using National Surgical Quality Improvement Project (NSQIP) database between 2007 and 2010 to predict stroke, cardiac, and mortality risk has yet to be externally validated (https://qxmd.com/calculate/calculator_823/woo-perioperative-risk).[10]

Timing of Noncardiac Surgery After Ischemic Stroke

The timing of elective surgery in patients who had a recent ischemic stroke is crucial. A study using the Danish registry reported that the perioperative risk of major adverse cardiovascular events and mortality was highest in patients who underwent elective noncardiac surgery within the first 3 months after an ischemic stroke. The increased risk of subsequent stroke declined with time and stabilized at 9 months after the ischemic stroke but was still higher compared to patients with no history of stroke.[11] However, there was no control group to evaluate the baseline risk of subsequent stroke in patients with a stroke who did not undergo surgery. Based on this data, the 2020 SNACC guidelines[5] recommend delaying elective surgery for 9 months after a stroke, and the 2021 American Heart Association/American Stroke Association (AHA/ASA) scientific statement[2] recommended delaying elective surgery for at least 6 months (possibly up to 9 months) after a stroke. In contrast to the Danish study, a more recent, larger study evaluating Medicare beneficiaries reported

that the risk of stroke was highest in the first month but leveled off when ≥3 months elapsed between a previous ischemic stroke and elective nonneurologic, noncardiac surgery.[12] Authors of this study, who were also authors of the AHA/ASA statement, concluded that their recommendations to delay elective surgery for at least 6 months was too conservative.[12]

The risk of recurrent stroke seems to be highest in the first 3 months, which may be explained, in part, by impaired cerebral autoregulation. Cerebral perfusion is very sensitive to blood pressure fluctuations, as may occur during anesthesia and surgery, and elective procedures should be avoided during this period. Ultimately, the decisions on the timing of surgery are often individualized based on the risks and benefits.

Carotid Bruits and Asymptomatic Carotid Artery Stenosis

Currently, in the context of preoperative evaluation prior to noncardiac surgery, there is no established guideline suggesting preoperative screening or revascularization of extracranial carotid stenosis to reduce the incidence of perioperative stroke.[1] There is no established correlation between carotid bruit and ipsilateral perioperative strokes.

Extracranial carotid stenosis is a marker of atherosclerotic disease. The 2021 AHA/ASA guidelines recommend CEA within 6 months of TIA or non-disabling ischemic stroke in patients with severe (70–99%) and moderate (50–69%; depending on patient-specific factors) ipsilateral carotid stenosis, if the estimated risk of perioperative morbidity and mortality is <6% (class I recommendation).[13] The recommendations for carotid artery revascularization in asymptomatic patients with carotid stenosis are based on dated trials (Veterans Affairs Cooperative Study [VACS in 1993], Asymptomatic Carotid Atherosclerosis Study [ACAS in 1995], and Asymptomatic Carotid Surgery Trial [ACST-1 in 2004]), and medical management has significantly improved since these trials. The results of the Carotid Revascularization and Medical Management for Asymptomatic Carotid Stenosis Trial (CREST-2; NCT02089217) comparing carotid revascularization with intensive medical therapy to intensive medical therapy alone for primary prevention of stroke in asymptomatic patients with >70% carotid stenosis are awaited.

PERIOPERATIVE MANAGEMENT AND RISK REDUCTION STRATEGIES

Multiple strategies have been proposed for perioperative stroke risk reduction besides optimization of modifiable cardiovascular risk factors (Figure 27-1).

Beta-blockers should be continued perioperatively in patients who have been taking them chronically.[14] If beta-blockers are newly initiated, it should be done at least 7 days prior to the noncardiac surgery, with preference to cardioselective beta-blockers such as atenolol or bisoprolol over noncardioselective beta-blockers. Guideline-directed protocols to minimize interruption of anticoagulants and/or bridging therapy should be followed (see Chapter 5).[1,3] There is insufficient evidence to conclude whether aspirin reduces stroke risk for the majority of patients undergoing noncardiac surgery, although it may reduce perioperative cardiac risk, especially in patients with coronary stents in whom it should be continued.[2,5] Perioperative statins may not decrease stroke risk but may decrease mortality and major morbidity after noncardiac surgery.[2,5] In patients with a history of stroke, PFO closure may be considered for secondary stroke prevention in selected patients. Patients with

PFO undergoing noncardiac surgery should have careful hemodynamic management to minimize right to left shunting, interruption of home antithrombotics should be minimized, and venous thromboprophylaxis should be implemented.[15]

Hypotension avoidance may or may not reduce the risk of stroke, and the evidence for this is still evolving. For surgeries performed in the sitting or beach chair position, blood pressure should be measured on the nonoperative upper arm (as opposed to the lower extremity) and with the understanding that the mean arterial pressure may be 12–24 mmHg lower in the brain compared to the nonoperative upper extremity.[1,5]

The association between anemia and perioperative stroke also remains unclear. The 2020 SNACC guidelines recommended a relatively high transfusion threshold of hemoglobin ≥ 9 g/dL in patients already taking a beta-blocker to reduce the perioperative stroke risk given the theoretical risk of reduced cerebral perfusion and cerebral hypoxia if the cardiac output is reduced and is combined with impaired beta-2-mediated cerebrovascular vasodilatation.[5] The 2021 AHA/ASA scientific statement recommends that it is reasonable to consider a transfusion threshold of 8 g/dL for patients with a history of recent stroke or

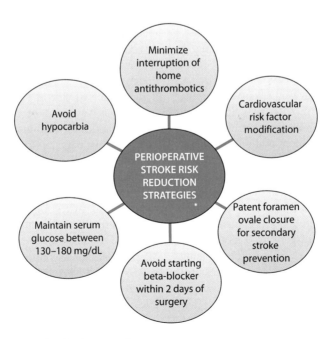

FIGURE 27-1. Perioperative stroke risk reduction strategies.

significant cerebrovascular disease; a higher transfusion threshold of 8–9 g/dL may be considered in those with an acute stroke, ongoing bleeding, hemodynamic instability, and known cerebrovascular insufficiency attributable to stenosis or occlusion.[2]

MANAGEMENT OF PERIOPERATIVE STROKE

Stroke is a clinical diagnosis, and imaging is obtained to confirm and localize the area of stroke. Identification of stroke is time-critical but may be challenging in the perioperative period when the patient may be sedated, have postoperative delirium, or be unable to participate in motor examination due to restrictions after surgery or due to pain. In the event of a stroke, a stroke code should be activated. A stroke neurologist should be consulted immediately to expedite guideline-directed management and eligibility for reperfusion therapy. Physiological perturbations such as hypotension, hypovolemia, hypoxia, hyperthermia, and hypo- or hyperglycemia should be corrected. Risk factors for stroke (e.g., atrial fibrillation) should be worked up.

Clinical pearls

- The most important risk factors for perioperative stroke are the type of surgery (highest in cardiac, carotid, and neurological surgery) and prior history of stroke or TIA.

- Carotid bruits are not a reliable indicator of the presence or severity of carotid stenosis and do not predict ipsilateral stroke.

- Elective surgery should probably be delayed for at least 3 months after an acute stroke.

- If a beta-blocker is being started in a high-risk patient, it should not be started within 24 hours of the surgery. Cardioselective beta-blockers (e.g., bisoprolol) may be preferable to noncardioselective beta-blockers (e.g., metoprolol).

- Alteplase is contraindicated within 14 days of intracranial or intraspinal surgeries, but a risk-benefit discussion should occur for other surgical patients with acute ischemic stroke who may be eligible. Mechanical thrombectomy within 24 hours of perioperative acute ischemic stroke may be considered in eligible patients.

REFERENCES

1. Fanning JP, Campbell BCV, Bulbulia R, et al. Perioperative stroke. *Nat Rev Dis Primers.* 2024 Jan 18;10(1):3. PMID: 38238382

2. Benesch C, Glance LG, Derdeyn CP, et al., American Heart Association Stroke Council; Council on Arteriosclerosis, Thrombosis and Vascular Biology; Council on Cardiovascular and Stroke Nursing; Council on Clinical Cardiology; Council on Epidemiology and Prevention. Perioperative neurological evaluation and management to lower the risk of acute stroke in patients undergoing noncardiac, nonneurological surgery: a scientific statement from the American Heart Association/American Stroke Association. *Circulation.* 2021;143:e923-e946. PMID: 33827230

3. Xin W, Yang S, Li Q, Yang X. Endarterectomy versus stenting for the prevention of periprocedural stroke or death in patients with symptomatic or asymptomatic carotid stenosis: a meta-analysis of 10 randomized trials. *Ann Transl Med.* 2021 Feb;9(3):256. PMID: 33708883

4. NeuroVISION Investigators. Perioperative covert stroke in patients undergoing non-cardiac surgery (NeuroVISION): a prospective cohort study. *Lancet.* 2019;394:1022-1029. PMID: 31422895

5. Vlisides PE, Moore LE, Whalin MK, et al. Perioperative care of patients at high risk for stroke during or after non-cardiac, non-neurological surgery: 2020 guidelines from the Society for Neuroscience in Anesthesiology and Critical Care. *J Neurosurg Anesthesiol.* 2020;32: 210-226. PMID: 32433102

6. POISE Study Group, Devereaux PJ, Yang H, Yusuf S, et al. Effects of extended-release metoprolol succinate in patients undergoing non-cardiac surgery (POISE trial): a randomised controlled trial. *Lancet.* 2008;371: 1839-1847. PMID: 18479744

7. Marcucci M, Painter TW, Conen D, et al., POISE-3 Trial Investigators and Study Groups. Hypotension-avoidance versus hypertension-avoidance strategies in noncardiac surgery: an international randomized controlled trial. *Ann Intern Med.* 2023;176:605–614. PMID: 37094336

8. Smilowitz NR, Subashchandran V, Berger JS. Atrial septal defect and the risk of ischemic stroke in the perioperative period of noncardiac surgery. *Am J Cardiol.* 2019;124:1120-1124. PMID: 31375244

9. Wilcox T, Smilowitz NR, Xia Y, Berger JS. Cardiovascular risk scores to predict perioperative stroke in noncardiac surgery. *Stroke.* 2019;50:2002-2006. PMID: 31234757

10. Woo SH, Marhefka GD, Cowan SW, Ackermann L. Development and validation of a prediction model for stroke, cardiac, and mortality risk after non-cardiac

surgery. *J Am Heart Assoc.* 2021;10(4):e018013. PMID: 33522252

11. Jørgensen ME, Torp-Pedersen C, Gislason GH, et al. Time elapsed after ischemic stroke and risk of adverse cardiovascular events and mortality following elective noncardiac surgery. *JAMA.* 2014;312:269-277. PMID: 25027142

12. Glance LG, Benesch CG, Holloway RG, et al. Association of time elapsed since ischemic stroke with risk of recurrent stroke in older patients undergoing elective nonneurologic, noncardiac surgery. *JAMA Surg.* 2022;157:e222236. PMID: 35767247

13. Kleindorfer DO, Towfighi A, Chaturvedi S, et al. 2021 Guideline for the prevention of stroke in patients with stroke and transient ischemic attack: a guideline from the American Heart Association/American Stroke Association. *Stroke.* 2021;52:e364-e467. PMID: 34024117

14. Writing Committee Members; Thompson A, Fleischmann KE, Smilowitz NR, et al. 2024 AHA/ACC/ACS/ASNC/HRS/SCA/SCCT/SCMR/SVM Guideline for Perioperative Cardiovascular Management for Noncardiac Surgery: A Report of the American College of Cardiology/American Heart Association Joint Committee on Clinical Practice Guidelines. *J Am Coll Cardiol.* 2024;84(19):1869-1969. PMID: 39320289

15. Rohatgi N, Smilowitz NR, Lansberg MG. Perioperative stroke risk reduction in patients with patent foramen ovale. *JAMA Neurol.* 2020;77:1479-1480. PMID: 32744603

28

Seizure Disorder, Parkinson's Disease, and Myasthenia Gravis

Nidhi Rohatgi, MD, MS, SFHM

COMMON CLINICAL QUESTIONS

1. How do you manage medications prescribed for these conditions?
2. What measures can be taken to prevent perioperative decompensation of these conditions?

Patients with known neurological conditions require special attention during the perioperative period. Sometimes, clinicians may newly diagnose neurological conditions during the perioperative period. In this chapter, we will focus on three neurological conditions: seizure disorder, Parkinson's disease, and myasthenia gravis.

SEIZURE DISORDER

Epilepsy usually refers to a condition in which there is a risk of recurrent seizures related to a nontransient chronic etiology. *Seizure* can be an isolated event with a transient precipitant. The term "convulsion" is no longer recommended. The 2017 International League Against Epilepsy Commission on Classification and Terminology classified seizure types into: (a) focal onset with or without impaired awareness (the terms "partial," "simple," or "complex" seizures are no longer preferred), (b) generalized onset, and (c) unknown onset (for tonic-clonic or behavior arrest seizures where focal versus generalized onset is unknown).[1]

Myoclonus is a sudden brief muscle contraction(s) of one part of the body or the entire body. It is one of the more common involuntary movements noted in the perioperative period. They are colloquially referred to as "twitches" and sometimes "myoclonic jerks." Patients with epilepsy may have myoclonic seizures. In the perioperative period, myoclonus may be triggered by hypoxia, hypercarbia, liver or kidney failure, medications (e.g., tramadol, quinolones, benzodiazepines, anticholinergics, gabapentin, opiates, propofol, etomidate), infection, or stroke.

Fasciculations, myoclonus, and waxing-waning delirium or consciousness may be observed in the intra- and postoperative period and be occasionally misclassified as a seizure. Sometimes patients with epilepsy may have a psychogenic nonepileptic seizure in the postoperative period. Common triggers of seizure in the perioperative period are listed in Table 28-1.

Seizures can manifest in a variety of ways and it is important for perioperative physicians to have knowledge of the common manifestations of seizures if they were to witness or manage such an event. A few key considerations in managing patients with seizure disorders in the perioperative setting are shown in Figure 28-1.

Preoperative Considerations

In patients with a prior history of seizure disorder, detailed history should be obtained regarding the type of seizure, any known triggers, last seizure occurrence,

TABLE 28-1. Potential Triggers of Seizures in the Perioperative Period

• Nonadherence	Missed home antiseizure medications or drug interactions
• Drugs	Quinolones, meperidine, tramadol, fentanyl, local anesthetics, sevoflurane, antipsychotics, iodinated contrast agents, ketamine, etomidate, high-dose penicillin, cephalosporins, and imipenem, illicit drugs (cocaine, amphetamine)
• Drug withdrawal	Benzodiazepines, barbiturates, alcohol, baclofen, zolpidem
• Metabolic	Hypoxia, hypoglycemia, hyperglycemia, hyponatremia, hypocalcemia
• Cerebrovascular disease	Stroke, central nervous system infections
• Other	Sleep deprivation, loud noises, flashing lights, pain, stress, fever

home antiseizure drugs (ASDs), and any known side effects. The most common cause of seizures in the perioperative period is a missed dose of ASD. Patients should take their home ASD on the morning of the surgery. If a patient has poor seizure control or is having significant or worsening adverse effects that are thought to be due to the patient's ASD, a discussion with the patient's outpatient neurologist should occur. A baseline complete blood count and a comprehensive metabolic profile should be obtained if the patient is on ASD that may cause adverse effects such as red cell aplasia (e.g., lamotrigine), pancytopenia (e.g., phenytoin), thrombocytopenia (e.g., carbamazepine, oxcarbazepine, valproate, phenytoin), hyponatremia (e.g., carbamazepine, oxcarbazepine), acidosis (e.g., topiramate), or hepatic failure (e.g., valproate, phenytoin). Blood levels of ASD are not required unless there is a concern for toxicity or nonadherence. Pregnancy status should be assessed in women of childbearing age

to guide the choice of ASD. If a patient is on a ketogenic diet to manage epilepsy, appropriate measures should be taken perioperatively to avoid carbohydrate and dextrose in diet and medications and to monitor serum electrolytes, glucose, and acid-base status, especially if long procedures are planned or a prolonged fasting state is expected.[2]

Intraoperative Considerations

Surgery and anesthesia can significantly alter the serum levels of ASD. Drug interactions between ASD and multiple medications should be noted as several new medications are administered in the intra- and postoperative period. Most commonly, these drug interactions are through the inhibition or activation of cytochrome P450 isoenzymes.

Postoperative Considerations

Known triggers of seizures should be avoided or promptly managed (Table 28-1). If home ASD cannot be given enterally and a parenteral formulation is not available, as a temporary measure, a benzodiazepine can be considered. If a patient has a seizure, then benzodiazepines are the first-line medication. In the event of status epilepticus (seizure lasting > 5 minutes) and/or if there is concern for airway protection, the patient should be transferred to the intensive care unit for close monitoring, ventilatory support, intravenous benzodiazepines, and ASD. Seizure and fall precautions should be implemented.

If a patient has a first seizure during the postoperative period or experiences worsening of a known seizure disorder, neurology consultation should be obtained to decide the need for continuous electroencephalographic monitoring, initiation of new ASD, or dose titration of home ASD.

PARKINSON'S DISEASE

Parkinson's disease (PD) is an age-related neurodegenerative disorder with clinical presentation varying from mild disease to advanced disease with disabling motor and nonmotor symptoms. Patients with PD are extremely vulnerable to medical complications in the perioperative period. A few considerations in managing patients with PD in the perioperative setting are shown in Figure 28-2.

PREOPERATIVE

Obtain detailed history (frequency of seizure, last seizure occurrence, manifestation of seizure [e.g., focal or generalized onset, characteristic of aura, postictal phase], history of status epilepticus, home antiseizure medications regimen and any adverse effects, compliance with antiseizure medications).

Obtain drug/alcohol history and history of withdrawal seizures.

(a) Obtain complete blood count and a comprehensive metabolic profile. Blood levels of antiseizure medications are not required unless concerned about toxicity or nonadherence. Surgery and anesthesia can significantly alter serum levels of antiseizure medications.

(a) If patient is strict NPO or having an intestinal surgery → Give parenteral formulation of home antiseizure medication.
(b) If parenteral formulation of home antiseizure medication not available → Discuss alternate regimen with a neurologist.
(c) The following antiseizure medications are available parenterally: Phenytoin, phenobarbital, valproic acid, levetiracetam, lacosamide, lorazepam, and midazolam.

When relevant, assess pregnancy status to guide the choice of antiseizure medication.

On the morning of surgery, allow patient to take home antiseizure medications with small sips of water.

INTRAOPERATIVE

(a) Select anesthetic medications carefully → Avoid medications that interact with home antiseizure medications or those that could cause seizures. (Note this is only a relative contraindication if other factors argue for a particular anesthetic. Most anesthetics, with the possible exceptions of ketamine and etomidate, usually suppress seizures.)

(a) Rarely seizures may occur under general anesthesia (e.g., neurosurgical patients or poorly controlled epilepsy). These are difficult to diagnose and patients may have an increase in the end-tidal CO_2, elevation in their blood pressure or heart rate, mydriasis, or increased oxygen requirement. If a seizure is suspected, anesthesia is deepened and any reversible precipitants such as hypoxia or hypoglycemia are corrected.

(a) POSTOPERATIVE

(a) Avoid interruption of home antiseizure medication or changes in the medication schedule. If home antiseizure medication cannot be given enterally and a parenteral formulation is not available, as a temporary coverage, a benzodiazepine, such as intravenous lorazepam, can be considered or neurology consultation should be obtained.

(a) Avoid triggers of seizures (e.g., sleep deprivation, loud noises, flashing lights, pain, stress, fever, or any known prior triggers for that patient). Avoid medications that may be associated with seizures (Table 28-1). Implement seizure and fall precautions (e.g., low-height bed, raise up and pad side rails of bed, set up suction and oxygen at bedside).

If patient is at high risk of drug/alcohol withdrawal seizures, prophylactic benzodiazepines and gabapentin are sometimes considered.

FIGURE 28-1. Perioperative considerations in the management of patients with seizures.

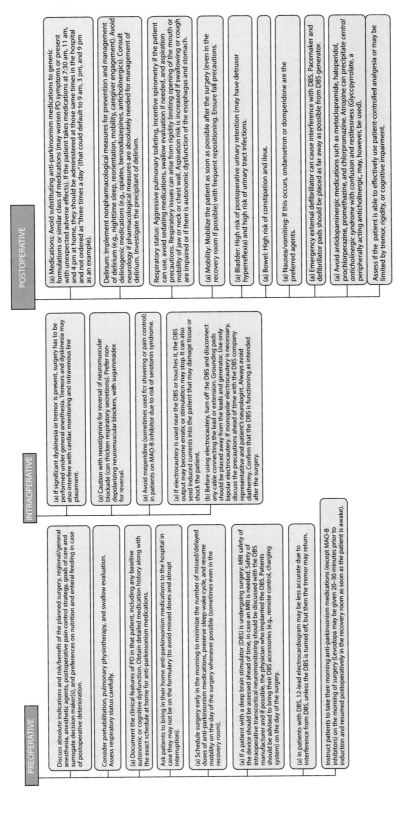

FIGURE 28-2. Perioperative considerations in the management of patients with Parkinson's disease.
PD, Parkinson's disease; DBS, deep brain stimulator; MAO-B, monoamine oxidase-B.

Preoperative Considerations

Careful and comprehensive preoperative evaluation in patients with PD is key. There should be a thorough discussion about the benefits and risks of the planned surgical procedure, type of anesthesia and anesthetic agents, postoperative pain control strategy, goals of care and surrogate decision maker(s), and preferences on nutrition and enteral feeding in case of postoperative deterioration. Surgery should be scheduled earlier in the morning. This can minimize the number of missed/delayed doses of anti-parkinsonism medications, preserve the sleep-wake cycle to reduce the risk of postoperative delirium, and create time to mobilize the patient in the evening of postoperative day 0 whenever possible. If a patient with a deep brain stimulator (DBS) is undergoing surgery, magnetic resonance imaging (MRI) safety of the device should be assessed, if an MRI is needed. Throughout the perioperative period, ensure that the DBS is charged and turned off only for the minimum duration necessary.

Detailed history and examination should be conducted with multisystem risk assessment as in all patients, with special consideration of discussion with the patient's neurologist about the clinical features and management of PD in that patient. Based on the patient's clinical status, prehabilitation, pulmonary physiotherapy, and swallow evaluation may be beneficial prior to surgery. One of the most critical historical details during preoperative evaluation of a patient with PD is their medication history; this includes the drug names, dose, exact schedule, and any known adverse effects or history of symptoms with transient interruption in the past. Patients should be asked to bring in their home anti-parkinsonism medications to the hospital to avoid missed doses, abrupt interruption, or unknown efficacy and tolerance for any medications that may be substituted for that patient based on the hospital formulary. Common classes of medications used in the management of PD and their adverse effects are shown in Table 28-2.[3]

Patients should be instructed to take their morning anti-parkinsonism medications on the day of the surgery (except monoamine oxidase-B [MAO-B] inhibitors, which should be held 2 weeks prior to the surgery after discussion with the patient's neurologist). Levodopa may be given 20–30 minutes prior to induction.

Intraoperative Considerations

If significant dyskinesia or tremor is present, surgery has to be performed under general anesthesia. Tremors and dyskinesia may also interfere with electrocardiography, cardiac monitoring, and intravenous line placement. Neostigmine should be used with caution for reversal of neuromuscular blockade as it may thicken the respiratory secretions. Nondepolarizing neuromuscular blockers are preferred as sugammadex could be used for reversal. If a patient with a DBS is undergoing surgery, monopolar electrocautery should be avoided as DBS may cause interference. Diathermy should always be avoided because tissue damage can lead to neurological injury or death.[4]

Postoperative Considerations

Patients with PD are at risk of several postoperative complications, especially if they have advanced PD and are undergoing a complicated surgery. The timing of anti-parkinsonism medications should be strictly adhered to, similar to their home schedule, in order to minimize the distressing motor symptoms of PD (except MAO-B inhibitors that can be resumed on postoperative day 1 or 2 if the blood pressure is stable). This is particularly challenging in patients who are strict NPO, have prolonged surgery, or are having gastrointestinal surgeries, as most of these medications can only be given orally.

Patients with PD are at high risk of pulmonary complications (e.g., aspiration, retention of secretions, mucus plugging, pneumonia, atelectasis, postextubation laryngospasm) with drooling, dysphagia, obstructive lung defect, restrictive pattern due to chest wall rigidity, sleep apnea, and a feeling of dyspnea during their "off" period. Aggressive pulmonary toileting, incentive spirometry, avoidance of sedating medications, swallow evaluation if needed, and aspiration precautions are vital.

These patients are at high fall risk with postural instability, gait freezing, shuffling, and orthostatic hypotension. Difficulties with mobility predispose them to venous thromboembolism, deconditioning, and pressure ulcers. Mobilize these patients as soon as possible after surgery with frequent repositioning, sometimes even in the postoperative recovery room if safely possible.

TABLE 28-2. Common Classes of Anti-Parkinsonism Medications and Their Adverse Effects

ANTI-PARKINSONISM MEDICATION	ADVERSE EFFECTS
Dopamine precursors (e.g., carbidopa-levodopa)	• Dyskinesia, orthostasis, hallucinations, nausea, and vomiting • These medications have a short half-life (60–90 min) and discontinuation for 6–12 hours can cause an abrupt loss of therapeutic effect; worsened skeletal muscle rigidity can interfere with ventilation • A rare but potentially life-threatening manifestation of abrupt withdrawal or rapid reduction in dose of dopamine precursors or agonists is Parkinsonism-Hyperpyrexia Syndrome (PHS). The symptoms of PHS mimic neuroleptic malignant syndrome and include high fever, severe muscle rigidity, autonomic instability, sedation, and rarely, multisystem involvement with acute kidney injury, disseminated intravascular coagulation, aspiration pneumonia, and other infections
Dopamine agonists (e.g., pramipexole, ropinirole, rotigotine, apomorphine)	• Nausea and vomiting, dyskinesia, orthostasis, impulse control disorder, and cognitive impairment • With abrupt discontinuation, dopamine acute withdrawal syndrome (DAWS) may occur. DAWS may present with panic attacks, agitation, orthostasis, or diaphoresis
Monoamine oxidase B (MAO-B) inhibitors (e.g., selegiline, rasagiline)	• Hypotension • Caution on serotonin syndrome with concurrent meperidine, selective serotonin receptor inhibitors, and serotonin-norepinephrine receptor inhibitors • Multiple drug interactions: Some medications that are contraindicated with MAO-B inhibitors include tramadol, methadone, dextromethorphan (risk of psychosis or bizarre behavior), St John's wort, cyclobenzaprine, or another (selective or nonselective) MAO inhibitor (risk of hypertensive crisis)
Catechol-O-methyl transferase (COMT) inhibitors (e.g., entacapone, tolcapone)	• Can exacerbate the adverse effects associated with levodopa • May cause dark discoloration of urine • Hepatic toxicity has been reported with tolcapone
N-methyl-D-aspartate (NMDA) receptor antagonist (e.g., amantadine)	• Cognitive impairment • Abrupt discontinuation may cause amantadine withdrawal syndrome that can manifest with delirium, delusions, hallucinations, dysarthria, depression, paranoia, worsening parkinsonian symptoms, or even stupor
Anticholinergics (e.g., trihexyphenidyl)	• Avoid in older adults or those with cognitive impairment as they are more susceptible to confusion or hallucinations with these medications

Patients with PD are at high risk of postoperative delirium. As the disease progresses, some patients with PD may develop cognitive impairment, either due to disease progression or as an adverse effect of some anti-parkinsonism medications. This may be confounded by difficulty in communication due to hypophonia. Often these patients have anxiety, depression, sensory disturbance (e.g., pain, paresthesia), and altered sleep-wake cycle. Change in the timing of home anti-parkinsonism medications or missed doses of medications are the most common precipitants of acute worsening of cognitive symptoms in these patients. Nonpharmacological delirium prevention measures (e.g., nighttime sleep, reorientation, mobility, caregiver engagement) should be implemented, and deliriogenic medications (e.g., opiates, benzodiazepines, anticholinergics) should be avoided. These patients may not be able to effectively use patient-controlled analgesia due to tremor, rigidity, or cognitive impairment. If the patient develops severe hyperactive delirium and pharmacological measures are absolutely needed, a neurology consultation should be considered, especially if there is a concern for Lewy body dementia. Typical and most atypical antipsychotics (such as haloperidol, olanzapine, aripiprazole, ziprasidone, and risperidone) should be avoided in patients with PD. If absolutely needed, quetiapine may be preferable at the lowest dose, for the shortest duration, though the evidence is lacking. Antidopaminergic medications such as metoclopramide, haloperidol, prochlorperazine, promethazine, and chlorpromazine should be avoided.

The risk of postoperative urinary retention is higher in these patients as they may have detrusor hyperreflexia. Urine output and postvoid residuals should be tracked. These patients may also have higher rates of urinary tract infections, and urinary catheter, if placed, should be removed as soon as possible. There is a higher risk of constipation and ileus in patients with PD, and aggressive bowel regimen should be prescribed.

Patients Undergoing DBS Placement

Placement of DBS typically occurs in two parts. First, a lead is placed in the basal ganglia (requiring at least an overnight stay post-procedure to monitor for intracranial hemorrhage, infarction, or seizures). Then after 1–2 weeks, a pulse generator is placed in the chest wall (similar to a pacemaker) that sends electrical impulses through the lead in the basal ganglia to regulate brain activity. Patients/caregivers can adjust the DBS settings within the set parameters based on their symptoms.

Since DBS lead placement is typically an awake procedure under monitored anesthesia care (to maximize the tremors to aid lead placement), levodopa is held on the morning of the procedure, and the patient is advised to skip 1–2 doses of home beta-blockers (propranolol, atenolol, metoprolol) prior to DBS lead placement. These medications are then resumed immediately after the procedure. If the patient is on beta-blockers for cardiac disease and holding a few doses before DBS lead placement may be potentially detrimental, these patients may need to be transitioned to a calcium channel blocker or alternate beta-blocker such as labetalol, carvedilol, nebivolol, or bisoprolol. Esmolol could be used if needed. Ophthalmic formulations with beta-blockers (e.g., timolol) can be continued.

Medications such as propofol and benzodiazepines are avoided intraoperatively to maximize the tremors to aid lead placement. Excessive sedation should be avoided as airway access may be limited due to the head frame and may also interfere with the microelectrode recordings for lead placement. Sometimes, general anesthesia may be required for DBS lead placement and always for pulse generator placement. As these surgeries are done in a sitting position, there is also a risk of air embolism.

MYASTHENIA GRAVIS

Myasthenia gravis (MG) is an autoimmune disorder of the neuromuscular junction with resulting skeletal muscle weakness. Clinical presentation varies from mild to severe disease involving bulbar and respiratory muscles. Treatment may include anticholinesterase agents, immunosuppressants, or thymectomy.

Patients with MG (especially those with bulbar symptoms) are at high risk of perioperative morbidity and mortality, if not carefully managed. A high index of clinical suspicion is warranted in the perioperative period in case of clinical deterioration. A few key considerations in managing patients with MG in the perioperative setting are shown in Figure 28-3.[5]

POSTOPERATIVE

(a) Respiratory status should be carefully monitored. Careful extubation at the end of the procedure can be carried out in many patients, depending on the type of surgery, residual anesthesia, and pulmonary comorbidities.

(a) Careful monitoring for myasthenic or cholinergic crisis. Medications that may exacerbate MG should be avoided.

(a) If patient is unable to tolerate orally or oral intake is contraindicated → Parenteral formulation of anticholinesterase agent or immunosuppressant (if the patient is on one) will need to be administered (with dose adjustment for route) to avoid interruption in the postoperative period.

INTRAOPERATIVE

(a) When possible, general anesthesia should be avoided. Regional and local anesthesia and spinal and epidural anesthesia with bupivacaine can be used. Scalene and intercostal muscle blocks should be avoided.

(a) Extreme caution should be exercised in the choice of anesthetic agents. Avoid nondepolarizing neuromuscular blockers even in those with mild MG, especially long-acting formulations. Close intraoperative monitoring (pulse oximetry, blood pressure, cardiac monitoring, end-tidal CO_2, neuromuscular) should be conducted as these patients can have a more rapid onset of block and a slower recovery time. If neuromuscular blockers are used, sugammadex is favored for reversal (instead of neostigmine that can precipitate a cholinergic crisis).

(a) May have resistance to depolarizing neuromuscular blockers such as succinylcholine. Inhaled anesthetics are likely safe.

(a) Surgical antibiotic prophylaxis should be carefully selected while avoiding medications that may exacerbate MG.

(a) If the patient has a thymoma in the anterior mediastinum, intrathoracic airway or vascular obstruction may occur.

PREOPERATIVE

Discuss the absolute indications and risk/benefit of the planned surgery, prehabilitation, pulmonary physiotherapy, regional/general anesthesia, anesthetic agents, postoperative pain control strategy, goals of care and surrogate decision maker(s), and preferences on nutrition and enteral feeding in case of postoperative deterioration. Elective surgery should be scheduled once myasthenic symptoms are optimally controlled.

Obtain detailed history and exam (clinical features of MG in that patient, disease severity, duration, treatment(s) pursued and compliance with medications, recent exacerbations). Patient's experience with any prior surgeries (e.g., reaction with certain anesthetics, timing of extubation postoperatively, any postoperative complications) should be enquired.

Assess respiratory status carefully. If the patient is on noninvasive ventilation at home, the settings should be recorded. Weak cough and swallowing difficulties may increase the risk of aspiration.

(a) If planning general anesthesia, surgery should be conducted in a location with access to ventilatory support and intensive care monitoring ability. Overnight stay for observation postoperatively should be planned.

When possible, surgery should be scheduled in the morning when muscle strength is the best.

On the morning of the surgery, home pyridostigmine may be held on a case-by-case basis (if this is agreed upon by the patient's neurologist and anesthesiologist).

FIGURE 28-3. Perioperative considerations in the management of patients with myasthenia gravis.

Several medications that may be added in the perioperative period can worsen muscle weakness in patients with MG and should be avoided. These medications include antibiotics (quinolones, macrolides, aminoglycosides, sulfonamides, vancomycin, clindamycin, penicillin), beta-blockers, calcium channel blockers, magnesium, muscle relaxants, nondepolarizing neuromuscular blockers (e.g., pancuronium, vecuronium), ester anesthetics, procainamide, phenytoin, carbamazepine, gabapentin, lidocaine, and iodinated contrast agents. Statins can aggravate or unmask MG, but they are not contraindicated and can be used cautiously if indicated.

Preoperative Considerations

Since patients with MG are at high risk for postoperative pulmonary complications, preoperative evaluation should focus on a thorough discussion about the benefits and risks of the planned surgical procedure, prehabilitation, pulmonary physiotherapy, type of anesthesia and anesthetic agents, pain medications, goals of care and surrogate decision maker(s), and nutrition and enteral feeding consideration in case of postoperative deterioration. If general anesthesia is planned, surgery should be conducted in a location with access to ventilatory support and intensive care monitoring ability. When possible, surgery should be scheduled earlier in the day when muscle strength is the best.

Detailed history and examination should be done preoperatively, including a discussion with the patient's neurologist about the clinical features of MG in that patient, history of exacerbations, disease severity, duration, treatment(s) pursued, and prognosis. Elective surgery should be scheduled once the symptoms of MG have achieved optimum control. If the patient is on noninvasive ventilation (NIV) at home, the settings should be noted, and a discussion with the patient's pulmonologist should be considered.

A recent pulmonary function test (PFT) including an arterial blood gas, ideally within the month prior to the surgery, should be obtained. Forced vital capacity (FVC) of less than 2.9 liters (<50% of predicted) portends a worse prognosis and higher risk of prolonged intubation postoperatively. These patients would benefit from consultation with a pulmonologist specializing in neuromuscular disorders and potential initiation of NIV several weeks prior to the planned surgery. Negative inspiratory force (NIF) or maximal inspiratory pressure (MIP or PI_{max}) reflects the strength of the diaphragm. MIP < 40 cmH$_2$O with good respiratory effort in a patient with no other known lung disease indicates severe respiratory muscle weakness. Maximal expiratory pressure (MEP or PE_{max}), on the other hand, reflects the strength of the expiratory muscles (e.g., abdominal muscle) and the ability for effective airway clearance. MEP < 30 cmH$_2$O indicates higher risk of respiratory failure.

In general, interruption of home medications for MG should be avoided unless recommended by the patient's neurologist. The decision to hold or continue pyridostigmine on the night before or the morning of the surgery should be individualized on a case-by-case basis and requires a discussion between the patient's neurologist and anesthesiologist, as pyridostigmine may interfere with the metabolism of some neuromuscular blockers.

Intraoperative Considerations

Extreme caution should be exercised in the choice of anesthetic agents for patients with MG, especially avoiding long-acting nondepolarizing neuromuscular blockers. Close intraoperative monitoring (pulse oximetry, blood pressure, cardiac monitoring, end-tidal CO$_2$, neuromuscular) should be conducted as these patients may have a more rapid onset of block and a slower recovery time. When possible, regional anesthesia should be favored over general anesthesia.

Postoperative Considerations

In the event of respiratory deterioration, other causes such as pneumonia, pulmonary edema, or pulmonary embolism should be ruled out first, similar to patients without MG. Patients should be carefully monitored for myasthenic or cholinergic crisis, and medications that may exacerbate MG should be avoided as noted above.[6,7]

Myasthenic crisis is a life-threatening situation that presents as acute respiratory failure caused by weakness of the diaphragmatic and intercostal muscles. Diagnosis requires a high degree of clinical suspicion. Rapid clinical deterioration can occur during myasthenic crisis. Careful monitoring in the intensive care unit, sometimes with ventilatory support and treatment of any underlying infection in these potentially immunocompromised patients, aggressive respiratory physiotherapy, and plasmapheresis or intravenous immunoglobulin may need to be considered.

Excess of anticholinesterase agents (e.g., pyridostigmine) may result in *cholinergic crisis*. This may manifest with muscarinic symptoms such as miosis (in contrast to mydriasis in myasthenic crisis) and "SLUDGE" symptoms (salivation, lacrimation, urinary urgency or incontinence, diarrhea, gastrointestinal upset and abdominal cramps, and emesis), and/or nicotinic symptoms such as twitching, fasciculations, and muscle weakness.

Home medications for MG should continue without interruption. If the patient is unable to tolerate orally or oral intake is contraindicated, a parenteral formulation of anticholinesterase agent or immunosuppressant (if the patient is on one at home) will need to be administered (with dose adjustment for route) to avoid interruption.

Careful extubation at the end of the surgery can be carried out in many patients with MG, depending on the type of surgery, residual anesthesia, and cardiopulmonary comorbidities. Respiratory status should be closely monitored thereafter, with careful attention to three aspects: oxygenation, ventilation, and airway clearance. If the oxygen saturations are lower than 94% on room air, careful multidisciplinary assessment should be performed to assess if oxygen supplementation should be given with bilevel NIV. Patients should ideally be extubated to bilevel NIV unless there is a history of chronic obstructive pulmonary disease (COPD) with bullous disease or pneumothorax. If the patient is on NIV at home, their home settings can be used. In patients who do not have a history of COPD with bullous disease or pneumothorax, a mechanical cough assist device or intrapulmonary percussive ventilator can be used along with scheduled ipratropium treatments to facilitate airway clearance. Patients with MG usually cannot use incentive spirometry or flutter/acapella devices effectively. Aspiration precautions should be maintained, and mobility should be encouraged if the patient can tolerate. Sedating medications (especially the combination of benzodiazepines with opiates) should be avoided, and muscle relaxants should not be given.

Routine spirometry in the postoperative period in the absence of clinical deterioration is usually not necessary. Daily FVC may be obtained at the bedside. MIP and MEP are usually not helpful in the acute setting and are limited by availability of masks in the inpatient setting (many patients cannot make a tight seal around the mouthpiece) and patient effort in the postoperative setting.

Clinical pearls

- The most common causes of seizures in the perioperative setting are missed doses of home ASD or drug interactions between home ASD and new medications that are administered intra- and postoperatively.

- Effective discharge planning and patient/caregiver education are of utmost importance for patients with a new seizure.

- Even a brief interruption of carbidopa-levodopa can, in rare instances, precipitate parkinsonism-hyperpyrexia syndrome that mimics neuroleptic malignant syndrome.

- Missed doses or change in the timing of the anti-parkinsonism medications (compared to their schedule at home) or prolonged interruption of DBS (in those with DBS for PD) are the most common precipitants of acute worsening of cognitive symptoms in the postoperative period in patients with PD.

- One exception when the patient should not take levodopa on the morning of surgery is before DBS lead placement.

- In patients with MG, closely monitor respiratory status with attention to oxygenation, ventilation, and airway clearance. Monitor patients for cholinergic and myasthenic crisis in the postoperative period.

REFERENCES

1. Fisher RS, Cross JH, French JA, et al. Operational classification of seizure types by the International League Against Epilepsy: Position Paper of the ILAE Commission for Classification and Terminology. *Epilepsia*. 2017;58(4):522-530. PMID: 28276060

2. Conover ZR, Talai A, Klockau KS, et al. Perioperative management of children on ketogenic dietary therapies. *Anesthesia & Analgesia.* 2020;131(6):1872-1882. PMID: 32769381

3. Chambers DJ, Sebastian J, Ahearn DJ. Parkinson's disease. *BJA Educ.* 2017;17(4):145-149. https://doi.org/10.1093/bjaed/mkw050.

4. Morano J, Uejima J, Tung A, Rosenow J. Management strategies for patients with neurologic stimulators during nonneurologic surgery: an update and review. *Current Opinion in Anaesthesiology.* 2023;36(5):461-467. PMID: 37552004

5. Daum P, Smelt J, Ibrahim IR. Perioperative management of myasthenia gravis. *BJA Educ.* 2021;21(11):414-419. PMID: 34707886

6. Abel M, Eisenkraft JB. Anesthetic implications of myasthenia gravis. *Mt Sinai J Med.* 2002;69(1-2):31-37. PMID: 11832968

7. Gilhus NE. Myasthenia gravis. *N Engl J Med.* 2016;375(26):2570-2581. PMID: 28029925

Rheumatoid Arthritis, Lupus, and Other Systemic Autoimmune Diseases

29

Linda A. Russell, MD

COMMON CLINICAL QUESTIONS

1. What are the risks of surgery in patients with rheumatic diseases?
2. What is the perioperative management of antirheumatic medications in patients with rheumatic diseases?

INTRODUCTION

Patients with rheumatic diseases often have multiple comorbidities that can affect surgical outcomes. In addition, these patients are often on medications that can cause immunosuppression and increase the risk of infection. It is critical that these patients be evaluated preoperatively so that the patient's health can be maximized and a plan with medicine, anesthesia, and surgery be coordinated preoperatively.

RHEUMATOID ARTHRITIS (RA)

Preoperative Evaluation and Specific Concerns

RA is a systemic inflammatory disorder that can result in joint deformity but also affects other organ systems (Table 29-1). Patients can develop pulmonary disease including interstitial lung disease and pulmonary hypertension. Cardiac disease can include pericardial effusion and conduction disease due to rheumatoid nodules. Cricoarytenoid involvement can present with hoarseness and be problematic for anesthesia.

Cervical spine instability can result in cervical spine compromise if not recognized during intubation. Both active rheumatoid arthritis and glucocorticoid (GC) exposure are associated with osteoporosis.

Although fewer RA patients seem to require orthopedic surgery due to better treatment, studies suggest up to 50% of RA patients will have an orthopedic procedure of any type over the course of their illness.[1] RA patients are at higher risk of total hip arthroplasty (THA) and total knee arthroplasty (TKA) infection compared to osteoarthritis patients (4.2% vs. 1.4%) over a 5-year period.[2]

There is an increased risk of cardiovascular disease in inflammatory disorders, which has been best studied in RA and systemic lupus erythematous (SLE). The risk is greater in poorly controlled disease and probably comparable to patients with diabetes.

The use of biologic therapy and biologic therapy combined with DMARD therapy has greatly increased since the late 1980s. These medications are associated with immunosuppression and a greater risk of infection perioperatively. Patients on GCs may have the highest risk of infection. One study demonstrated the RA patients on anti-TNF therapy were statistically more likely to be colonized with MSSA and MRSA than OA patients and RA patients on DMARD therapy.[3]

One study that examined 68,348 patients undergoing THA compared patients with OA to those with inflammatory arthritis. Those with inflammatory arthritis had a greater risk of transfusion, mechanical

TABLE 29-1. Perioperative Considerations for Rheumatic Diseases

PATIENTS WITH RHEUMATOID ARTHRITIS	PATIENTS WITH SYSTEMIC LUPUS ERYTHEMATOUS
Interstitial lung disease	Antiphospholipid syndrome
Pulmonary hypertension	Raynaud's phenomena
Pericardial effusion	Interstitial lung disease
Conduction disease	Pericardial effusion
Cricoarytenoid involvement	Vasculitis
Cervical spine instability	Acute or chronic kidney disease
Cardiovascular disease	Immunosuppression
Immunosuppression	Frailty
Staph colonization	Osteoporosis
Frailty	
Osteoporosis	

complications, infection, and readmission following THA.[4] Many patients with inflammatory arthritis have anemia of chronic disease, and this may account for the greater need for transfusion. When undergoing spinal surgery, patients with RA have a greater risk of operative complications and infection.[5]

Perioperative Management/Risk Reduction Strategies

Due to the increased risk of interstitial lung disease and pulmonary hypertension, the patient should have a room air O_2 saturation and auscultation of the chest. If hypoxia is present or there is an abnormal lung exam, appropriate imaging should be considered. If there is a suspicion for pulmonary hypertension, an echo should be considered. This is particularly important in orthopedic procedures as during surgery pieces of bone and marrow can lodge in the lungs, which can lead to hemodynamic compromise.

It is worth considering cervical spine films (AP, lateral, flexion, extension) in patients with severe RA (Figure 29-1). Older literature suggests that cervical spine disease correlates with the destruction of shoulder and peripheral joints.[6] More recent literature suggests that patients treated early and aggressively with intensive, remission-targeted treatment have a much

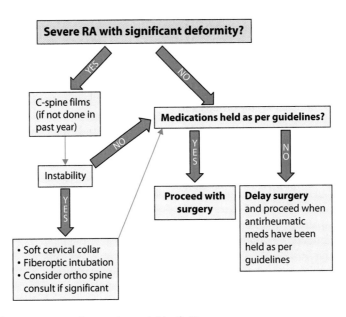

FIGURE 29-1. Perioperative management of severe rheumatoid arthritis.

lower incidence of cervical spine disease.[7] Films can help diagnose cervical instability, which is helpful for anesthesia. Fiberoptic intubation would be a better option when instability is noted. Taking all of this into account, it seems reasonable to obtain cervical spine films within 1 year in patients with RA with significant deformity on physical exam.

Medication management can be challenging, trying to balance control of disease activity and risk of infection. The American College of Rheumatology (ACR) and the American Association of Hip and Knee Surgeons (AHKS) created a revised evidence-based guideline for the perioperative management of antirheumatic medication in patients undergoing elective THA or TKA.[8] For patients with rheumatic diseases undergoing THA and TKA who are receiving GCs, the guideline recommends continuing their current daily dose of GCs, rather than administering supraphysiologic doses of GCs, on the day of surgery. Although it was written for this specific patient population, the guidelines are often considered when making decisions about other surgery types. However, recent evidence has emerged suggesting it may be safe to continue the biologics for patients with inflammatory bowel disease undergoing abdominal surgery as opposed to the ACR recommendation to stop them before orthopedic surgery (see Chapter 4). The recommendations are outlined in Table 29-2.

PSORIATIC ARTHRITIS

Preoperative Evaluation

Psoriatic arthritis, another type of inflammatory arthritis, poses the unique problem of plaque psoriasis. If these lesions are over the surgical site, there can be an increase in surgical site infections. Plaque psoriasis elsewhere can be the nidus for entry of pathogens into the circulation, and this can be especially problematic for arthroplasty patients. An older study noted the rate of prosthetic joint infection can be as high as 9–17% in patients with psoriatic arthritis,[9] although a more recent study suggests the risk of infection may not be as high as previously thought.[10]

Perioperative Management

Aim to control psoriatic plaques over the surgical site as well as psoriatic plaques over other areas as much as possible. Consideration for antibiotic-laden cement for patients undergoing arthroplasty may help reduce the risk of prosthetic joint infection.

TABLE 29-2. Suggested Medication Considerations for Inflammatory Arthritis Patients

MEDICATION	PREOPERATIVE RECOMMENDATION
MTX	Continue
Sulfasalazine	Continue
Hydroxychloroquine	Continue
Leflunomide	Continue
Doxycycline	Continue
Apremilast	Continue
Glucocorticoids	Continue current daily dose rather than supraphysiologic doses
Biologic agents	Stop these medications prior to surgery and schedule surgery at the end of the dosing cycle. Resume medications at minimum 14 days after surgery in the absence of a surgical site infection or systemic infection
Tofacitinib	Stop 3 days preop

ANKYLOSING SPONDYLITIS

Preoperative Evaluation

Ankylosing spondylitis, a spondyloarthropathy, is often associated with decreased cervical spine motion, which can have implications during intubation. Poor chest wall expansion can contribute to postoperative pulmonary complications.

Perioperative Management

Anesthesia should consider fiberoptic intubation when general anesthesia is required. Due to the increased risk of pulmonary complications, regional anesthesia should be performed when possible. Aim to prevent postoperative ileus and constipation, which may interfere with diaphragm function, further compromising pulmonary function.

Patients are at increased risk for heterotopic ossification after THA. This is most common in young men, revision surgery, and a trans trochanter approach. Consider treating at-risk patients with indomethacin for 2–4 weeks and/or a single dose of postoperative radiation.

SYSTEMIC LUPUS ERYTHEMATOSUS (SLE)

Preoperative Evaluation and Specific Concerns

SLE is a systemic inflammatory condition that can have manifestations that are mild to those that are severe and life-threatening, resulting in death. There are concerns unique to this group of patients (Table 29-1). A subset of patients with SLE have antiphospholipid (APL) syndrome, which can increase the risk of both arterial and venous thromboembolism as well as stroke. Raynaud's phenomena can be exaggerated by cold operating rooms and cool IV fluids and blood products. This can contribute to vasospasm of the small vessels in the hands and feet as well as the coronary arteries.

Traditionally, there have been few studies on patients with SLE undergoing surgery. In a very small study of 29 patients undergoing surgery for a total of 36 procedures (19 had active disease at the time of surgery), 37 complications occurred, which were mostly infectious. Patients with infections had higher doses of prednisone, higher number of organ systems involved, and more frequent renal involvement.[11] In another study assessing for complications in patients with SLE undergoing surgery, risk factors included lymphopenia and hypoalbuminemia.[12] A more recent study evaluating 28,269 SLE patients (matched to controls) undergoing major surgery noted an increase in renal complications and inhospital mortality, but not cardiac events.[13] A recent study noted more complications after cardiac valve surgery in SLE patients with a higher ACR damage index.[14]

It is generally recommended that patients with lupus be screened with a thorough history, physical examination, and laboratory evaluation. SLE patients with recent hospitalization seem to be at increased risk for renal failure, VTE, sepsis, stroke, and 30-day mortality.

Perioperative Management

Patients with SLE should be thoroughly assessed for disease activity and the number of organ systems involved. It is particularly important to assess the degree of renal insufficiency and if there is active renal disease. For patients with APL syndrome, a preoperative plan must include management of anticoagulation perioperatively; for these patients, we like to err on the side of bleeding over clotting (i.e., requiring a transfusion postop over a stroke). Whenever possible, elective surgery should be postponed until disease activity is low or in remission, and medications should be managed based on recommendations from the 2022 ACR/AHKS guidelines for severe SLE and non-severe SLE (Table 29-3).

MYOSITIS

Preoperative Evaluation

Patients with myositis or inflammatory muscle disease can have unique perioperative considerations. These patients can have interstitial lung disease and respiratory muscle weakness, which is problematic if general anesthesia is required. Patients can have esophageal dysmotility and are at increased risk for aspiration and pneumonia. Cardiomyopathy can occur. Generalized weakness can complicate postoperative mobilization.

Perioperative Management

In the literature, there is very little guidance on how to manage patients with myositis perioperatively. It makes inherent sense to try and control disease activity preoperatively as much as possible, while decreasing the dose of GC to the lowest dose possible. Regional anesthesia should be used whenever possible

TABLE 29-3. Suggested Medication Considerations for SLE Patients

	SEVERE SLE	NON-SEVERE SLE
MEDICATION TYPE	PREOPERATIVE RECOMMENDATION	PREOPERATIVE RECOMMENDATION
Mycophenolate mofetil	Continue	Discontinue 7 days preop
Azathioprine	Continue	Discontinue 7 days preop
Cyclosporine	Continue	Discontinue 7 days preop
Voclosporin*	Continue	(Not used for mild SLE)
Tacrolimus	Continue	Discontinue 7 days preop
Rituximab	Continue	Discontinue 6 months preop
Belimumab	Continue	Discontinue 4 weeks (IV)
Anifrolumab†	Continue	1 week (sq) preop
Glucocorticoids	Continue current daily dose rather than supraphysiologic doses (discuss dosing with rheumatologist)	(Not used for mild SLE) Continue current daily dose rather than supraphysiologic doses

*FDA-approved for active lupus nephritis.

†FDA-approved for moderate to severe lupus.

due to a concern of prolonged intubation with general anesthesia. Assessment by a dysphasia team postoperatively may help prevent aspiration pneumonia. Due to muscle weakness, many patients are at greater fall risk, and perioperative physical therapy may be helpful in this regard.

Clinical pearls

- RA: In general, biologic medications should be stopped at the end of the dosing cycle and be restarted 14 days postop if there is no evidence of a surgical site infection. The dose of GC should be tapered to the lowest dose preoperatively that can control disease activity to a manageable level.

- SLE: Patients with SLE who are in remission or have mild disease activity can generally tolerate holding immunosuppressive medications. Those with moderate to severe disease activity would probably benefit most from continued use of immunosuppressive medications. In addition, the use of perioperative GCs to prevent disease activation is not recommended. The dose of GC should be tapered to the lowest dose to control disease activity preoperatively.

REFERENCES

1. Massardo L, Gabriel SE, Crowson CS, et al. A population-based assessment of the use of orthopedic surgery in patients with rheumatoid arthritis. *J Rheumatol.* 2002;29(1):52. PMID: 11824971

2. Bongartz T, Halligan CS, Osmon DR, et al. Incidence and risk factors of prosthetic joint infection after total hip or knee replacement in patients with rheumatoid arthritis. *Arthritis Care Res.* 2008;59(12):1713. PMID: 19035425

3. Goodman SM, Nocon AA, Selemon NA, et al. Increased *Staphylococcus aureus* nasal carriage rates in rheumatoid arthritis patients on biologic therapy. *J Arthroplasty.* 2019;34(5):954. PMID: 30733073

4. Richardson SS, Kahlenberg CA, Goodman SM, et al. Inflammatory arthritis is a risk factor for multiple complications after total hip arthroplasty: a population-based comparative study of 68,348 patients. *J Arthroplasty.* 2019;34(6):1150. PMID: 30853155

5. Zhang S, Wang L, Bao L, et al. Does rheumatoid arthritis affect the infection and complication rates of spinal surgery? A systemic review and meta-analysis. *World Neurosurg.* 2021;145:260. PMID: 32977033

6. Neva MH, Kotaniemi A, Kaarela K, et al. Atlantoaxial disorders in rheumatoid arthritis associate with the destruction of peripheral and shoulder joints, and decreased bone mineral density. *Clin Exp Rheumatol.* 2003;21(2):179. PMID: 12747271

7. Sandström T, Rantalaiho V, Yli-Kerttula T, et al. Cervical spine involvement is very rare in patients with rheumatoid arthritis treated actively with treat to target strategy. Ten-year results of the NEORACo study. *J Rheumatol.* 2020;47(8):1160-1164. PMID: 3173258

8. Goodman SM, Springer B, Chen AF, et al. 2022 American College of Rheumatology/American Association of Hip and Knee Surgeons guideline for the perioperative management of antirheumatic medication in patients with rheumatic diseases undergoing elective total hip or total knee arthroplasty. *Arthritis Care Res.* 2022;74(9):1399. PMID: 35718887

9. Stern SH, Insall JN, Windsor RE, et al. Total knee arthroplasty in patients with psoriasis. *Clin Orthop Relat Res.* 1989;248:108. PMID: 2805466

10. Schnaser EA, Browne JA, Padgett DE, et al. Perioperative complications in patients with inflammatory arthropathy undergoing total hip arthroplasty. *J Arthroplasty.* 2016;31(10):2286. PMID: 27133160

11. Papa MZ, Shiloni E, Vetto JT, et al. Surgical morbidity in patients with systemic lupus erythematosus. *Am J Surg.* 1989;157(3):295. PMID: 2919734

12. Takahashi T, De La-Garza L, Ponce-De-Leon S, et al. Risk factors for operative morbidity in patients with systemic lupus erythematosus: an analysis of 63 surgical procedures. *Am Surg.* 1995;62(3):260. PMID: 7887543

13. Babazade R, Yilmaz HO, Leung SM, et al. Systemic lupus erythematosus is associated with increased adverse postoperative renal outcomes and mortality: a historical cohort study using administrative health data. *Anesth Analg.* 2017;124(4):1118. PMID: 28319545

14. Hu SY, Cheng CF, Yang KJ et al. Association between SLICC/ACR damage index and outcomes for lupus patients after cardiac valve surgery. *Interact Cardiovasc Thorac Surg.* 2022;35(4):221. PMID: 35997571

## 30

Substance Use Disorder

Avital Y. O'Glasser, MD, FACP, SFHM, DFPM and Christine E. Boxhorn, MD, DABA

COMMON CLINICAL QUESTIONS

1. How does marijuana impact perioperative risk, and should patients be advised to stop use before surgery?

2. Is active stimulant intoxication or recent use a contraindication to surgery?

3. How should a patient on pharmacologic treatment for opioid use disorder be instructed to handle their therapy preoperatively?

EVALUATION/RISK FACTORS

Introduction

"Substance use" and "substance use disorder" (SUD) are broad terms that encompass a spectrum of patterns of use and results to overall health. Multiple substances fall under the umbrella of SUD, including illicit/illegal agents such as nonprescription opioids or stimulants (Table 30-1). The potential for misuse also occurs with legally regulated agents such as alcohol, prescription opioids, prescription stimulants, and cannabis (recreational or medical legalization varies by state). Rates of illicit substance use are increasing, with over 46 million Americans over 12 years old reporting use in the prior month, increasing the potential that patients who use substances will present for surgery.[6] Certain surgical subspecialties are more likely to encounter patients with an SUD, such as otolaryngology and trauma.[1]

SUDs are best viewed as medical conditions with available treatments rather than choice, poor willpower, or moral failure. The term "substance use disorder" rather than "substance abuse" or "substance dependence" reflects a shift toward more scientifically based, patient-centered language. Discriminatory language like "addict," "intravenous drug user," or "alcoholic" should also be avoided in favor of more medical descriptions.

Appropriately assessing and managing SUD in the perioperative period is an opportunity for high value, patient-centered care that also draws attention to preoperative optimization of modifiable risk factors and harm reduction. Preoperative management may also facilitate the chance to initiate sustained recovery or prevent perioperative relapse.

Medical Complications of SUD

SUD can increase perioperative risk due to the medical sequelae of current or former use. Some of these risks may include interactions between the agent used and anesthetic agents and risk of perioperative medical complications such as myocardial infarction. In addition to complications of intoxication or chronic use, withdrawal syndromes may add to perioperative risk.

Medical complications of use vary by agent as well as route and duration of use (Tables 30-1 and 30-2). Patients may use more than one illicit substance, so it is important to get a complete history. Complications

TABLE 30-1. Complications of Chronic and/or Long-Term Use of Illicit Substances, Which Can Increase the Risk of Perioperative Respiratory, Cardiac, Infectious, or Neuropsychiatric Postoperative Complications[1-5]

CLASS	LONG-TERM EFFECTS OF USE
Marijuana	Chronic bronchitis/emphysema Airway hyperreactivity Atheromatous disease Orthostasis Cerebral vasospasm Memory dysfunction Psychiatric symptoms Hyperemesis Impaired central thermoregulation Bleeding risk
Stimulants • Cocaine • Methamphetamine • Amphetamine • Prescription stimulants	Cardiovascular -Coronary ischemia, coronary vasospasm, accelerated CAD, arrhythmias, cardiomyopathy, hypertension Stroke Psychosis Infectious complications Poor dentition Nasal septal perforation

Alcohol	Gastrointestinal
	  -Alcoholic hepatitis, cirrhosis, gastritis, pancreatitis
	Cardiovascular
	  -Cardiomyopathy, arrhythmias, hypertension
	Anemia
	Malnutrition
	Electrolyte abnormalities

Opioids • Heroin • Fentanyl • Prescription opioids	Infectious complications Skin/soft tissue infections Endocarditis Arrhythmias
Hallucinogens • Lysergic acid diethylamide (LSD) • Phencyclidine (PCP)	Dissociative state Agitation Aggression

TABLE 30-2. Representative Signs/Symptoms of Both Intoxication and Withdrawal, with Emphasis on Perioperative Implications[1,2,4,5]

CLASS	INTOXICATION	WITHDRAWAL
Marijuana	Anxiolysis Anxiety Psychosis Paranoia Euphoria Dizziness Analgesia Memory impairment Tachycardia	Anxiety Restlessness Irritability Depression Agitation Insomnia Anorexia Nausea Abdominal cramping
Stimulants	Euphoria Tachycardia Hypertension Anxiety Hyperactivity Respiratory depression Psychosis Stroke Coronary ischemia Sudden death	Fatigue Somnolence Depression
Alcohol	Sedation Disinhibition	Autonomic hyperactivity Tremors Agitation Insomnia Tachycardia Hypertension Hallucinations Seizures Delirium tremens
Opioids	Sedation Respiratory suppression Bradycardia Hypotension Constipation Urinary retention	Diaphoresis Vomiting Diarrhea Tachycardia Hyperthermia Myalgias
Hallucinogens	Agitation Aggression Delirium Hallucinations Sympathetic activation Tachycardia Respiratory depression	Anxiety Shaking Diaphoresis Palpitations

relevant to the perioperative period include cardiac complications, infectious complications (HIV, hepatitis B or C), liver disease, or neuropsychiatric symptoms.

In addition to being physically stressful, surgery can be emotionally and psychologically stressful. Patients facing the challenges of active substance use or maintaining remission may also face unique perioperative psychosocial challenges. A holistic, addiction medicine-based approach to their perioperative care may avoid relapse as well as identify opportunities for risk reduction. Attention to substance use may provide an opportunity to identify other social determinants of health that could negatively impact perioperative outcomes, such as unstable housing, underinsurance or lack of insurance, or impaired access to resources.

Perioperative Complications

Marijuana or cannabis is derived from species of the *Cannabis* plant. Marijuana contains nearly 500 known chemical compounds, the most relevant of which are the main psychoactive compound delta-9-tetrahydrocannabinol (THC) and the less psychoactive cannabidiol (CBD). Legal medical and recreational marijuana use has expanded, and approximately 62 million American adults over 12 years old used marijuana at least once in 2022, an increase from 53 million the previous year.[6] Between 2006 and 2015, marijuana use in patients presenting for surgery has increased from 21.1 to 71.0 per 1,000,000 surgical admissions.[2] Marijuana can be used in multiple forms (inhaled, vaped, oral, topical) and with varying THC/CBD ratios. Patients can experience both acute intoxication and withdrawal perioperatively. Preoperative marijuana use has been linked to increased doses needed for procedural sedation but an unclear effect on general anesthesia,[7] as well as respiratory complications due to airway hyperreactivity, hemodynamic instability, and potentially more challenging pain control.[7] Marijuana use has been linked with an increased risk of postoperative myocardial infarction, especially when used within 2 hours of surgery, but not overall perioperative morbidity, mortality, length of stay, or costs.[2] Marijuana use is also associated with higher rates of postoperative nausea and vomiting.

Stimulants include cocaine and methamphetamine. Cocaine is a sympathomimetic agent that inhibits the presynaptic uptake of neurotransmitters, increasing available catecholamine levels. Amphetamines, including methamphetamine, have sympathomimetic activity by inducing the release of neurotransmitters. Approximately 5 million Americans over 12 years old used cocaine and 2.7 million used methamphetamine in the preceding year.[6] The potential for inappropriate use of prescription stimulants or psychotherapeutics also exists. Cocaine has a much shorter half-life than methamphetamine (60–90 minutes vs. approximately 12 hours),[3,8] which may affect timing of nonelective surgery after usage. One study did not show differences in the administered doses of inhaled anesthetic agents or propofol for patients using cocaine.[3] Perioperative concerns include hemodynamic instability, myocardial infarction, and arrhythmias with acute intoxication.

Illegal *opioids* include heroin and illicit fentanyl. Opioid misuse can also occur with prescription opioids, both by the individual who prescribed the therapy as well as through diversion to others. Nearly 9 million Americans over 12 years old misused prescription or nonprescription opioids in the prior year.[6] Methadone, buprenorphine (with or without naloxone), and naltrexone are FDA-approved to treat opioid use disorder.

Clinicians should also be aware of additional illicit agents, including but not limited to hallucinogens, such as lysergic acid diethylamide (LSD) and phencyclidine (PCP), as well as agents such as MDMA (Ecstasy or Molly).

Alcohol is legally available but misuse and heavy use can lead to perioperative complications.[1,9] High-risk or excessive drinking is defined as ≥3 drinks in a day or ≥7 drinks per week for women or men older than 65 years of age, and ≥4 drinks in a day or ≥14 drinks per week for men under the age of 65.[4] Alcohol withdrawal can be life-threatening and cause delirium tremens or seizures. Data support 4–8 weeks of preoperative alcohol cessation to lower postoperative complications.[10]

Preoperative Evaluation

The preoperative history and physical examination for all patients should include a social history that inquires about tobacco, alcohol, marijuana, or other illicit agent use. Asking all patients these questions in a structured format helps the clinician prepare for this in a nonjudgmental manner.

If patients acknowledge substance use, the clinician should then ask about usage and complications. Ask about route of use, as complications might vary based on formulation (inhaled, intranasal, intravenous, intramuscular, ingested, topical), as well as overall duration, frequency, amount, and timing of last use. Amount of use might also be expressed in dollar amount purchased over weight or "unit" (e.g., number of marijuana cigarettes). For certain substances, structured questionnaires can be utilized—for example—AUDIT (https://auditscreen.org/using-audit) or CAGE (https://www.mdcalc.com/cage-questions-alcohol-use#next-steps) for alcohol use. AUDIT-C scores $\geq$ 5 (out of a maximum of 12 points) were associated with increased risk of perioperative complications.[4]

Inquire about a history of withdrawal symptoms. Explore the current state of sobriety as well as details of prior attempts at sobriety, as these might provide valuable clues as to how sobriety might be maintained or initiated in the upcoming perioperative period. Obtain prescriber information for medication-assisted treatment (MAT) or medication for opioid use disorder (MOUD), as well as information regarding addiction treatment support such as mental health/community resources or methadone dispensing clinics. For patients not currently abstinent, ask about readiness to pursue SUD treatment and support preoperatively.

If patients have a history of current or former substance use, ask about known complications anticipated by the agent of use (Table 30-1). Elicit signs and symptoms of potential complications on the review of systems and exam (e.g., stigmata of chronic liver disease, cardiac findings, sinus damage, skin/soft tissue inspection for infections).

Check labs in a patient-centered fashion based on the pretest probability of abnormalities and have a low threshold to check a comprehensive metabolic profile, which includes liver function tests over a basic metabolic profile, as well as an INR if there are concerns for liver disease related to alcohol use disorder or intravenous drug use. The benefit of urine drug screening likely varies by clinical situation. A positive drug screen does not confirm timing of last use given detection times (including inactive metabolites) that extend past acute intoxication windows, though the test may have a role in confirming suspected or unclear use, especially for an acutely impaired patient or for a patient one is concerned is not forthcoming with substance use.[8] On the other hand, performing a urine drug screen the morning of surgery may lead to unnecessary cancellations; for example, a positive screen for cocaine alone does not appear to be associated with cardiovascular complications.[11]

Consider a baseline EKG for patients with a history of stimulant use disorder given the potential for cardiac complications. A preoperative EKG to evaluate the QT interval might also be valuable for patients on certain pharmacotherapies used for MOUD, such as methadone and, to a lesser extent, buprenorphine, especially if additional QT-prolonging agents, such as antiemetic medications, will be administered perioperatively.

MANAGEMENT/RISK REDUCTION

Preoperative Management

Preoperative management should focus on lowering complications, promoting sobriety, and managing addiction treatment while minimizing the risk of relapse. Where available, community resources, psychosocial support, and formal addiction treatment should be utilized.

Patients with opioid use disorders have several available pharmacotherapies for MOUD. Main classes are the opioid agonist methadone, partial agonist buprenorphine (as monotherapy or in combination with naloxone), or antagonist naltrexone (see Chapter 45). Methadone should be continued perioperatively. Historically, much controversy existed in the literature regarding optimal preoperative management of the partial agonist buprenorphine, especially as old information led to the belief that acute pain control could not be achieved in the presence of that agent.[5,12-14] However, the partial agonism can be overcome by a strong mu receptor agonist such as fentanyl or hydromorphone. The literature now indicates that holding buprenorphine perioperatively can lead to SUD relapse, and that effective perioperative analgesia can be achieved without stopping or lowering the dose preoperatively.[5,12-14] With this in mind, several societies have published guidelines regarding the perioperative management of buprenorphine, all of which recommend buprenorphine continuation without routine preoperative dose reduction or cessation.[14] However, clinician comfort level for continuing MOUD preoperatively may vary depending on available access to addiction medicine specialists as well as inpatient and outpatient resources. The antagonist naltrexone should be held preoperatively, with oral dosing stopped 3 days preoperatively and surgery timed as close to the end of the 4-week dosing window for intramuscular naltrexone.[12] The MOUD prescriber should be engaged in the perioperative care team before and after surgery.

Patients with alcohol use disorder might utilize the opioid antagonist naltrexone for MAT; the oral form should be stopped 3 days and the intramuscular form 4 weeks before surgery.[12] Other MAT options for alcohol use disorder include disulfiram and acamprosate; optimal hold times for these agents are unclear with minimal guidance in the literature, although some recommend holding disulfiram for up to 2 weeks due to its potential reaction with alcohol-containing medications and topical preparations utilized in the perioperative setting.[15]

Recent Use or Intoxication on the Day of Surgery

Patients may also arrive for emergency or urgent surgeries while acutely intoxicated. If possible, surgery should be delayed until the patient is no longer acutely intoxicated.[8] Cocaine has a short half-life.[3] The optimal timing of surgery from the last intake of marijuana is unclear, though most recent evidence suggests waiting at least 2 hours after last use.[7] Clinicians should be aware of the potential need for modified anesthetic dosing requirements as well as the potential for hemodynamic instability. The decision to proceed with surgery for a patient with very recent substance use must weigh the risks of surgical delay versus perioperative complications due to the illicit agent (Figure 30-1).

Postoperative Management

Patients should be monitored closely both for complications of intoxication and for withdrawal symptoms (Table 30-2). Marijuana withdrawal occurs for heavy or daily users within 1–2 days after last use and symptoms can last 2–4 weeks, albeit symptoms tend to be milder when compared to opioid or alcohol withdrawal.[7,8] Alcohol withdrawal begins 6–12 hours

from the last drink, though potential intraoperative benzodiazepine use should be considered when calculating the window for onset of withdrawal symptoms. Benzodiazepines are first-line treatment for alcohol withdrawal, which can be life-threatening. Cocaine withdrawal is usually minor and self-limited, although it can present beginning with the "crash period" hours to days after last use; methamphetamine withdrawal lasts longer.[8] Patients should be monitored closely for potential cardiac complications.

Depending on the agent of use, postoperative analgesia may be more difficult to achieve. Multimodal analgesia including acetaminophen, NSAIDs, gabapentinoids, and regional and/or local anesthesia should be utilized when possible.[5,7,12–14] Depending on local resources, a multidisciplinary team should be utilized, such as pain medicine or addiction medicine experts. Outpatient care teams including MOUD prescribers and community resources should be updated, especially if any dosing changes or new prescriptions for analgesia are issued.

Patients with opioid use disorder may have higher tolerance to opioids, and they can experience postoperative pain from the surgery itself in addition to withdrawal symptoms. The timeframe and duration of withdrawal symptoms depends on the specific opioid but can begin within 8–12 hours and last for several weeks.[8] Pain should be viewed as genuine rather than immediately regarded as "drug-seeking" behavior. MOUD should be continued, but it should not be assumed that it confers any acute pain relief. MOUD does not preclude the use of additional opioid dosing, though patients need to be monitored for respiratory depression. Short-acting opioids can be dosed in addition to maintenance methadone doses. Additional short-acting analgesia can also be given for those on buprenorphine, ideally choosing an opioid with a high affinity for the mu-opioid receptor, such as hydromorphone or fentanyl[5,13,14] because the analgesic effect of buprenorphine has a shorter half-life, a postoperative strategy for less-painful procedures is to increase the total buprenorphine dose and/or divide the total daily dose into TID dosing from daily dosing, thereby providing more effective analgesia without requiring additional postoperative opioid agonists.[12] Naltrexone should be resumed only once patients are abstinent from all opioids for 7 to 10 days to avoid precipitating withdrawal.[12]

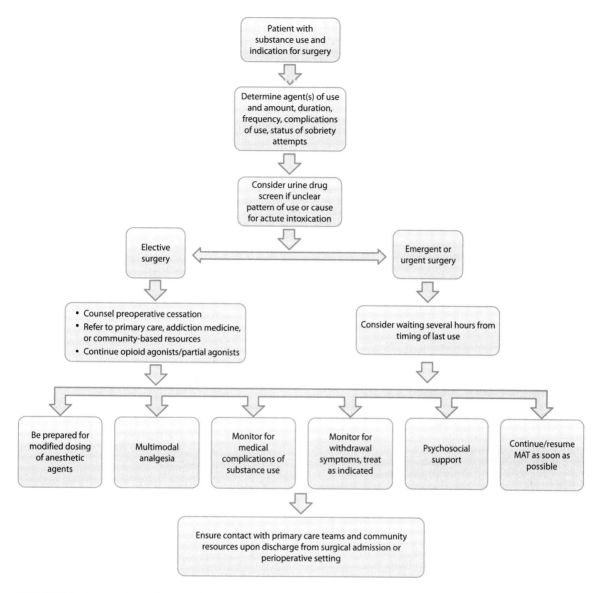

FIGURE 30-1. Preoperative evaluation and management pathway for patients with substance use disorder presenting for surgery.

SUMMARY

SUD, which continues to increase in prevalence, increases the risk of perioperative complications. A patient-centered, comprehensive assessment that fosters trust by using tenants of addiction medicine through the lens of harm reduction may serve as an opportunity to engage patients with SUD in reduced use, sobriety, or sustained remission perioperatively. MAT (and MOUD) should be appropriately managed perioperatively, and patients should be monitored closely for complications of intoxication as well as withdrawal and medical complications of substance use in the perioperative setting.

REFERENCES

1. Harris AHS, Frey MS, DeBenedetti AF, et al. Alcohol misuse prevalence and associations with post-operative complications in US surgical patients: a review. *Open Surg J.* 2008;2:50-58.

2. Goel A, McGuinness B, Jivraj NK, et al. Cannabis use disorder and perioperative outcomes in major elective surgeries: a retrospective cohort analysis. *Anesthesiology.* 2020;132(4):625-635. PMID: 31789638

3. Moon TS, Gonzales MX, Sun JJ, et al. Recent cocaine use and the incidence of hemodynamic events during general anesthesia: a retrospective cohort study. *J Clin Anesth.* 2019;55:146-150. PMID: 30660093

4. Patel AK, Balasanova AA. Unhealthy alcohol use. *JAMA.* 2021;326(2):196. PMID: 34255006

5. Warner NS, Warner MA, Cunningham JL, et al. A practical approach for the management of the mixed opioid agonist-antagonist buprenorphine during acute pain and surgery. *Mayo Clin Proc.* 2020;95(6):1253-1267. PMID: 32061413

6. Center for Behavioral Health Statistics and Quality. 2022 National Survey on Drug Use and Health: detailed tables. Substance Abuse and Mental Health Services Administration, Rockville, MD, 2023.

7. Shah S, Schwenk ES, Sondekoppam RV, et al. ASRA pain medicine consensus guidelines on the management of the perioperative patient on cannabis and cannabinoids. *Reg Anesth Pain Med.* 2023;48(3):97-117. PMID: 36596580

8. Beaulieu P. Anesthetic implications of recreational drug use. *Can J Anaesth.* 2017;64(12):1236-1264. PMID: 28956316

9. Bradley KA, Rubinsky AD, Sun H, et al. Alcohol screening and risk of postoperative complications in male VA patients undergoing major non-cardiac surgery. *J Gen Intern Med.* 2011;26(2):162-169. PMID: 20878363

10. Egholm JW, Pedersen B, Møller AM, et al. Perioperative alcohol cessation intervention for postoperative complications. *Cochrane Database Syst Rev.* 2018;11(11):CD008343. PMID: 30408162

11. Satish S, Freeman C, Culhane J. Urine drug screen positive for cocaine and amphetamine is not an adverse risk factor for cardiovascular morbidity or mortality in trauma. *Trauma Surg Acute Care Open.* 2021;6(1):e000749. PMID: 34514174

12. Harrison TK, Kornfeld H, Aggarwal AK, Lembke A. Perioperative considerations for the patient with opioid use disorder on buprenorphine, methadone, or naltrexone maintenance therapy. *Anesthesiol Clin.* 2018;36(3):345-359. PMID: 30092933

13. Kohan L, Potru S, Barreveld AM, et al. Buprenorphine management in the perioperative period: educational review and recommendations from a multisociety expert panel. *Reg Anesth Pain Med.* 2021;46(10):840-859. PMID: 34385292

14. Hickey T, Abelleira A, Acampora G, et al. Perioperative bprenorphine management: a multidisciplinary approach. *Med Clin North Am.* 2022;106(1):169-185. PMID: 34823729

15. Hill, L. Preoperative drug management. In: Evers AS, Maze M, Kharasch ED, eds. *Anesthetic pharmacology: basic principles and clinical practice.* 2nd ed. Cambridge University Press; 2011:998.

## 31

Surgery and the Older Adult

Heather E. Nye, MD, PhD, SFHM, FACP and Daniel I. McIsaac, MD, MPH, FRCPC

COMMON CLINICAL QUESTIONS

1. What is frailty?
2. What screening tools are available to assess frailty?
3. What measures can be implemented to reduce risk of postoperative complications in the older adult?

INTRODUCTION

As the population ages, greater numbers of older adults are undergoing major surgery. Adults over the age of 65 are more likely to have medical comorbidities, functional or cognitive deficits, and other geriatric states such as frailty, placing them at higher risk for postoperative complications and poor outcomes. Increased rates of delirium, mortality, cardiac, pulmonary, and infectious complications, and prolonged cognitive and functional decline have all been described following surgery in older adults. Using available literature, best practices have been delineated by experts in geriatrics, anesthesia, and surgery for the optimization of older adults before surgery and for their perioperative care.[1,2]

PREOPERATIVE EVALUATION AND RISK REDUCTION

It is recommended that older adults undergo a standard medical preoperative assessment with several important additions. Heightened focus is emphasized in domains of function, cognition, socioenvironmental surroundings, goals of care, and nutrition. Screening for common geriatric conditions, especially frailty, is widely recommended.[1] The older adult also merits an extended discussion of overall health goals, incorporating expectations, values, and preferences to inform any decision about surgery. Patients, their families, and caregivers should also be educated on specific risks and mitigation strategies for geriatric patients. Exploring the role of surgery in satisfying a patient's goals and priorities can help ensure that risks incurred do not outweigh anticipated benefits and improvement in quality of life.[2]

Geriatric states and syndromes commonly encountered in older adults, especially frailty, sarcopenia, and cognitive impairment, can negatively impact surgical outcomes. Ideally, modifiable risk factors can be detected and addressed well in advance of major surgery. At the preoperative visit, validated screening tools may help identify important deficits and should be employed as time and resources allow. Frailty assessment and linked communication to the perioperative team should be prioritized and are supported by high-quality evidence in improving postoperative outcomes.[3] Individual screens for cognitive impairment, functional dependence, delirium risk, polypharmacy, Beers "potentially inappropriate medications," and malnutrition prior to surgery are also recommended to guide perioperative management.[2] Additional areas of evaluation can include mental health, alcohol use, urinary retention, constipation, hearing and vision impairment, and adequacy of social supports. A comprehensive geriatric assessment (CGA) is the gold standard for evaluation of geriatric syndromes. In surgical patients, randomized trial and comparative effectiveness data demonstrate meaningful decreases in length of stay and delirium, as well as increased survival when a CGA is performed.[4] As multiple disciplines and extended visits are required to complete a CGA, this approach is often not feasible. Shortened screening instruments in the preoperative period may be a more realistic approach to identifying vulnerable patients who could benefit from more in-depth geriatric evaluations or consideration of less invasive treatment options. Recommended screening tools can be found in Table 31-1.

Frailty

Frailty is a state of multidimensional loss of reserve resulting in vulnerability to stressors and places older adults at greater risk of adverse health outcomes. Estimates suggest that 20% to 40% of adults over 65

TABLE 31-1. Suggested Frailty Instruments for Preoperative Use

FRAILTY INSTRUMENT	DESCRIPTION	CONSIDERATIONS
Risk Analysis Index (RAI) https://efrailty.hsl.harvard.edu/ToolRiskAnalysisIndex.html	Weighted scale based on responses to 14 survey items	• Requires no subscales or physical measurements • Can be calculated electronically • Has been implemented at health system level • When used to trigger best practice advisories is associated with decreased mortality
Clinical Frailty Scale (CFS) https://rise.articulate.com/share/deb4rT02lvONbq4AfcMNRUudcd6QMts3#/lessons/07kjAp–OngOuNH1ko514Y4XL28y4w1-	Ordinal scale based on clinical assessment, enhanced by vignettes and images	• Requires no subscales or physical measurements • Can be completed in <1 min • As, or more accurate in predicting patient-important outcomes than more resource-intensive instruments • More feasible than Fried Phenotype when compared head-to-head
Fried Phenotype (FFP) https://hopkinsfrailtyassessment.org/(S(53xfjftnrnihmjdjn0w3ucqx))/Default.aspx	Based on the identification of 5 deficits (2 points by history, 2 physical measurements, and 1 subscale)	• Directly aligns with Phenotype model of frailty • Requires space for walking tests and a handheld dynamometer • Most widely studied tool in perioperative setting
Frailty Index (FI)	A count of multidimensional deficits present divided by the number assessed (minimum 30)	• Directly aligns with Accumulating Deficits model of frailty • Assessment of 30 multidimensional deficits may not be clinically feasible • Can be operationalized electronically
Edmonton Frail Scale (EFS) https://edmontonfrailscale.org/	Assessment of 8 multidimensional deficits	• Operationally a condensed frailty index • Requires completion and assessment of a clock draw • Generally feasible in most clinical settings

years of age live with a meaningful degree of frailty before surgery. Compared to the general population of older adults, frailty prevalence is much higher in surgical patients, which partly reflects the fact that the indication for surgery is often a concurrent driver of frailty.[5] Among older adults with frailty who undergo surgery, the risk of postoperative morbidity, patient-reported disability, and mortality is at least twofold higher. Almost half of older adults with frailty experience a complication after surgery and 1 in 5 go on to develop a new or worsened disability 3 months after surgery.[6] Importantly, the odds of delirium and nonhome discharge are increased by factors of 4 and 5, respectively.[5,6] Because frailty is a multidimensional condition, recognizing it before surgery may help to identify domains where optimization is possible. As such, frailty assessment for all adults 65 years or older is a recommended best practice from multiple national and international guidelines. These guidelines also stress the importance of using a frailty instrument that assesses multiple domains, including physical function, cognition, nutrition, and mental health.[1] Systematic reviews demonstrate

that the Clinical Frailty Scale and the Risk Analysis Index are most accurate and feasible for preoperative use, although clinicians can also consider the Freid Phenotype, Frailty Index, Edmonton Frail Scale, and related variants.[5] Once the presence of frailty has been determined, frailty status should be communicated to the entire perioperative team. However, the presence of frailty should not preclude consideration of surgery, as multicenter cohort studies suggest that despite high rates of early adverse outcomes, older adults with frailty may achieve greater improvements in long-term function than those who do not have frailty.[7] To increase the likelihood of positive outcomes, interventions such as CGA, exercise and/or nutritional prehabilitation, and institution of delirium prevention bundles should be considered. While the evidence for prehabilitation is promising, adherence is often a challenge for older adults with frailty, who often have pain and fatigue that act as barriers to participation. Ensuring adequate support and motivation is there to achieve efficacy. Suggested frailty instruments are provided in Table 31-2.

TABLE 31-2. Suggested Screens and Interventions for Geriatric Syndromes

GERIATRIC SYNDROME	PREOPERATIVE SCREEN(S)	PREOPERATIVE INTERVENTION(S)
Single-Component Screen		
Cognitive impairment	**Mini-COG** 1. Three-word recall (0–3 pts) *Apple Chair Nickel* *Have patient repeat words, then recall each after clock draw* 2. Draw a clock (0 or 2 pts) *Instruct to start by drawing a large circle, then put all the numbers in the circle and set the hands at 10 past 11. (11:10)* https://mini-cog.com/	**Impairment suggested if < 3** • Do full MMSE or MoCA • If above ++, full neuropsychological testing is recommended • Educate on periop delirium risks • Ensure capacity for decision making around surgery • Geriatric referral, comanagement
Functional deficits	*Do you need any help with …* **ADLs** **IADLs** Dressing Shopping Bathing Paying Bills Getting up Cooking Eating Med Management	• Enhanced conversations around postoperative supports needed, possible worsening of functional status

(Continued)

TABLE 31-2. Suggested Screens and Interventions for Geriatric Syndromes *(Continued)*

GERIATRIC SYNDROME	PREOPERATIVE SCREEN(S)	PREOPERATIVE INTERVENTION(S)
Mobility	**Timed Up and Go** (TUG-test) *Patient stands from sitting position in chair, walks 10 feet, turns around, and sits back down*	**If > 15 seconds, higher risk for falls, functional decline, increased 1-yr mortality after surgery** • PT/OT intervention preoperatively
Polypharmacy	>5 medications	Discontinue unnecessary medications
Potentially inappropriate medications	Cross-check meds list with AGS Beers List*	Counsel to stop or taper inappropriate meds as possible
Depression	**Patient Health Questionnaire-2** *In past year have you …* 1. Had little interest or pleasure in doing things 2. Felt down, depressed, or hopeless *… for a period of 2 weeks or more?*	• If YES to either question, warrants full depression evaluation • Enhanced conversation with patients on higher risk for postoperative complications, including delirium, loss of functional independence, poor surgical outcomes, difficulty with pain control, and higher mortality
Hearing impairment	Hearing aids, reports of difficulty with hearing	Ensure inhospital presence of hearing aids or pocket-talker
Visual impairment	Eyewear, reports of difficulty with eyesight	• Ensure inhospital presence of eyewear • Awareness of medication management affected by vision
Falls	Ask about # of falls in the past 12 months	• If elevated, higher fall risk following surgery and predicts functional decline • Take appropriate fall precautions in the hospital, consult PT/OT • Educate patients and families
Malnutrition	>10% unintended weight loss in 6 months BMI < 20.5 Albumin < 3.0 *If one or more of the above are present, concern for malnutrition* Nutritional Risk Screening 2002 https://www.mdcalc.com/nutrition-risk-screening-2002-nrs-2002	• Nutritional counseling • Consider 10–14 days high-protein intake prior to surgery • Limit the preoperative fasting period • Multimodal prehab programs with exercise and nutritional components if available

*See Table 31-3.

Cognitive Function

Studies estimate that ~10% of adults over 65 years of age have mild cognitive impairment (MCI), a percentage that doubles in subsequent decades. In addition,

~14% over 71 years of age have overt dementia (above and beyond those with MCI). Many adults with cognitive impairment (CI) continue to live independently and are unaware of the diagnosis until deficits are unmasked in the setting of a major stressor such as surgery. Cognitive impairment is a strong predictor of postoperative delirium, prolonged hospitalization, increased mortality, worse surgical outcomes, and functional decline.[8] Following noncardiac surgery, adults with dementia or MCI experience 1-year mortality rates over twice as high as patients without cognitive issues, and have nearly twice as many complications in the first 1–3 months after surgery.[9] A cognitive baseline should be established before surgery and providers, patients, and families educated on delirium risk and risk reduction strategies. When cognitive impairment is suspected, decision-making capacity may also be compromised. In such circumstances, it is necessary to ensure that patient understands their disease, the planned surgery, its risks, potential outcomes, and alternatives. Involving a friend or family member in the preoperative visit can be helpful in providing collateral information and in reiterating perioperative instructions. The Mini-Cog assessment (https://mini-cog.com/download-the-mini-cog-instrument/) is recommended as an initial cognitive screen due to excellent sensitivity and specificity as well as reduced bias among different literacy and education levels. It consists of a three-item recall exercise and clock draw. A score of <3 suggests cognitive impairment and should prompt more comprehensive testing with the Mini Mental Status Exam (https://compendiumapp.com/post_4xQIen-Ly) or Montreal Cognitive Assessment (https://www.mocatest.org/app/).

Functional Status

Functional status is another strong predictor of perioperative outcomes. After surgery, patients with lower functional status, even after adjusting for medical comorbidity, are at greater risk for medical complications, increased length of stay, and long-term mortality.[2,8] Studies estimate threefold higher mortality rates after carotid endarterectomy and over double the risk of major complications after hip arthroplasty for adults with functional dependence. Even patients with partial dependence experienced five times higher rates of discharge to a nonhome setting than independent patients in a mixture of orthopedic, general, and vascular patients.

Functional status is comprised of a person's ability to perform activities of daily living (ADLs), such as eating, bathing, and dressing, instrumental activities

of daily living (IADLs), such as shopping, paying bills, and doing laundry, their mobility, and presence of sensory deficits. Screening can be achieved by targeted questions about ADLs/IADLs, hearing and vision impairment, and performance of the Timed Up and Go Test (TUGT). Some functional deficits can be addressed preoperatively by strength and balance exercises and ensuring presence of appropriate hearing and/or visual aids. Since adequate functional status is critical for independent living, a discussion around possible loss of function and need for nursing facility postoperatively is warranted in those at highest risk. Ideally, consideration should be given to building functional reserve prior to surgery, which moderate certainty evidence suggests can be achieved through prehabilitation, especially in cancer patients.[10] Planning for adequate home supports during the transition from hospital is also strongly recommended as this represents a key challenge for older patients and their families.

Medication Review

A standard review of medications and guidance on perioperative management of drugs is warranted for all patients preoperatively. In the older adult, there should also be special attention paid to identifying potentially harmful or unnecessary medications, although limited data are available to inform the safety of discontinuation prior to surgery. Polypharmacy, typically defined as taking five or more concurrent medications, is associated with delirium, increases the risk of drug-drug interactions and noncompliance, and may predict poor outcomes.[11] Currently, anticholinergic medications demonstrate the strongest associations with adverse postoperative outcomes. The American Geriatrics Society Beers List (Table 31-3) identifies agents that are more likely to cause undesirable side effects in older adults, such as delirium, kidney dysfunction, and bleeding. Other medications, while not harmful per se, may have been continued indefinitely with unclear indications. The perioperative period presents an opportunity to thoroughly review medications and evaluate need for ongoing use. The discontinuation of medications, however, is more appropriately overseen by a primary prescriber—and ideally is not done during the immediate perioperative period, to avoid precipitating withdrawal or clinical instability.

TABLE 31-3. Highlighted Medications to Avoid or Use with Caution from AGS Beers List

DELIRIOGENIC MEDS, FALL RISK, RENAL OR BLEEDING RISKS IN OLDER ADULTS

Medications with anticholinergic properties
    Antihistamines
    Antispasmodics
    Tricyclic antidepressants
    Antipsychotics
Benzodiazepines
Non-benzodiazepine hypnotics (e.g., zolpidem)
Opioids
NSAIDs
Other psychotropic or sedating meds (muscle relaxants, gabapentinoids)

Nutrition

As many as two-thirds of older adults in the hospital, nursing home, and community have or are at risk for malnutrition. Surgery induces a catabolic state in response to stress and inflammation to mobilize factors for tissue repair. Absence of adequate nutritional stores may compromise surgical outcomes. Increased rates of complications, such as surgical site infection, pneumonia, urinary tract infection, and wound dehiscence, are more common following surgery in individuals with poor nutritional status.[12] Single-point screens (>10% loss of body weight over 6 months, BMI < 20.5, albumin < 3.0) or composite screens (e.g., Nutrition Risk Screen [NRS] https://www.mdcalc.com/nutrition-risk-screening-2002-nrs-2002) can be used to identify patients at risk for malnutrition who may benefit from preoperative nutritional interventions. Interventions may include referral to a dietician, high-protein oral nutrition supplementation (ONS), reduced duration of preoperative fasting, and early postoperative feeding.[12] A simple target for patients is to aim to achieve more than 1.2 g/kg of daily protein intake which can often be achieved with the addition of a single daily scoop of protein supplement. In fact, as little as 1–2 weeks of protein supplementation is linked to a >1 day reduction in length of stay.

Delirium Risk

Delirium is an acute, reversible confusional state marked by fluctuations in attention, cognition, and consciousness. It is common in older patients after surgery and associated with increased costs, length of stay, medical complications, poor outcomes, and increased mortality. Up to 40% of cases can be prevented with simple behavioral interventions. Preoperative screening for delirium risk is an important step in reducing modifiable risks and educating patients and families on prevention strategies in the hospital.[13] Unfortunately, no multivariable risk calculators provide adequate predictive accuracy; however, individual risk factors such as a history of delirium, frailty, and preexisting cognitive impairment increase the odds of delirium more than fourfold.[14] Many aspects of the procedure itself or hospitalization are also associated with delirium, but may not be modifiable. Emerging techniques (such as avoidance of deep general anesthesia using processed electro-encephalography [EEG]), optimal choice of intraoperative sedatives (such as dexmedetomidine over propofol), and avoidance of unnecessary benzodiazepines also appear to help reduce delirium risk. Table 31-4 highlights delirium risk factors and key interventions that may mitigate risk throughout the perioperative period.[13,15]

Goals of Care/Shared Decision Making

The preoperative evaluation serves as an opportunity to better understand patients' overall health goals and expectations about how surgery may help them. It also is a time to ensure patients and families appreciate the risks of surgery beyond specific medical complications. These might include the possibility of prolonged hospitalization, ICU stay, skilled rehab facility at discharge, or loss of function and/or independence. Eliciting an individual's unique expectations, values, and preferences is critical to guide shared decision making (SDM). While clinicians routinely cite time constraints as barriers to SDM, evidence supports its efficacy in fostering optimal patient decisions. Use of simple approaches such as "BRAN" (Benefits, Risks, Alternatives, do Nothing) can facilitate efficient SDM. A preferred surrogate decision maker should be identified and documented prior to any surgery, even if already within an advanced directive. Suggested questions for older adults preparing for surgery are in

TABLE 31-4. Delirium Risk Factors and Prevention Strategies	
DELIRIUM RISK FACTORS	**PREVENTION STRATEGIES**
PATIENT-RELATED	PREOP

DELIRIUM RISK FACTORS — PATIENT-RELATED

Nonmodifiable	Modifiable
Age ≥ 65	Depression
Cognitive impairment	Sensory impairment
	Poor functional status
	Excessive alcohol use
	Polypharmacy
	Renal insufficiency
	Poor nutrition

PREVENTION STRATEGIES — PREOP

- Reduce or eliminate alcohol intake
- Stop unnecessary or inappropriate medications
- Treat depression
- Educate patients and families on delirium
- Prehabilitation strategies with nutrition and exercise interventions
- Ensure hearing and visual aids available

DELIRIUM RISK FACTORS — PROCEDURE AND HOSPITAL-RELATED

Nonmodifiable	Modifiable
Type of surgery	Type of anesthesia
Surgical duration	Medication effect
Postoperative	Sleep deprivation complications
	Poor pain control
	Constipation (infection, cardiopulmonary)
	Dehydration
Surgical stress	Urinary retention > 3 new medications
	Bladder catheters/tethers

PREVENTION STRATEGIES — INTRAOP AND POSTOP

- Avoid medications on Beers list
- Regional anesthesia when possible
- Ensure hearing and visual aids present
- Remove bladder catheters/tethers
- Adequate pain control
- Limit overnight disturbances to enhance sleep/wake cycle
- Good bowel regimen
- Attention to adequate fluid intake
- Monitor for urinary retention
- Promote mobilization, PT/OT
- Frequent reorienting communication
- Nutritional assistance
- Encourage family at bedside

Table 31-5. While not exhaustive, these cover the most salient topics to discuss.

Prehabilitation

Prehabilitation is an intervention that aims to build reserve before surgery to improve postoperative outcomes and recovery.[10] Prehabilitation programs typically include one or more components, with exercise and nutrition being most common, and cognitive and psychosocial aspects emerging as important considerations. Data specific to older surgical patients, or those with geriatric conditions like frailty or sarcopenia, are limited, yet many such patients have been enrolled in existing prehabilitation trials. Currently, data supporting prehabilitation's efficacy are promising, but of low certainty. It appears that in cancer surgery patients, prehabilitation likely improves functional recovery. Across different types of surgery, prehabilitation may also decrease complication rates and reduce length of stay.[10]

No single approach to prehabilitation exists as a gold standard. In general, exercise appears to be a foundational component, with most efficacious programs combining moderate-intensity aerobic exercise and strength training. The optimal duration of exercise prehabilitation remains unclear, but at least 3–5 weeks are likely required. For older patients who are often at risk of malnutrition at baseline, experts suggest that nutritional intake be carefully supported when increasing exercise participation. Nutritional prehabilitation, with or without concurrent exercise, can potentially improve postoperative outcomes in

TABLE 31-5. Key Questions for Older Adults Undergoing Major Surgery

GOALS/EXPECTATIONS

What are you hoping this surgery will do for you?

What are your biggest concerns?

Would you regret having this surgery if it resulted in you no longer being able to live independently?

ADVANCED CARE PLANNING

If you were too sick to make a medical decision after surgery, who would you trust to decide for you?

Have you discussed your preferences with them?

HOME SUPPORT

After your surgery, who might help you with cooking, cleaning, shopping, or any other needs in the weeks after returning home?

as little as 1–2 weeks, and should primarily focus on achieving target protein intake of >1.2 g/kg each day. For older adults with frailty, adherence to prehabilitation can be a challenge; therefore, programs should ideally include personalization, motivational strategies, and psychosocial support to ensure adequate participation to achieve benefit. While few data exist regarding cognitive prehabilitation, promising data suggest that preoperative brain training may decrease delirium with adequate participation.[16] Overall, consideration of prehabilitation is recommended by several guidelines when resources are available.

POSTOPERATIVE RISK REDUCTION

While some of the most important efforts at minimizing postoperative complications in the older adult take place in advance of surgery, additional measures can be implemented postoperatively. Postoperative delirium prevention strategies (Table 31-3) are often bundled together in order sets and involve consultation with geriatrics services when possible. Key interventions include limiting tethers/catheters, ensuring hearing and visual aids are available, early mobilization, and frequent orientation (including family members or caregivers at bedside).[13] Medications should be prescribed with an eye to potential complications in geriatric patients. Evidence-based strategies include

avoidance of gabapentinoids, optimal use of local anesthetic–based techniques, and consistent use of nonopioid analgesics such as acetaminophen and nonsteroidal anti-inflammatories when not contraindicated. In addition to limiting nighttime interruptions, melatonin may help foster good sleep hygiene; whether melatonin reduces the risk of delirium remains uncertain, with systematic reviews finding some evidence of reduced risk, but without resulting improvements in delirium duration or length of hospital stay.[17,18] A Cochrane systematic review noted strong evidence supporting multicomponent interventions to prevent delirium in hospitalized patients, but no clear evidence for cholinesterase inhibitors or antipsychotic medications. In hip fracture patients, use of peripheral nerve blocks likely reduces delirium risk,[19] but the role of drugs and other anesthetic techniques to prevent delirium in other surgical populations is uncertain. Ideally, postoperative care for higher risk older patients should include comanagement with a hospitalist or geriatric medicine team. This approach can facilitate earlier identification and treatment of medical complications as well as thoughtful use of medications, and serve as an important layer of communication with families and surgeons to revisit goals of care when necessary. Where resources are available, this approach to geriatric comanagement should be informed by a preoperative CGA, and includes proactive discharge planning prior to hospital admission for elective surgery.[4]

Resource-Intensive Assessment and Interventions

The full complement of screening tools and potential risk reduction interventions for older adults undergoing surgery requires extensive time and resources not available in all settings. As such, there is considerable heterogeneity in preoperative programs for such patients. We suggest a tiered approach to assessment and optimization based on both the amount of time available prior to surgery and the specific resources at a given hospital program (Figure 31-1). In any case, a specialized, often multidisciplinary approach to preoperative evaluation is warranted to ensure optimal outcomes in older adults. Consistent and thorough communication among providers about the plan of care is essential across the perioperative period.

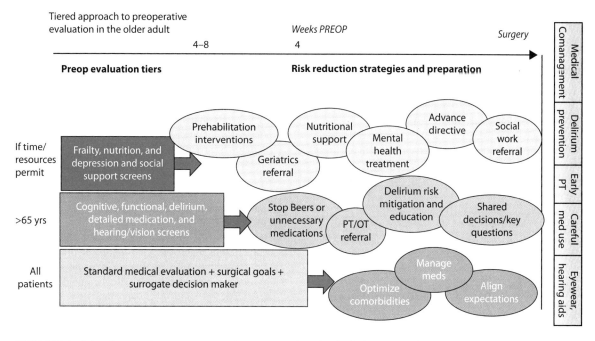

FIGURE 31-1. A tiered approach to assessment and optimization based on both the amount of time available prior to surgery and the specific resources available at a given hospital program.

SUMMARY

Optimal care of the older surgical patient is truly a perioperative undertaking, beginning at the time of surgical consultation and continuing through the transition out of hospital after surgery. Early identification of key geriatric risk factors like frailty, sarcopenia, and cognitive impairment can allow the multidisciplinary team to personalize preoperative optimization, perioperative comanagement, and discharge planning.

Clinical pearls

- In addition to the standard medical evaluation, preoperative assessment of the older adult should focus on frailty, function, cognition, socioenvironmental surroundings, goals of care, and nutrition.

- Use feasible and validated screening tools where indicated, including multidimensional frailty instruments and brief cognitive screeners.

- Where available, comprehensive geriatric assessment should be used to provide a personalized assessment and management plan for the perioperative period.

- Identify and limit use of drugs that are more likely to cause undesirable side effects (using references such as American Geriatrics Society Beers List), such as gabapentanoids and anticholinergics.

- Use bundled nursing and behavioral interventions to prevent postoperative delirium and other complications.

- Comanagement with a hospitalist or geriatrician can facilitate earlier identification and treatment of medical complications, judicious use of new medications, and augmented communication with the patient's family.

REFERENCES

1. Engel JS, Tran J, Khalil N, et al. A systematic review of perioperative clinical practice guidelines for care of older adults living with frailty. *Br J Anaesth*. 2023;130(3): 262-271. PMID: 36707368
2. Colburn JL, Mohanty S, Burton JR. Surgical guidelines for perioperative management of older adults: what geriatricians need to know. *J Am Geriatr Soc*. 2017;65(6):1339-1346. PMID: 28323335

3. Varley PR, Buchanan D, Bilderback A, et al. Association of routine preoperative frailty assessment with 1-year postoperative mortality. *JAMA Surg.* 2023;158(5): 475-483. PMID: 36811872

4. Partridge JSL, Harari D, Martin FC, et al. Randomized clinical trial of comprehensive geriatric assessment and optimization in vascular surgery. *Br J Surg.* 2017;104(6):679-687. PMID: 28198997

5. Aucoin SD, Hao M, Sohi R, et al. Accuracy and feasibility of clinically applied frailty instruments before surgery. *Anesthesiology.* 2020;133(1):78-95. PMID: 32243326

6. McIsaac DI, Taljaard M, Bryson GL, et al. Frailty as a predictor of death or new disability after surgery: a prospective cohort study. *Ann Surg.* 2020;271(2):283-289. PMID: 30048320

7. McIsaac DI, Taljaard M, Bryson GL, et al. Frailty and long-term postoperative disability trajectories: a prospective multicentre cohort study. *Br J Anaesth.* 2020;125(5):704-711. PMID: 32778405

8. Oresanya LB, Lyons WL, Finlayson E. Preoperative assessment of the older patient: a narrative review. *JAMA.* 2014;311(20):2110-2120. PMID: 24867014

9. Chen L, Au E, Saripella A, et al. Postoperative outcomes in older surgical patients with preoperative cognitive impairment: a systematic review and meta-analysis. *J Clin Anesth.* 2022;80:110883. PMID: 35623265

10. McIsaac DI, Gill M, Boland L, et al. Prehabilitation in adult patients undergoing surgery: an umbrella review of systematic reviews. *Br J Anaesth.* 2022;128(2): 244-257. PMID: 34922735

11. Maher RL, Hanlon J, Hajjar ER. Clinical consequences of polypharmacy in elderly. *Expert Opin Drug Saf.* 2014;13(1):57-65. PMID: 24073682

12. Weimann A, Braga M, Carli F, et al. ESPEN guideline: clinical nutrition in surgery. *Clin Nutr Edinb Scotl.* 2017;36(3):623-650. PMID: 28385477

13. American Geriatrics Society Expert Panel on Postoperative Delirium in Older Adults. Postoperative delirium in older adults: best practice statement from the American Geriatrics Society. *J Am Coll Surg.* 2015;220(2):136-148.e1. PMID: 25535170

14. Watt J, Tricco AC, Talbot-Hamon C, et al. Identifying older adults at risk of delirium following elective surgery: a systematic review and meta-analysis. *J Gen Intern Med.* 2018;33(4):500-509. PMID: 29374358

15. Mohanty S, Rosenthal RA, Russell MM, Neuman MD, Ko CY, Esnaola NF. Optimal perioperative management of the geriatric patient: a best practices guideline from the American College of Surgeons NSQIP and the American Geriatrics Society. *J Am Coll Surg.* 2016;222(5):930-947. PMID: 27049783

16. Humeidan ML, Reyes JC, Mavarez-Martinez A, et al. Effect of cognitive prehabilitation on the incidence of postoperative delirium among older adults undergoing major noncardiac surgery: the neurobics randomized clinical trial. *JAMA Surg.* 2021;156(2):148-156. PMID: 33175114

17. Khaing K, Nair BR. Melatonin for delirium prevention in hospitalized patients: a systematic review and meta-analysis. *J Psychiatr Res.* 2021;133:181-190. PMID: 33348252

18. Ng KT, Teoh WY, Khor AJ. The effect of melatonin on delirium in hospitalised patients: a systematic review and meta-analyses with trial sequential analysis. *J Clin Anesth.* 2020;59:74-81. PMID: 31279283

19. Guay J, Kopp S. Peripheral nerve blocks for hip fractures in adults. *Cochrane Database Syst Rev.* 2020;11(11):CD001159. PMID: 33238043

## 32

Enhanced Recovery Programs

Jeffrey W. Simmons, MD, MSHQS, FASA and Sunil K. Sahai, MD, FAAP, FACP, SFHM

COMMON CLINICAL QUESTIONS

1. How does preoperative nutrition management differ in ERP versus traditional management?
2. How is multimodal analgesia employed in ERP?
3. What are the main goals of intravenous fluid therapy in ERP?

INTRODUCTION

Enhanced recovery programs (ERPs) seek to improve the quality of surgical care by decreasing costs, decreasing complications, and increasing patient satisfaction and outcomes. It is well known that variations in surgical and anesthetic practice lead to variable outcomes, and as such, enhanced recovery programs seek to combine evidence-based recommendations to reduce complications by standardizing aspects of perioperative care. Additionally, a major tenet of ERP is to minimize physiologic disruption for the patient by using minimally invasive techniques and allowing for the return to homeostasis as soon as possible after surgery. Enhanced recovery programs are considered "modular," in that practices may adopt parts of the program that suit their needs and incorporate others as they evolve. Enhanced recovery programs are divided into three distinct phases: preoperative, intraoperative, and postoperative.

HISTORY

Enhanced recovery programs initially started as "fast track" recovery programs after colorectal surgery in the mid-1990s. Formal studies were conducted in the early part of the millennium, and enhanced recovery after surgery (ERAS) programs were started in Europe. With the success of the early collaboratives, the ERAS Society was founded in 2010.[1] Since then, the ERAS Society has pioneered the development of protocols for numerous types of surgery. They have partnered with numerous medical societies around the world. Additionally, many institutions have undertaken their own initiatives, which collectively fall under the concept of enhanced recovery programs.

PREOPERATIVE PHASE

The preoperative phase incorporates many concepts central to the perioperative medicine principle of "medical optimization" and incorporates them into a single framework. A successful ERP addresses modifiable risks to the patient for weeks to months before surgery. Central lifestyle modification concepts include the use of prehabilitation, smoking cessation, and limiting alcohol intake. In addition to these lifestyle changes, ERPs also focus on optimizing nutritional status and managing comorbid medical conditions in the preoperative phase. Another central tenet of ERP is patient education. Establishing perioperative assessment clinics staffed in a multidisciplinary fashion with anesthesiologists, internists, and allied health providers such as nutritionists can help standardize preoperative care among numerous surgical specialties at an institution.

In line with the philosophy of minimal disruption of physiologic functions, preoperative management in ERP protocols also targets the following three areas: bowel preparation, preoperative fasting, and carbohydrate loading.

Thoughtful Use of Mechanical Bowel Preparation

For years, patients have dreaded the bowel preparation they must undergo before elective abdominal surgery. Mechanical bowel preparations have the unintended effect of being uncomfortable and increasing the likelihood of preoperative dehydration, in contravention with ERPs that seek to minimize physiologic disturbance with no difference in outcomes. As such, ERPs call for the judicious use of mechanical bowel preparations. A bowel preparation with intravenous and oral antibiotics without mechanical bowel prep is gaining acceptance as a standard of care in elective colorectal surgery.[2]

Preoperative Fasting

Despite new guidelines in 2017, the standard order of "NPO after midnight" remains pervasive. ERP encourages limited fluid intake in line with the 2023 modular update by the American Society of Anesthesiologists (Table 32-1).[3] The ASA recommends that healthy adults drink carbohydrate containing clear liquids until 2 hours before elective surgery. Up to 400 mL of clear liquid is considered an appropriate volume. Trials provided participants with a median of 400 mL of clear liquids 2 hours before anesthesia administration without adverse consequences such as aspiration of gastric contents.

Carbohydrate Loading

Carbohydrate loading has several advantages: minimizing the postsurgical catabolic state, reducing insulin resistance, and, from a patient perspective, reducing hunger, thirst, and anxiety.[4] While immunonutrition is still controversial, some evidence suggests it may benefit moderate-to-high-risk abdominal surgeries. Immunonutrition reportedly enhances

TABLE 32-1. Fasting Recommendations

INGESTED MATERIAL	MINIMUM FASTING PERIOD
Clear liquids	2 hours
Breast milk	4 hours
Infant formulas	6 hours
Nonhuman milk	8 hours
Light meal	6 hours
Fried foods, fatty foods, or meat	Additional fasting time (e.g., 8 or more hours) may be needed

Source: Reproduced with permission from Practice guidelines for preoperative fasting and the use of pharmacologic agents to reduce the risk of pulmonary aspiration: Application to healthy patients undergoing elective procedures: An updated report by the American society of anesthesiologists task force on preoperative fasting and the use of pharmacologic agents to reduce the risk of pulmonary aspiration. *Anesthesiology.* 2017;126(3):376-393.

immune response, decreases inflammatory response, and improves protein synthesis after surgery.

A summary of recommendations in the preoperative phase and the strength of evidence is shown in Table 32-2.

INTRAOPERATIVE PHASE

What are the major components of intraoperative enhanced recovery? Principles of enhanced recovery should be applied in the intraoperative phase with the knowledge that hemodynamics during surgery and anesthesia are dynamic and may require tailored intervention. Proponents of ERP do not argue treating every patient the same (i.e., cookbook medicine) but that the principles of enhanced recovery are broadly applicable. When the principles are bundled into a protocol, high compliance or adherence has proven more beneficial in outcomes than low compliance.[5] The six beneficial practices incorporated into most ERPs are listed in Figure 32-1.

Multimodal Analgesia

Multimodal analgesia (MMA) is defined as using multiple analgesic agents with different mechanisms of action at lower doses to effectively lower pain versus

TABLE 32-2. ERAS Society Recommendations

RECOMMENDATIONS	TYPE OF SURGERY	STRENGTH OF EVIDENCE	ERAS RECOMMENDATION GRADE
Preadmission education and testing	All	Low	Strong
Prehabilitation	All	Very low	None (ongoing studies)
Smoking cessation	All	High	Strong
Abstinence from alcohol	All	Low	Strong
No mechanical bowel preparation	All	High	Strong
Preoperative fasting	All	Moderate	Strong
Carbohydrate treatment	Major abdominal, head, and neck	Low-moderate	Strong: nondiabetic patients
			Weak: diabetic patients
Immunonutrition	All	Low	Weak
No routine preanesthetic/ premedication	All	High	Strong

Source: Reproduced with permission from Jankowski CJ. Preparing the patient for enhanced recovery after surgery. *Inter Anesthesiology Clinics*. 2017;55(4):12-20.

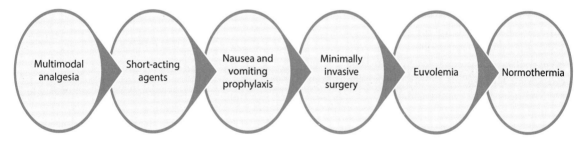

FIGURE 32-1. Intraoperative enhanced recovery principles.

using any one single agent at higher doses. These include neuraxial or regional nerve blocks, dexmedetomidine or lidocaine infusions, ketamine/magnesium, dexamethasone, acetaminophen, NSAIDs, or gabapentinoids. Multimodal analgesia limits the side effects of single agents while acknowledging the complexity of pain networks and receptors. In enhanced recovery, MMA is also used to limit overall opioid consumption, reduce the surgical stress response, and aid in a quick return to normal activities of daily living.[6] Multimodal analgesia has theoretical advantages of decreased postoperative pain, faster emergence from anesthesia, reduced postoperative delirium and nausea, and faster discharge from the postoperative

care unit. The sparing of opioids during the intraoperative phase reduces respiratory depression and helps prevent gut immobility. Of the multimodal medications commonly used in ERP, gabapentenoids should be used cautiously in patients with renal disease, advanced age, and high-risk for sleep apnea as adverse events have been recognized in these populations and risk may outweigh benefits.[7]

Short-Acting Agents

Anesthetic agents with short half-lives aid in the earlier recovery of patients after surgery. These agents include both inhaled and intravenous agents. Inhaled anesthetics such as sevoflurane and desflurane are rapidly cleared from circulation and considered short-acting inhaled agents. Intravenous opioids such as morphine or hydromorphone have longer half-lives compared to either fentanyl or remifentanil; the latter two are sometimes preferred in ERPs.[8] Anesthesia providers should use intravenous antiemetics such as ondansetron and dexamethasone in favor of longer-acting haloperidol and promethazine, which have unfavorable sedating properties.

Nausea and Vomiting Prevention

Current guidelines advocate for the use of at least two antiemetics from different classes for any patient at risk for nausea and three to four agents for patients considered high risk.[9] PONV risk factors include female, type of surgery, younger age, nonsmokers, history of postoperative nausea or motion sickness, use of inhaled anesthesia, duration of general anesthesia, and use of intraoperative opioids. Dexamethasone and 5-HT3 antagonists (such as ondansetron) provide adequate prophylaxis for low-risk patients. For patients with extreme postoperative nausea and vomiting, a total intravenous anesthesia technique may be employed, avoiding inhaled agents. Aprepitant, a medication previously reserved for chemotherapy-induced nausea, is now available for preoperative prophylaxis and has very high efficacy against PONV.[10] Aprepitant 40 mg should be taken orally approximately 3 hours before induction of anesthesia. When patients have PONV despite prevention measures, rescue treatment should utilize an agent from a different class of medication not already used. See Chapter 43 for more information.

Minimally Invasive Surgery

Enhanced recovery surgeons utilize laparoscopic (including robotic) techniques versus open surgical techniques to improve time to ambulation by limiting tissue damage. Multiple studies demonstrate that minimally invasive surgery in enhanced recovery is more effective than open procedures combined with ERP principles.[11]

Euvolemia

The goal of intraoperative fluid therapy is to avoid infusion of excess salt and water intake that will eventually shift into the interstitium, causing bowel edema and ileus. A balanced salt solution may be used for low cardiovascular-risk patients, aiming for zero balance at the end of the procedure. Higher cardiovascular risk patients or patients having more complex procedures may require goal-directed hemodynamic therapy (GDHT). GDHT, which monitors cardiac output, helps guide fluid replacement. It is essential not to restrict fluids or attempt to achieve a negative balance, as restrictive techniques may be associated with increased kidney injury.[12]

Normothermia

Maintaining normal body temperature is essential for wound healing, reduced bleeding, and prevention of shivering, and aids in faster emergence from anesthesia. Hypothermia occurs quickly in cold operating rooms, especially in uncovered patients also receiving unwarmed intravenous fluids. Thus, the mechanisms to warm the patients must be quickly employed once the patient arrives in the OR (forced air warmers, warm ambient room temperature, warmed intravenous fluids).[13]

POSTOPERATIVE PHASE

Multimodal Analgesia (Figure 32-2)

The postoperative use of multimodal analgesia techniques is vital to reduce postoperative delirium, augment the patient's ability to begin rehabilitation, reduce nausea and bowel ileus, and promote better respiratory mechanics. Conventional regional techniques include epidural anesthesia and continuous catheter nerve blocks. When utilizing epidural anesthesia, special care must be taken with deep vein thrombosis (DVT) prevention strategies. Coordination with the anesthesia pain service is necessary before the removal of the epidural catheter when patients are treated with DVT prophylaxis medications (e.g., unfractionated heparin, low molecular weight heparin, fondaparinux). Infusions of drugs such as lidocaine or ketamine provide excellent analgesia while avoiding routine opioids when regional techniques are not used. Finally, scheduled acetaminophen and ibuprofen are mainstays of enhanced recovery pain protocols.

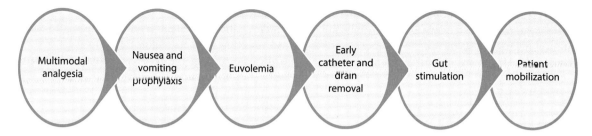

FIGURE 32-2. Postoperative enhanced recovery principles.

Nausea and Vomiting Prevention

A strong correlation exists between nausea and increased length of stay in the postoperative recovery.[14] Postoperative nausea and vomiting (PONV) are best treated with prevention, as described in the intraoperative phase. Nausea and vomiting may also persist in some unfortunate patients, lasting 72 hours to 1 week after surgery, known as Post Discharge Nausea and Vomiting (PDNV). PDNV affects approximately 37% of patients after outpatient surgery, even when treated with prophylaxis.[15] Predictors of PDNV are female gender, age less than 50, opioid administration, and the presence of PONV in the recovery room. The essential treatment for PDNV is again prevention by avoiding opioids with the use of multimodal analgesia. When PDNV is encountered, 5-HT receptor antagonists such as Ondansetron can be administered in sublingual form. Oral dexamethasone attenuates the symptoms of PDNV. Finally, promethazine (oral or suppository) may be necessary as a rescue agent.

Euvolemia

Intraoperative hypotension strongly correlates with postoperative acute kidney injury. It is, therefore, essential for patients to begin *oral* fluid intake immediately after surgery (the goal for a patient without ongoing fluid losses is 1.75 L/day). Intravenous fluids should be continued only for essential medications. In high cardiovascular-risk patients still requiring intravenous fluids after surgery, consideration should be given to noninvasive cardiac output monitoring to achieve GDHT.[16] These patients should have a balanced crystalloid (e.g., lactated Ringer's [LR], Plasma-Lyte, or Normosol-R) administered in favor of higher sodium fluids such as normal saline.

Removal of Catheters, Drains, and Nasogastric Tubes

The routine use of surgical drains, nasogastric tubes, and catheters hinders patient ambulation and is associated with increased hospital length of stay.[17] Naso/orogastric tubes and urinary catheters should be removed as soon as possible to reduce the risk of pulmonary and urinary tract infections. Nurse-driven protocols for removing naso/orogastric tubes and Foley catheters may improve compliance with early removal.

Gut Stimulation

Enhanced recovery places particular emphasis on returning the patient to a normal oral diet within 24 hours of surgery to promote peristalsis and increase patient satisfaction. Gut stimulation is also promoted by early mobilization and avoidance of opioid medications. Additionally, it is recognized that a significant percentage of surgical patients are malnourished, so the replacement of protein calories is given priority over total calories. A disadvantage of early oral nutrition after surgery is increased nausea and vomiting; however, severe complications are rare. As protein replacement is essential for wound healing, feeding tube or parenteral nutrition should be considered if the patient cannot tolerate food orally.[18]

Early Mobilization

Early mobilization after surgery (ranging from sitting up in a chair to ambulation) is associated with decreased length of hospital stay, reduced pulmonary complications, reduced incidence of venous thromboembolism, improved bowel stimulation, and improved orthostatic tolerance.[19] Most enhanced recovery protocols incorporate protocolized strategies to ambulate the patient early after surgery. Additionally, those patients who require extended venous thromboembolism prophylaxis are identified, and appropriate education is provided along with medication.

OUTCOMES

Compliance and Auditing

After implementing an enhanced recovery program, measuring outcomes is essential for long-term sustainment. Clearly, labeling or marking a case as "ERP" is the first step toward accurate data collection. Next, nurses and physicians must pay careful attention to consistent documentation practices. Enhanced recovery protocols routinely encompass 20–25 individual best practices, each requiring discreet documentation. For example, a standard documentation practice for ambulation must be in place if an organization is to

measure the benefit of early mobilization. Likewise, standard and consistent documentation of nausea and vomiting must be engineered into the electronic medical records in the recovery room and postsurgical floor to capture the effectiveness of the ERP intervention. Only with standardized, discreet field documentation will efficacy and return on investment be realized through data. Thus, successful enhanced recovery programs emphasize data collection early in developing their enhanced recovery protocol.

Many enhanced recovery programs base success on reduced hospital length of stay, reduced overall complications, and reduced cost (measures consistently demonstrated with successful program implementation).[20] Enhanced recovery programs also provide the capability to install quality initiatives into routine surgical care. A list of commonly measured outcomes is presented in Table 32-3.

TABLE 32-3. Commonly Measured Outcomes and Metrics for Enhanced Recovery Programs

Patient comfort	PONV incidence	Return of bowel flatus
	Pain scores	Sleep quality
Clinical quality	Hypothermia prevention measures	Pressure ulcer prevention measures
	DVT prophylaxis compliance	Unplanned admission to ICU
Cognition	Postoperative delirium incidence	Postoperative cognitive decline
	Postoperative stroke	
Cardiovascular	Perioperative hypotension	Venous thromboembolism rate
	Myocardial injury	Composite incidence of major adverse cardiac event
Pulmonary	Postoperative pneumonia	Unplanned reintubation
Infectious disease	Wound infection rate	Bloodstream infections
Renal	Acute kidney injury	Rate of new postoperative hemodialysis
Hematology	Blood loss	Rate of transfusion
Patient-reported	Return to work	Patient satisfaction
	Disability-free survival	Quality of recovery
Resource management	Hospital length of stay	Total and variable cost
	Reduction in gender and ethnic healthcare disparity	

Outcomes can be described as clinician-versus patient-reported, clinical versus resource management, adverse events, and composite versus single event. Recently, national organizations have attempted to standardize endpoints and definitions for enhanced recovery programs, identifying over 30 parameters without standardized definitions.

FUTURE OF ENHANCED RECOVERY PROGRAMS

There is increasing research on using technologies to improve ERP delivery. This includes using technologies to improve ERP adherence (patient engagement technologies), monitoring patients remotely (step counters), and delivering education better. ERPs also improve metrics beyond traditional ones (LOS, readmissions, costs, complications). These nontraditional metrics being studied include improvements in opioid utilization, patient-reported outcomes, and surgical disparities. Finally, ERPs are increasingly utilized for cutting-edge surgical advances such as outpatient colectomy and other same-day surgeries.

Clinical pearls

- For ERPs to be effective, refer patients at least 2–4 weeks before surgery.
- Preoperatively, medical optimization focuses on lifestyle modifications, nutritional status, and optimizing treatment of medical comorbidities.
- Minimize disruption of physiologic function by following protocols for bowel preparation, preoperative fasting, and carbohydrate loading.
- Intraoperatively, ERP bundles include multimodal analgesia, use of short-acting agents, prevention of nausea/vomiting, minimally invasive surgery, maintenance of euvolemia, and normothermia.
- Postoperatively, components of ERPs include multimodal analgesia, prevention of nausea/vomiting, euvolemia, removal of catheters, drains, and nasogastric tubes, gut stimulation, and early mobilization.

REFERENCES

1. Tanious MK, Ljungqvist O, Urman RD. Enhanced recovery after surgery: history, evolution, guidelines, and future directions. *Int Anesthesiol Clin.* 2017;55(4): 1-11. PMID: 28901977
2. Tan J, Ryan ÉJ, Davey MG, et al. Mechanical bowel preparation and antibiotics in elective colorectal surgery: network meta-analysis. *BJS Open.* 2023;7(3):zrad040. PMID: 37257059
3. Joshi GP, Abdelmalak BB, Weigel WA, et al. 2023 American Society of Anesthesiologists practice guidelines for preoperative fasting: carbohydrate-containing clear liquids with or without protein, chewing gum, and pediatric fasting duration—a modular update of the 2017 American Society of Anesthesiologists practice guidelines for preoperative fasting. *Anesthesiology.* 2023;138(2):132-151. PMID: 36629465
4. Jankowski CJ. Preparing the patient for enhanced recovery after surgery. *Int Anesthesiol Clin.* 2017;55(4):12. PMID: 28858906
5. Gustafsson UO, Hausel J, Thorell A, et al. Adherence to the enhanced recovery after surgery protocol and outcomes after colorectal cancer surgery. *Arch Surg.* 2011;146(5):571-577. PMID: 21242424
6. McEvoy MD, Raymond BL, Krige A. Opioid-sparing perioperative analgesia within enhanced recovery programs. *Anesthesiol Clin.* 2022;40(1):35-58. PMID: 35236582
7. Verret M, Lauzier F, Zarychanski R, et al. Canadian Perioperative Anesthesia Clinical Trials (PACT) Group. Perioperative use of gabapentinoids for the management of postoperative acute pain: a systematic review and meta-analysis. *Anesthesiology.* 2020;133(2):265-279. PMID: 32667154
8. Feldheiser A, Aziz O, Baldini G, et al. Enhanced recovery after surgery (ERAS) for gastrointestinal surgery, part 2: consensus statement for anaesthesia practice. *Acta Anaesthesiol Scand.* 2016;60(3):289-334. PMID: 26514824
9. Gan TJ, Belani KG, Bergese S, et al. Fourth consensus guidelines for the management of postoperative nausea and vomiting [published correction appears in *Anesth Analg.* 2020 Nov;131(5):e241]. *Anesth Analg.* 2020;131(2):411-448. PMID: 32467512
10. Parrish RH 2nd, Findley R, Elias KM, et al. Pharmacotherapeutic prophylaxis and post-operative outcomes within an Enhanced Recovery After Surgery (ERAS®) program: a randomized retrospective cohort study. *Ann Med Surg (Lond).* 2021;73:103178. PMID: 35003725

11. Pache B, Hübner M, Jurt J, et al. Minimally invasive surgery and enhanced recovery after surgery: the ideal combination? *J Surg Oncol.* 2017;116(5):613-616. PMID: 29081065

12. Drakeford PA, Tham SQ, Kwek JL, et al. Acute kidney injury within an Enhanced Recovery after Surgery (ERAS) Program for colorectal surgery. *World J Surg.* 2022;46(1):19-33. PMID: 34665309

13. Billeter AT, Hohmann SF, Druen D, et al. Unintentional perioperative hypothermia is associated with severe complications and high mortality in elective operations. *Surgery.* 2014;156(5):1245-1252. PMID: 24947647

14. Ganter MT, Blumenthal S, Dübendorfer S, et al. The length of stay in the post-anaesthesia care unit correlates with pain intensity, nausea and vomiting on arrival. *Perioper Med (Lond).* 2014;3(1):10. PMID: 25485103

15. Schlesinger T, Meybohm P, Kranke P. Postoperative nausea and vomiting: risk factors, prediction tools, and algorithms. *Curr Opin Anaesthesiol.* 2023;36(1):117-123. PMID: 36550611

16. Jessen MK, Vallentin MF, Holmberg MJ, et al. Goal-directed haemodynamic therapy during general anaesthesia for noncardiac surgery: a systematic review and meta-analysis. *Br J Anaesth.* 2022;128(3):416-433. PMID: 34916049

17. Kallen AN. Perioperative pathways: enhanced recovery after surgery. *Obstet Gynecol.* 2018;132(3):E120-E130. PMID: 30134426

18. Lewis SJ, Andersen HK, Thomas S. Early enteral nutrition within 24 h of intestinal surgery versus later commencement of feeding: a systematic review and meta-analysis. *J Gastrointest Surg.* 2009;13(3):569. PMID: 18629592

19. Kehlet H, Wilmore DW. Multimodal strategies to improve surgical outcome. *Am J Surg.* 2002;183(6):630-641. PMID: 12095591

20. Lau CS, Chamberlain RS. Enhanced recovery after surgery programs improve patient outcomes and recovery: a meta-analysis. *World J Surg.* 2017;41(4):899-913. PMID: 27822725

## 33

The Obese Patient

Christopher M. Whinney, MD, FACP, SFHM and Sunil K. Sahai, MD, FAAP, FACP, SFHM

COMMON CLINICAL QUESTIONS

1. Are morbidly obese patients at greater risk of perioperative medical complications?
2. At what BMI should bariatric surgery be offered to patients?
3. Which cardiac diagnostic tests have the best predictive value for postoperative cardiac events?

INTRODUCTION

Obesity is a prevalent medical condition, and its incidence has tripled worldwide since 1975. By 2030, nearly 1 in 2 Americans will be considered obese and 1 in 4 will be projected to have severe obesity.[1] The Body Mass Index (BMI), a person's weight in kilograms divided by the square of height in meters, is the most commonly accepted measure of obesity. Using BMI as the sole criteria for measuring obesity is controversial, especially in light of the "obesity paradox"—the finding that overweight (BMI 25–29.9 kg/m²) and obese (BMI 30–34.9 kg/m²) patients with established cardiovascular disease have a better prognosis when compared to lean patients with the identical cardiovascular disease burden[2]; however, it remains the most widely accepted measure in use. In general, morbid obesity is defined as a BMI greater than 40 kg/m², a BMI of greater than 35 kg/m² with at least one serious obesity-related condition, or being more than 100 pounds over ideal body weight (IBW).

PREOPERATIVE RISK ASSESSMENT/ RISKS FOR SURGERY WITH OBESITY

During the preoperative evaluation of an obese patient, it must be recognized that targeted/goal-directed weight loss will be a challenge. Only those patients who are extremely motivated and have time to achieve significant weight loss will benefit from delaying surgery to lose weight. For most patients, the perioperative clinician should focus on recognizing and, if possible, optimizing comorbid medical issues. The recent FDA approval of glucagon-like peptide-1 (GLP-1) receptor agonists for weight loss is revolutionizing our ability to medically manage obesity, and their role in the perioperative space has yet to be determined.

As the patient's BMI increases, the risk of comorbid medical conditions increases. Most of these comorbid conditions and their preoperative evaluation and optimization are addressed in detail in other chapters.

Cardiac Risk Assessment

While some consensus guidelines do not consider obesity alone as an independent risk factor for postoperative complications, the ESC guidelines suggest cardiorespiratory fitness testing and evaluation for obesity hypoventilation syndrome.[3] In a recent study, obese patients who were unable to complete a six-minute-walk test had poorer outcomes.[4] Obesity is associated with other cardiac and pulmonary comorbidities that do predict complications and influence preoperative assessment and management. These include atherosclerotic cardiovascular disease, heart failure, arrhythmias, hypertension, poor exercise capacity, pulmonary hypertension, obstructive sleep apnea/hypoventilation, and history of venous thromboembolism. Please see the corresponding chapters for detailed discussions of these individual risk comorbidities.

An electrocardiogram (ECG) is commonly done preoperatively but should not be routinely requested for obesity per se without other risk factors. ECG changes that are present in higher rates in obese patients include left shifts of the P, QRS, and T axes; low QRS amplitude; flattening of the T wave; and prolonged QT and QTc intervals. However, these ECG findings typically are not independent predictors of postoperative cardiac complications and do not usually change management.

Additional diagnostic testing for coronary artery disease may be limited in obese patients. Diminished aerobic capacity and/or degenerative joint disease will limit the ability of the patient to achieve target heart rates during stress testing, and general fatigue, leg pain, or dyspnea often lead to early test termination. Coronary CT angiography has been shown to have excellent negative predictive value for major adverse cardiac events in the postoperative period.[5]

Echocardiography may be indicated for LV function assessment if heart failure is suspected based on significant dyspnea, and it is unclear whether it is due to obesity and deconditioning or cardiac disease. There is an association between obesity and pulmonary hypertension, and if pulmonary hypertension is suspected, an echocardiogram to determine right ventricular systolic pressures may assist in perioperative planning, especially if large volume shifts are expected. Patients with obesity may also have cardiomyopathy, thought to be due to increased blood volume and a high cardiac output state lasting for many years, which eventually leads to congestive heart failure (left and right) and associated conditions, including coronary atherosclerosis. An algorithm from the AHA Science Advisory for preoperative evaluation of the severely obese patient undergoing noncardiac surgery is seen in Figure 33-1.

Pulmonary Risk Assessment and Risk Reduction

Postoperative pulmonary complications (atelectasis, pneumonia, and respiratory failure) are more common than cardiac complications and have a worse long-term prognosis. Obese individuals have an increased demand for ventilation and breathing workload, respiratory muscle inefficiency, decreased functional reserve capacity and expiratory reserve volume, and closure of peripheral lung units. These often result in a ventilation-perfusion mismatch, especially when in the supine position.

Obese patients have a higher rate of obstructive sleep apnea (OSA) and obesity hypoventilation syndrome (OHS), both of which are associated with worse outcomes after surgery.[6] Patients with undiagnosed sleep apnea are potentially at greater risk for postoperative complications than those with known sleep apnea and on treatment with CPAP. Preoperative evaluation should focus on identifying OSA and OHS using clinical tools such as the STOP-BANG score and arterial blood gas assessment and chemistries. The presence of polycythemia, symptoms of habitual snoring, nocturnal gasping or choking, witnessed episodes of apnea, and daytime sleepiness should prompt further investigation.[6] (See Chapter 17.) Decisions to pursue testing to confirm the presence of OSA are especially important in procedures with prolonged anesthesia time and/or require thoracic or upper abdominal incisions that lead to splinting and impaired chest wall excursion.

Obesity is associated with increased risk of difficult intubation, difficult laryngoscopy, and a Mallampati score $\geq$ 3, and fiberoptic intubation may be necessary, but that decision should be individualized to the patient.[7] In a recent study, neck circumference more than 42 cm and BMI more than 50 were independent predictors of difficult intubation. Male sex and BMI more than 50 were independent predictors of difficult mask ventilation.

Other Obesity-Related Conditions

Metabolic Syndrome: A patient with metabolic syndrome (three of the following five criteria: elevated waist circumference, elevated triglycerides, reduced HDL-C, hypertension, and elevated fasting glucose/diabetes) should be evaluated for medical optimization of diabetes/insulin resistance, sleep apnea, cardiovascular disease, and risk of perioperative deep venous thrombosis. While these issues are addressed elsewhere in this book, it is important to note that the presence of metabolic syndrome may be an added independent risk factor for perioperative complications.

Comprehensive medical history, physical examination, and blood chemistry as clinically indicated

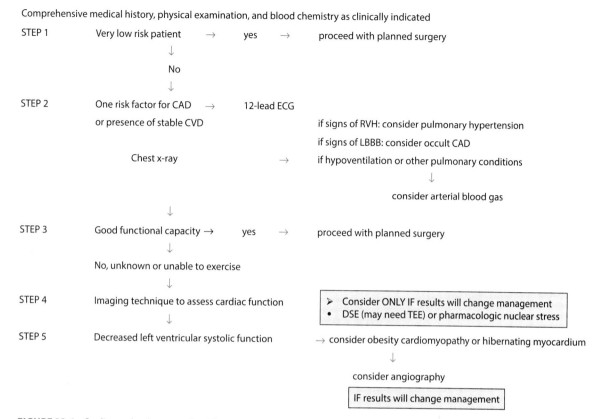

STEP 1   Very low risk patient   →   yes   →   proceed with planned surgery

        ↓

        No

        ↓

STEP 2   One risk factor for CAD   →   12-lead ECG

        or presence of stable CVD   if signs of RVH: consider pulmonary hypertension

                if signs of LBBB: consider occult CAD

        Chest x-ray   →   if hypoventilation or other pulmonary conditions

                  ↓

                  consider arterial blood gas

        ↓

STEP 3   Good functional capacity →   yes   →   proceed with planned surgery

        ↓

        No, unknown or unable to exercise

        ↓

STEP 4   Imaging technique to assess cardiac function   ➤ Consider ONLY IF results will change management

        ↓   • DSE (may need TEE) or pharmacologic nuclear stress

STEP 5   Decreased left ventricular systolic function   → consider obesity cardiomyopathy or hibernating myocardium

                  ↓

                consider angiography

                IF results will change management

FIGURE 33-1. Cardiac and pulmonary algorithm assessment for elective noncardiac surgery in severely obese patients. CAD, coronary artery disease; ECG, electrocardiogram; CVD, cardiovascular disease; RVH, right ventricular hypertrophy; and LBBB, left bundle-branch block.
Reproduced with permission from Poirier P, Alpert MA, Fleisher LA, et al. Cardiovascular Evaluation and Management of Severely Obese Patients Undergoing Surgery A Science Advisory From the American Heart Association. *Circulation.* 2009;120(1):86-95.

Liver Disease. The obese patient may have hepatic steatosis. Asymptomatic nonalcoholic fatty liver disease (NAFLD) has not been shown to increase perioperative complications, unlike cirrhosis of the liver,[8] which requires further evaluation (see Chapter 26).

RISK REDUCTION STRATEGIES

Preoperative evaluation should focus on identifying and managing obesity-related comorbid conditions when present. Assessment for end-organ dysfunction as well as optimizing blood glucose, blood pressure, and lipids with lifestyle and medications should be accomplished if time permits. If a patient with obesity is felt to be at significantly increased risk for postoperative cardiac or pulmonary complications, consider performing the procedure in a hospital-based setting with critical care or rapid response support as opposed to an ambulatory center. Postoperatively, weaning from the ventilator may be challenging, and noninvasive ventilation and continuous oximetry monitoring are appropriate in patients who have known OSA or OHS or have risk factors for the same.[6] Optimization of lung function with preoperative inspiratory muscle training has some benefits in patients with existing lung disease. Morbidly obese patients are at risk for venous thromboembolism. Consider weight-based dosing in this patient population with unfractionated heparin and/or low-molecular-weight heparin. Table 33-1 provides recommendations for preoperative, intraoperative, and postoperative management of obese patients undergoing noncardiac surgery.

Patients on GLP-1 agonists are theoretically at increased risk for the possibility of regurgitation and aspiration due to delayed gastric emptying. While a recent ASA consensus statement recommends holding the medication prior to an elective procedure,[9] more recent literature suggests this risk may be overstated, and the risks of poor perioperative glycemic control may outweigh the benefits of discontinuation (see Chapter 4).

Bariatric Surgery

Bariatric surgery is increasingly popular as a treatment choice for those with morbid obesity. In 2022, the American Society for Metabolic and Bariatric Surgery updated their guidelines to recommend bariatric surgery for any patient with a BMI greater than 35, regardless of the presence of comorbid conditions. Additionally, they provided an adjusted BMI cut-off of 27.5 for those of Asian descent.[10] In general, mortality for these procedures has been low—<0.5% for gastric banding, gastroplasty, and gastric bypass and approximately 1% for biliopancreatic diversion with duodenal switch. Patient and procedure selection for bariatric surgery are beyond the scope of this chapter. However, the Metabolic and Bariatric Surgery Accreditation and Quality Improvement Program (MBSAQIP) surgical risk/benefit calculator may help inform medical and surgical teams regarding specific perioperative risks for each procedure (https://riskcalculator.facs.org/bariatric/). The perioperative clinician may be consulted to help evaluate a patient for bariatric surgery, and in these situations, established guidelines should be followed[11] (Table 33-2).

TABLE 33-1. Perioperative Management of Obesity			
	PREOPERATIVE TO INDUCTION	**INTRAOPERATIVE**	**POSTOPERATIVE**
Cardiovascular	Evaluate for traditional risk factors Use preoperative scoring systems (RCRI, NSQIP) Assess LVH, LV/RV dysfunction w/EKG, ECHO Consider preop NTproBNP	Ensure stable vascular access (use US guidance if needed) Arterial line (cuff BP may not be reliable)	Telemetry monitoring in SDU or ICU for postop arrhythmias (Afib) Postop NTproBNP and/or troponin VTE Prophylaxis requires weight-based dosing; ensure IPCs are correct size
Pulmonary	Evaluate for OSA (STOP-BANG), OHS (ABG for pCO2), Pulm HTN Sleep study if time permits +/− PAP therapy Preop inspiratory muscle training Evaluate for difficult airway; consider fiberoptic intubation or LMA; preoxygenate +/− NIV	Aspiration risk not increased but higher rate of GERD: consider H2RA or PPI Use PEEP/lung recruitment maneuvers Attention to positioning and effect on pulmonary mechanics (Trendelenburg, Supine vs. Prone, Lateral) Consider regional/spinal when possible; may be technically more difficult; consider longer needles and/or US guidance	Reposition to sitting or reverse Trendelenburg at extubation, ensure awake, alert, and appropriate reversal; consider NIV postop; ICU or SDU admission for monitoring
Medication management	Optimize with GDMT if time permits (BB, ACE-I/ARB, statin preop) Continue BB but hold ACEI/ARB, diuretics on morning of surgery	Recognize pharmacokinetic issues: Use IBW for muscle relaxants except succinylcholine (TBW) and LBW for induction agents, opioids	Pain control with regional anesthetics, nonopioid modalities, opioids at lowest effective dose

Source: Data from Cullen A, Ferguson A, *Can J Anesth*, 2012;59:974-996.[10]

TABLE 33-2. Medical Evaluation for Bariatric Surgery

PREPROCEDURE CHECKLIST (INCLUDING LIFESTYLE MEDICINE)

✓Complete H & P (obesity-related comorbidities, causes of obesity, weight BMI, weight loss history, commitment, and exclusions related to surgical risk)

✓Routine labs (including fasting blood glucose and lipid panel, kidney function, liver profile, lipid profile, CBC)

✓Nutrient screening with iron studies, B_{12}, folic acid (RBC folate, homocysteine, methylmalonic acid optional), and 25-vitamin D (vitamins A and E optional); consider more extensive testing in patients undergoing malabsorptive procedures based on symptoms and risks

✓Cardiopulmonary evaluation with sleep apnea screening (ECG, CSR, echocardiography if cardiac disease or pulmonary hypertension suspected; deep-venous thrombosis evaluation, if clinically indicated)

✓GI evaluation (*H. pylori* screening in areas of high prevalence; gallbladder evaluation and upper endoscopy, if clinically indicated)

✓Endocrine evaluation (HbA1C with suspected or diagnosed prediabetes or diabetes; TSH with symptoms or increased risk of thyroid disease; androgens with PCOS suspicion [total/bioavailable testosterone, DHEAS, Δ_4-androstenedione]; screening for Cushing's syndrome if clinically suspected (1-mg overnight dexamethasone test, 24-hour urinary free cortisol, 11 PM salivary cortisol)

✓Lifestyle medicine evaluation: healthy eating index; cardiovascular fitness; strength training; sleep hygiene (duration and quality); mood and happiness; alcohol use; substance abuse; community engagement

✓Clinical nutrition evaluation by RD

✓Psychosocial-behavioral evaluation

✓Assess for individual psychological support/counseling

✓Document medical necessity for bariatric surgery

✓Informed consent

✓Provide relevant financial information

✓Continue efforts for preoperative weight loss

✓Optimize glycemic control

✓Pregnancy counseling

✓Smoking-cessation counseling

✓Verify cancer screening by primary care physician

H & P, history & physical; BMI, body mass index; INR, international normalized ratio; CBC, complete blood count; RBC, red blood cell; ECG, electrocardiogram; CSR, Cheyne Stokes respiration; GI, gastrointestinal; HbA1C, glycosylated hemoglobin; TSH, thyroid-stimulating hormone; PCOS, polycystic ovary syndrome; DHEAS, dehydroepiandrosterone-sulfate; RD, registered dietician.

Source: Reproduced with permission from Mechanick JI, Apovian C, Brethauer S, et al. Clinical Practice Guidelines For The Perioperative Nutrition, Metabolic, and Nonsurgical Support of Patients Undergoing Bariatric Procedures – 2019 Update: Cosponsored By American Association of Clinical Endocrinologists/American College of Endocrinology, The Obesity Society, American Society For Metabolic & Bariatric Surgery, Obesity Medicine Association, and American Society of Anesthesiologists. *Obesity* (Silver Spring). 2020;28(4):O1-O58.

Situations may arise, especially for those with BMIs over 60, that elective surgery may need to be delayed to have weight reduction surgery first. In these cases, limited studies in the spinal and orthopedic population have shown some benefits, but no clear conclusions can be reached.[12] In patients with type II diabetes, prior bariatric surgery was associated with a lower risk of major adverse cardiovascular and cerebrovascular events, mortality, acute kidney injury, and acute respiratory failure in a retrospective study using the Nationwide Inpatient Sample (NIS).[13] Thus, for patients with BMI over 60, it is reasonable to engage a frank discussion of the risks and benefits of elective surgery at a higher BMI, as opposed to bariatric surgery to optimize BMI prior to elective surgery when feasible.

Clinical pearls

- Obesity is a risk factor for multiple conditions including diabetes, hypertension, congestive heart failure, obstructive sleep apnea, and obesity hypoventilation syndrome that increase the risk of postoperative complications.
- Since weight loss surgery is challenging to achieve for nonobesity-related surgeries in the short term, the clinical focus should be on optimizing obesity-related comorbid conditions.
- A high index of suspicion should be maintained for "silent" comorbid conditions, that is, shortness of breath attributed to deconditioning versus heart failure.
- Cardiovascular testing to assess risk in the obese patient, when indicated, is best assessed with noninvasive testing such as cardiac CT scanning or echocardiography with contrast.
- Assess for obstructive sleep apnea and obesity hypoventilation syndrome in obese patients and ensure a higher level of postoperative monitoring in patients diagnosed with these conditions.
- Bariatric surgery should be considered for any patient with a BMI > 35 who has not been able to achieve targeted weight loss by other means, including medication.

REFERENCES

1. Ward ZJ, Bleich SN, Cradock AL, et al. Projected U.S. state-level prevalence of adult obesity and severe obesity. *N Engl J Med.* 2019;381:2440-2450. PMID: 31851800
2. Tutor AW, Lavie CJ, Kachur S, et al. Updates on obesity and the obesity paradox in cardiovascular diseases. *Prog Cardiovasc Dis.* 2023;78:2-10. PMID: 36481212
3. Halvorsen S, Mehilli J, Cassese S, et al. 2022 ESC guidelines on cardiovascular assessment and management of patients undergoing non-cardiac surgery. *Eur Heart J.* 2022;43:3826-3924. PMID: 36017553
4. Smith NA, Batterham M, Shulman MA. Predicting recovery and disability after surgery in patients with severe obesity: the role of the six-minute walk test. *Anaesth Intensive Care.* 2022;50:159-168. PMID: 35171060
5. Messerli M, Maywald C, Walti S, et al. Prognostic value of negative coronary CT angiography in severely obese patients prior to bariatric surgery: a follow-up after 6 years. *Obes Surg.* 2017;27:2044-2049. PMID: 28243857
6. Raveendran R, Wong J, Singh M, et al. Obesity hypoventilation syndrome, sleep apnea, overlap syndrome: perioperative management to prevent complications. *Curr Opin Anaesthesiol.* 2017;30:146-155. PMID: 27792079
7. Wang T, Sun S, Huang S. The association of body mass index with difficult tracheal intubation management by direct laryngoscopy: a meta-analysis. *BMC Anesthesiol.* 2018;18:79. PMID: 29960594
8. Mavilia MG, Wakefield D, Karagozian R. Nonalcoholic fatty liver disease does not predict worse perioperative outcomes in bariatric surgery. *Obes Res Clin Pract.* 2019;13:416-418. PMID: 31307925
9. Ushakumari DS, Sladen RN. ASA consensus-based guidance on preoperative management of patients on glucagon-like peptide-1 receptor agonists. *Anesthesiology.* 2024;140:346-348. PMID: 37982170
10. Eisenberg D, Shikora SA, Aarts E, et al. 2022 American Society of Metabolic and Bariatric Surgery (ASMBS) and International Federation for the Surgery of Obesity and Metabolic Disorders (IFSO) indications for metabolic and bariatric surgery. *Obes Surg.* 2023;33:3-14. PMID: 36336720
11. Mechanick JI, Apovian C, Brethauer S, et al. Clinical practice guidelines for the perioperative nutrition, metabolic, and nonsurgical support of patients undergoing bariatric procedures—2019 update: Cosponsored by American Association of Clinical Endocrinologists/American College of Endocrinology, The Obesity Society, American Society for Metabolic and Bariatric

Surgery, Obesity Medicine Association, and American Society of Anesthesiologists. *Obesity (Silver Spring).* 2020;28:O1-O58. PMID: 32202076

12. McLawhorn AS, Levack AE, Lee YY, et al. Bariatric surgery improves outcomes after lower extremity arthroplasty in the morbidly obese: a propensity score-matched analysis of a New York statewide database. *J Arthroplasty.* 2018;33:2062-2069 e2064. PMID: 29366728

13. Jin J, Deng Z, Xu L, et al. Prior bariatric surgery and perioperative cardiovascular outcomes following noncardiac surgery in patients with type 2 diabetes mellitus: hint from National Inpatient Sample Database. *Cardiovasc Diabetol.* 2020;19:103. PMID: 32631310

## 34

The Cancer Patient

Sunil K. Sahai, MD, FAAP, FACP, SFHM

COMMON CLINICAL QUESTIONS

1. What specific considerations need to be accounted for in the perioperative risk assessment of the cancer patient?

2. How is the assessment of functional status of the cancer patient different from that of the noncancer patient?

3. Are there any special considerations for postoperative VTE prophylaxis in the cancer patient undergoing major surgery?

INTRODUCTION

By the year 2030, it is estimated that over 17 million cancer patients will need a surgical procedure for diagnosis, treatment, or palliation.[1] With the rise in incidence of cancer, the number of therapeutic options has also increased over the years, with more patients undergoing multimodality treatment involving chemotherapy, radiotherapy, and surgery. In more recent years, the advent of immunotherapy has the promise of revolutionizing cancer treatment. The perioperative clinician needs to be aware of the unique issues that are involved in the perioperative evaluation and management of the cancer patient facing surgery.

PREOPERATIVE EVALUATION

For some cancer patients who have early tumors detected before the onset of symptoms, the preoperative evaluation and medical optimization is straightforward, following established criteria and guidelines. For the majority of cancer patients, delaying surgery to optimize medical and functional status is not a viable option due to tumor growth and disease progression. For cancer patients facing surgical treatment, a variety of comorbid conditions can affect the ability to provide a clear risk assessment. These conditions conspire to further decondition the patient, potentially increasing risk and complications.[2] Therefore, it is important for the perioperative clinician to have a comprehensive understanding of the cancer, cancer treatment, and their effects on the patient. In addition to the cancer, the patient's history and the planned procedure should be considered when evaluating a patient for surgery.

The patient's history of cancer, including presentation and treatments to date, will inform the perioperative risk assessment. A patient in good health with an incidental finding of a tumor on unrelated imaging will need a straightforward evaluation per current guidelines. However, the patient with a complicated cancer history with multiple prior treatments or history of other prior cancers requires closer evaluation.

The patient with cancer suffers from the metabolic and physiologic derangements from the disease itself. Fatigue, cachexia, malnutrition, pain, and other symptoms lead to deconditioning and frailty. It is important to assess how much a patient diagnosed with cancer has deviated from their usual state of health prior to diagnosis and treatment.

No cancer treatment is benign; the patient may experience complications from the treatment itself, such as surgery complications or organ dysfunction caused by chemotherapy and radiation therapy. Some side effects are seen immediately but others may take years to manifest.

Patient History

Unlike elective procedures, cancer surgery usually is urgent and delaying a surgery to optimize a medical condition like diabetes or hypertension may risk tumor and disease progression. Close communication with the surgical and anesthetic team is needed in such instances. Having an accurate medication list and medical problem list documented in the preoperative evaluation provides a single source of truth for all medical teams down the line.

Treatment History

Prior treatment with chemotherapy, radiotherapy, or surgery can lead to deconditioning of the cancer patient, which will adversely affect their ability to exercise and provide an accurate assessment of functional status.

Immunotherapy and Checkpoint Inhibitors. At the time of this writing, newer treatment modalities such as checkpoint inhibitors and other forms of immunotherapy are promising therapeutic options in the treatment of cancer. These agents may cause a myriad of complications that may persist into the perioperative period (Table 34-1). The timing of immune-related adverse events (IRAEs) can be highly variable from the date of treatment. In general, IRAEs onset from initial treatment are:

- Dermatologic: first few weeks
- Diarrhea and colitis: weeks 5–10
- Hepatitis: weeks 7–14
- Hypophysitis: week 6+
- Pneumonitis: week 12+
- Up to 24 weeks out, unpredictable

If an immune-related adverse event is suspected in the perioperative period, then we recommend urgent consultation with the treating oncologist as surgery may be delayed.

TABLE 34-1. Immune-Related Adverse Events (IRAEs)

SYSTEM	MEDICAL CONDITION
Eye	Uveitis, scleritis, retinitis, conjunctivitis
Pituitary	Hypophysitis
Thyroid	Thyroiditis
CNS	Guillain Barre syndrome, myasthenia gravis, meningitis, neuropathy
Lung	Pneumonitis, pleuritis, sarcoid-like granulomatosis
Heart	Myocarditis, pericarditis, vasculitis
Liver	Hepatitis
Pancreas	Type 1 diabetes, pancreatitis
Adrenal	Adrenal insufficiency
Gastrointestinal	Gastritis, colitis, ileitis
Kidney	Nephritis
Muscle	Myositis, dermatomyositis, myopathies
Rheumatologic	Vasculitis, arthritis
Skin	Vitiligo, alopecia, psoriasis, DRESS syndrome, rash, pruritus, Stevens-Johnson syndrome
Blood	Thrombocytopenia, hemolytic anemia, neutropenia, pancytopenia

Source: Data from Varricchi G, Galdiero MR, Marone G, et al. Cardiotoxicity of immune checkpoint inhibitors. *ESMO Open.* 2017;2(4): e000247-e000247; and Ventola, CL. Cancer immunotherapy, Part 2: efficacy, safety, and other clinical considerations. *P T.* 2017;42(7):452-463.

Cardiotoxicity. The perioperative clinician should be attuned to the development or exacerbation of cardiomyopathy, valvular disease, ischemia, and arrythmias after treatment for cancer. The prevalence of cardiotoxic side effects tends to be consistent within classes of chemotherapy. In other words, if cardiomyopathy is seen in those patients

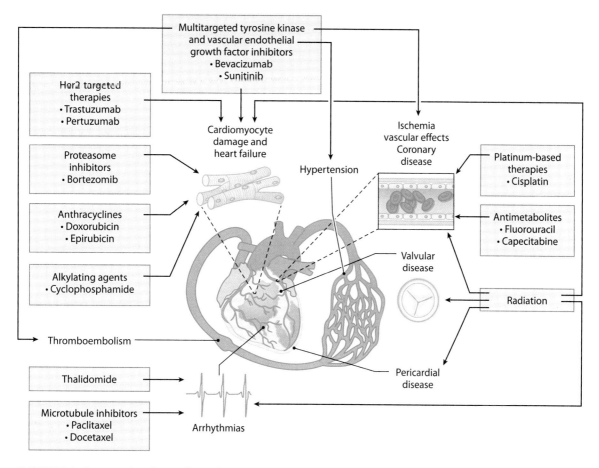

FIGURE 34-1. Summary the adverse effects of radiation therapy and chemotherapy on the cardiovascular system. Reproduced with permission from Babiker HM, McBride A, Newton M, et al. Cardiotoxic effects of chemotherapy: a review of both cytotoxic and molecular targeted oncology therapies and their effect on the cardiovascular system. *Crit Rev Oncol Hematol.* 2018; 126:186-200.

receiving imatibib, a tyrosine kinase inhibitor (TKI), then all TKIs will tend to have cardiomyopathy as a side effect. See Figure 34-1, which summarizes the adverse effects of radiation therapy and chemotherapy on the cardiovascular system.[3]

Pulmonary Toxicity. Radiation therapy to the chest and thorax can lead to the development of radiation pneumonitis, and subsequently pulmonary fibrosis, which may compromise lung function and predispose to postoperative pulmonary complications. See Table 34-2, which summarizes common pulmonary side effects of chemotherapy.

Frailty and Nutrition. As cancer is predominantly a disease of older people, issues of frailty need to take center stage, with assessments of cognition, mental health, nutrition, and physical performance in the perioperative period (see Chapter 31).

Cancer patients suffer from malnutrition to a disproportionate degree. The routine assessment of nutritional status prior to surgery is recommended as an albumin less than 3.5 g/dL is an independent risk factor for postoperative complications.[4]

PLANNED SURGERY

Preoperative Evaluation

The preoperative evaluation may uncover conditions that require altering the surgical or anesthetic plans that have been made. For example, a history of

TABLE 34-2. Common Pulmonary Side Effects of Chemotherapeutic Agents

ANTHRACYCLINES	TAXANES	MONOCLONAL ANTIBODIES	TYROSINE KINASE INHIBITORS	ALKALOIDS	ANTIMETABOLITES	ALYLATING AGENTS
Bronchospasm/hypersensitivity reactions						
Doxorubicin	Paclitaxel	Rituximab		Vinblastine	Fludarabine	Cyclophosphamide
	Docetaxel	Panitumumab		Vincristine		Busulfan
		Cetuximan		Vinorelbine		Procarbazine
Interstitial lung disease (Pneumonitis/Fibrosis)						
Epirubicen		Bevacizumab	Sorafenib		Capecitabine	Ifosfamide
		Trastuzumab	Sunitinib		Gemcitabine	Oxaliplatin
		Ofatumumab			5-Fluorouracil	
Pleural effusions						
Epirubicen	Paclitaxel		Dasatinib		5-Fluorouracil	Ifosfamide
	Docetaxel		Imatinib			

Source: Reproduced with permission from Sahai SK. Perioperative assessment of the cancer patient. *Best Pract Res Clin Anaesthesiol.* 2013;27(4):465-480.

significant medical comorbid conditions may put the patient at high risk for perioperative complications, causing the surgical team to alter the plan of care from a curative resection to a palliative one. Conversely, the preoperative evaluation may also reveal conditions that require closer monitoring after surgery in the intensive care unit as opposed to the regular ward. The patient will still proceed to the operating room; however, they may need alterations from normal care pathways to prevent complications.

For other medical comorbid conditions, routine assessment and optimization as outlined in the other chapters in this book should be followed. A thorough medical history and review of systems is warranted prior to surgery. For each medical condition present or uncovered, it is prudent to ask:

- Is this medical condition relevant to the planned procedure?

- If yes, is the medical condition optimized for the planned procedure?

- If not optimized, what can be done in the preoperative period to improve the condition?

Preoperative evaluation of the cancer patient, like that of most surgical patients, tends to focus on cardiovascular assessment. Many times, deconditioning and fatigue from cancer and treatments are confused with cardiac decompensation. Treatments that cause cardiotoxicity may unmask previously unknown cardiac issues. In Figure 34-2, we present a schema for approaching the patient with cancer who may have cardiac disease.

Pulmonary function testing is rarely helpful in the cancer patient unless they meet the criteria for PFT testing independently of the cancer diagnosis. Routine preoperative blood testing or chest imaging is also not indicated. For the patient with cancer who has undergone neoadjuvant treatment, there will be a plethora of laboratory and imaging results to review prior to surgery. Repeating them is unnecessary unless a clinical suspicion exists for a condition. For example, the patient that experiences prolonged nausea and vomiting after the last round of chemotherapy may benefit from checking electrolytes prior to surgery to avoid undiagnosed hyponatremia. Additionally, for those patients with anemia due to chemotherapy or cancer, repeating a CBC prior to surgery may reveal anemia or neutropenia that needs evaluation. Neoplastic-related

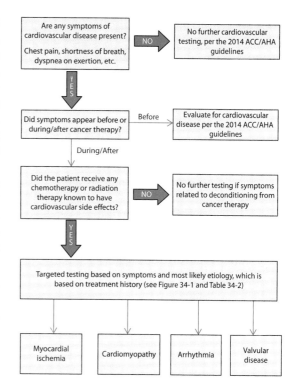

FIGURE 34-2. Schema for the perioperative cardiac evaluation of a cancer patient. Reproduced with permission from Sahai SK. Perioperative assessment of the cancer patient. *Best Pract Res Clin Anaesthesiol.* 2013;27(4):465-480.

anemia is closely followed by oncology teams, and as such, the patient may have already been treated with a blood transfusion prior to surgery.

On the other hand, it is important to remember that not all medical issues can be blamed on cancer and its treatment. A patient may have undiagnosed iron deficiency anemia that is exacerbated by chemotherapy, and as such the treatment is iron supplementation, not transfusion.

RISK REDUCTION

Recommendations for optimization of medical comorbid conditions that are presented elsewhere in this publication stand unchanged for patients with cancer. Deconditioning and other treatment side effects may preclude maximal medical optimization of the patient prior to surgery. However, we feel that even modest attempts at medical optimization in the perioperative period are beneficial. There is growing evidence that prehabilitation prior to surgery is beneficial and may improve outcomes.[5] With patients frequently undergoing preoperative chemotherapy or radiation therapy, the preoperative period is the ideal time to emphasize exercise and optimization of medical issues.

POSTOPERATIVE MANAGEMENT

Cancer patients in the postoperative period are at increased risk for venous thromboembolism. The American Society of Clinical Oncology guidelines recommend extended DVT prophylaxis with LMWH for up to 4 weeks postoperatively for patients undergoing major open or laparoscopic abdominal or pelvic surgery for cancer who have high-risk features, such as restricted mobility, obesity, history of VTE, or with additional risk factors.[6]

CONCLUSION

Surgery is no longer the only treatment modality for patients and is usually part of a continuum of care that involves neoadjuvant and adjuvant treatment. As such, patients experiencing postoperative complications and longer lengths of stay and recovery will experience delays in starting therapy after discharge. This delay in resumption of adjuvant therapy may allow for tumor growth and worse outcomes. Thus, the concept of Return to Intended Oncologic Treatment (RIOT) is gaining favor as a metric in cancer care.[7] For the perioperative clinician, the opportunity to anticipate and possibly mitigate postoperative complications, in order for the patient to resume intended postoperative therapy, should not be squandered.

Clinical pearls

- Cancer fatigue can masquerade as cardiovascular compromise and vice versa.
- Immune-related adverse events are highly varied and there should be a high index of suspicion for these conditions.

- Prior history of cancer and treatment may inform surgical decision making.
- Frailty and cancer are bedfellows, and the neoadjunctive period can be used to optimize medical issues and improve functional status.
- Cancer surgery is time-sensitive which may interfere with ideal medical optimization.

REFERENCES

1. Sullivan R, Alatise OI, Anderson BO, et al. Global cancer surgery: delivering safe, affordable, and timely cancer surgery. *Lancet Oncol.* 2015;16:1193-1224. PMID: 26427363
2. Sahai SK, Ismail H. Perioperative implications of neoadjuvant therapies and optimization strategies for cancer surgery. *Current Anesthesiology Reports.* 2015;5:305-317.
3. Babiker HM, McBride A, Newton M, et al. Cardiotoxic effects of chemotherapy: a review of both cytotoxic and molecular targeted oncology therapies and their effect on the cardiovascular system. *Crit Rev Oncol Hematol.* 2018;126:186-200. PMID: 29759560
4. Hu WH, Cajas-Monson LC, Eisenstein S, et al. Preoperative malnutrition assessments as predictors of postoperative mortality and morbidity in colorectal cancer: an analysis of ACS-NSQIP. *Nutr J.* 2015;14:91. PMID: 26345703
5. Fry BT, Hallway A, Englesbe MJ. Moving toward every patient training for surgery. *JAMA Surg.* 2018;153:1089. PMID: 30193332
6. Key NS, Khorana AA, Kuderer NM, et al. Venous thromboembolism prophylaxis and treatment in patients with cancer: ASCO guideline update. *J Clin Oncol.* 2023;41:3063-3071. PMID: 37075273
7. Kim BJ, Caudle AS, Gottumukkala V, Aloia TA. The impact of postoperative complications on a timely return to intended oncologic therapy (RIOT): the role of enhanced recovery in the cancer journey. *Int Anesthesiol Clin.* 2016;54:e33-e46. PMID: 27623128

COMMON POSTOPERATIVE PROBLEMS

## 35

Fever

J. Njeri Wainaina, MD, FACP, FHM, FIDSA

COMMON CLINICAL QUESTIONS

1. What causes fever after surgery?
2. How should postoperative fever be evaluated?

INTRODUCTION

Fever, defined as a temperature greater than 38°C (100.4°F), is common after surgical and nonsurgical procedures, with reported incidence in the literature ranging from 15% to 47%. A structured approach is necessary to separate physiological from pathological causes and to identify the need and urgency of further evaluation or intervention. This section reviews causes of fever after surgery and summarizes the approach to diagnosis and management.

THE SURGICAL INFLAMMATORY RESPONSE

Tissue damage triggers an inflammatory response that is primarily designed to promote healing, restore homeostasis, and eradicate microorganisms. This response is similar whether caused by hypoxia, ischemia, accidental trauma, or surgery and usually occurs early in the postoperative course.[1] The "danger theory" posits that injury to cells and tissues leads to the release of structurally diverse endogenous proteins, referred to collectively as alarmins, that activate effector cells such as macrophages, lymphocytes, endothelial cells, and stromal cells.[2] Activated cells expand the inflammatory process through systemic release of pyrogenic cytokines of which TNF-α, IL-1β, IL-6, IL-8, IL-12, and IFN-γ are the most well characterized.[3] TNF-α, IL-1, and IL-6 trigger increased production of prostaglandin E2 by the hypothalamus leading to elevation of the thermostatic set point. Systemic levels of IL-6 have been shown to correlate with temperature elevation in the postoperative period.[4] The duration and invasiveness of surgery thus are directly associated with the likelihood, magnitude, and duration of postoperative fever. This febrile response is benign and self-limiting.

CAUSES OF POSTOPERATIVE FEVER

The timing of fever after surgery is the most important predictive variable of the cause and is typically divided into immediate, early, late, or delayed. Consider a broad differential and do not assume all fever is due to infection. Table 35-1 lists frequently encountered etiologies classified according to timeline of usual manifestation. The rule of W's, an anecdotal mnemonic that has been validated and extended over time[5]— Wind (pneumonia, aspiration), Water (urinary tract infection), Wound (surgical site infection), Walking (venous thromboembolism), Wonder drugs (drug fever, withdrawal), Waves (myocardial ischemia), What did we do (iatrogenic causes), and others— serves as a starting point to investigating postoperative fever. Table 35-2 outlines common etiologies associated with specific types of surgery.

TABLE 35-1. Causes of Postoperative Fever

IMMEDIATE	EARLY	LATE	DELAYED
Within hours of surgery	*Postoperative day 0–3*	*Postoperative day 4–30*	*After day 30*
Malignant hyperthermia	Surgical inflammatory response	Nosocomial pneumonia	Deep surgical site infection
Drug reaction	Transfusion reaction	CLABSI	Device or implant-related infection
Transfusion reaction	Drug reaction	UTI	
Preexisting infection	Myocardial infarction	Surgical site infection	
	Venous thromboembolism	Anastomotic leak	
	Acute adrenal insufficiency	Acalculous cholecystitis	
	Thyroid storm	Venous thromboembolism	
	Drug or alcohol withdrawal	Sinusitis	
	Preexisting infection	*C. difficile* colitis	
	Acute pancreatitis	Acute gout	
	Hematoma	Drug reaction	
	Pneumonia (aspiration or nosocomial)	Hematoma	

TABLE 35-2. Common Non-SSI Etiologies of Postoperative Fever by Surgical Site

TYPE OF PROCEDURE	ASSOCIATED ETIOLOGIES
Vascular	Arterial embolization
Cardiothoracic	Pneumonia, central line–associated bloodstream infection, pericarditis (Dressler's syndrome)
Abdominal	Hematoma, pancreatitis, cholecystitis, anastomotic leak
Urologic	Catheter-associated UTI
Orthopedic	Hematoma, fat embolism, VTE
Neurosurgical	Chemical meningitis/ventriculitis, hypothalamic dysregulation, VTE

Misconceptions: Atelectasis and Fever

Both fever and atelectasis occur frequently after surgery and timing tends to overlap. Resolution of early postoperative fever was attributed to the treatment of atelectasis, leading to the historically entrenched association. However, atelectasis is not associated with fever outside the postoperative setting. Studies in laboratory models and in various postoperative populations have failed to show a causative association.[6–8] Conversely, incentive spirometry has not been shown to reduce the incidence of postoperative fever.[9]

Early postoperative fever is most commonly due to the surgical inflammatory response but there are other less common causes. While atelectasis during the postoperative period should be addressed, the danger of presuming this to be the cause of fever is a premature closure and a lack of vigilance for the less common causes.

EVALUATING THE PATIENT WITH FEVER AFTER SURGERY

While fever in the immediate and early postoperative phase is often benign and self-limiting, it is critical to identify serious etiologies that require immediate action or further workup. A systematic approach that includes a thorough review of history and physical examination with directed testing provides the most effective approach.

History

A detailed review of events prior to surgery should be undertaken to evaluate comorbidities, such as poorly controlled diabetes, that increase the risk of infection, and to identify exposures that may predispose to infection and potential infections that may have been incubating prior to surgery. Attention should be paid to comorbidities that can present with a fever when decompensated or exacerbated. Medications prescribed prior to surgery should be reviewed for omissions that could lead to fever, such as cessation of or missed stress-dosing of glucocorticoids leading to acute adrenal insufficiency. Fever onset relative to blood products and new medications administered during or after surgery should be reviewed for potential causative correlation. Details of the anesthetic and surgical course of the procedure may provide additional clues. A history of substance abuse, particularly alcohol, should raise suspicion for acute withdrawal.

Patients and family members should be interviewed for new symptoms that could point to an infectious or noninfectious cause of fever. Nursing staff can provide important additional information such as the presence of cough, sputum, diarrhea, and skin changes.

Physical Examination

A detailed physical examination that explores reported symptoms and other findings gleaned from the history should be undertaken. Close attention should be paid to the heart, lungs, surgical wound, and catheter sites. The skin should be evaluated for new rash and limbs for new swelling and joint inflammation.

Testing

The purpose of laboratory testing and imaging should be to rule in or rule out a suspected cause of fever and thus selection should be informed by history and physical examination findings. Fever related to infection in the immediate postoperative period is rare unless the patient has been operated on to treat a febrile illness (exceptions are necrotizing SSI from Streptococcus pyogenes or Clostridium species). The patient who is hemodynamically stable with no symptoms other than appropriate postoperative pain and a fever does not warrant "routine" testing.

SUMMARY

Fever after surgical and nonsurgical procedures is common and is due to a wide variety of infectious and noninfectious etiologies, the likelihood of which varies with the timing of onset. Clinicians who provide postoperative care need to be able to identify high-risk causes that require urgent intervention. A focused approach that starts with bedside evaluation and physical examination that directs testing is the most effective. Reflexive laboratory testing and imaging is wasteful as it is time-consuming, expensive, and yields little.

Clinical pearls

- Do not assume all fever is due to infection. Fever in the first 24–48 hours after surgery can be due to medications, the inflammatory response to tissue damage during the procedure, and other intraoperative events.
- Atelectasis does not cause fever.
- The timing of fever onset after surgery can aid with generating a differential diagnosis to guide evaluation. Remember the "W's"—Wind, Water, Wound, Walking, Wonder drugs, Waves, What did we do?
- Postoperative fever should be evaluated using a systematic approach that takes the timing of onset and new signs or symptoms into account. Empiric chest x-ray, urinalysis and culture, and blood cultures are not routinely indicated for all febrile postoperative patients.

REFERENCES

1. Cruickshank AM, Fraser WD, Burns HJG, et al. Response of serum interleukin-6 in patients undergoing elective surgery of varying severity. *Clin Sci (Lond)*. 1990;79(2):161-165. PMID: 2167805

2. Pugin J. How tissue injury alarms the immune system and causes a systemic inflammatory response syndrome. *Ann Intensive Care.* 2012;2:27. PMID: 22788849

3. Hsing CH, Wang JJ. Clinical implications of perioperative inflammatory cytokine alteration. *Acta Anaesthesiol Taiwan.* 2015;53(1):23-28. PMID: 25837846

4. Frank SM, Kluger MJ, Kunkel SL. Elevated thermostatic setpoint in postoperative patients. *Anesthesiology.* 2000;93(6):1426. PMID: 11149437

5. Hyder JA, Wakeam E, Arora V, et al. Investigating the "Rule of W," a mnemonic for teaching on postoperative complications. *J Surg Educ.* 2015;72(3):430-437. PMID: 25523129

6. Lansing AM, Jamieson WG. Mechanisms of fever in pulmonary atelectasis. *Arch Surg.* 1963;87:184-190. PMID: 13928705

7. Engoren M. Lack of association between atelectasis and fever. *Chest.* 1995;107(1):81-84. PMID: 7813318

8. Mavros MN, Velmahos GC, Falagas ME. Atelectasis as a cause of postoperative fever: where is the clinical evidence? *Chest.* 2011;140(2):418-424. PMID: 21527508

9. Do Nascimento Junior P, Módolo NS, Andrade S, et al. Incentive spirometry for prevention of postoperative pulmonary complications in upper abdominal surgery. *Cochrane Database Syst Rev.* 2014;(2):CD006058. PMID: 24510642

## 36

Hypotension and Hypertension

Alexander I.R. Jackson, BMedSci(Hons,) MBChB, MSc and Michael P.W. Grocott, BSc, MSc, MBBS, MD, FRCA, FRCP, FFICM, GChPOM

COMMON CLINICAL QUESTIONS

1. What values for blood pressure should I be worried about?
2. How do I approach the assessment of a patient with high or low blood pressure after surgery?
3. How can I establish if a patient with low blood pressure needs fluid or vasopressors?

INTRODUCTION

Perioperative haemodynamic instability, encompassing both hypo- and hypertension, is common. The recent Advanced Recovery Room Care (ARRC) Study found that systolic blood pressure was the most common trigger for a postoperative medical emergency response (MER) in a medium-risk surgical population.[1] The study also demonstrated that high acuity care with access to a multidisciplinary team able to detect and respond to these events could improve patient outcomes. It is therefore vital to be comfortable in the assessment and management of these common issues that can adversely affect our patients.

HYPERTENSION

Postoperative hypertension is independently associated with adverse outcomes including myocardial infarction, stroke, and bleeding.[2] Unfortunately there is no consensus on level of postoperative hypertension

likely to cause harm,[2] with thresholds of >190 mmHg systolic/>100 mmHg diastolic and >180 mmHg systolic/>110 mmHg diastolic proposed. The most widely accepted definition favors an approach based on the risk of harm: "a significant elevation in blood pressure during the immediate postoperative period that may lead to serious neurologic, cardiovascular, or surgical-site complications and that requires urgent management."[3] This suggests the clinician should evaluate the patient's individual circumstance and define the risk of harm. This will be influenced by several factors including severity, onset, and duration of hypertension. For example, many episodes of hypertension occurring in the immediate postoperative phase are short lived. Such episodes are likely to be less concerning than those which persist for prolonged periods without treatment.[2] Likewise, the risk profile will vary greatly between surgeries, both in terms of expected incidence and potential harm from hypertension.

When assessing the postoperative patient with hypertension it is vital to consider the underlying etiology (see Table 36-1). Many causes represent normal physiological responses to other stimuli. Therefore, before delving into advanced blood pressure management, the treating clinician must prioritize a thorough assessment to identify and treat issues of ventilation, homeostasis, and pain or discomfort.

Although detailed intraoperative management is the responsibility of the anesthetist, and beyond the scope of this chapter, it is important to consider how

TABLE 36-1. Etiologies of Intraoperative/Postoperative Hypertension

INTRAOP	EARLY POSTOP (FIRST 4 HOURS)	DELAYED POSTOP
Laryngoscopy/intubation	Emergence from anesthesia	Fluid shifts
"Too light" anesthesia (pain)	Reaction to endotracheal tube	Failure to restart usual BP meds
Surgical incision/manipulation	Pain/inadequate analgesia	Decreasing effects or dose of analgesics/sedatives (pain/anxiety)
Fluid overload (iatrogenic)	Urinary bladder distension	
Ventilatory inadequacy (hypoxemia/hypercarbia)	Ventilatory insufficiency (hypercarbia/hypoxia)	
Use of pressors	Hypothermia with shivering	
Extubation/arousal	Postop nausea/vomiting	
Antihypertensive medication withdrawal/drug withdrawal	Antihypertensive medication withdrawal/drug withdrawal	
	Delirium	

intraoperative events can impact the postoperative patient. A cohort study of >18,000 patients demonstrated that patients with intraoperative hypertension, excessive pain, and inadequate ventilation were more likely to have postoperative hypertension, critical care admissions, and a higher mortality.[4] Therefore, nonanesthetists should still familiarize themselves with the intraoperative course when trying to elucidate the cause of postoperative hypertension. Table 36-1 highlights both intraoperative and postoperative causes, with a degree of overlap seen.

Management should follow the principles outlined above and in Figure 36-1. If reversible causes are found, they should be a priority, for example, adequate analgesia in the case of acute pain or a forced air warmer in cases of hypothermia. Where no reversible causes are identified, antihypertensive agents may be considered. In patients who routinely take an antihypertensive drug that has been omitted in the perioperative setting, reintroduction is likely to be the most appropriate option. There is evidence of harm from withholding β-blockers and ACEIs/ARBs in the postoperative period, and restarting them within 48 hours of surgery is recommended, although caution should be exercised in selecting dose and in those with renal injury.[2] In patients not taking regular preoperative antihypertensives, an oral agent should be used where feasible. If a reduction in blood pressure is needed more urgently, or the oral route is not possible, then IV agents, such as those listed in Table 36-2, can be considered.

HYPOTENSION

Hypotension has been more tightly defined with clear evidence of postoperative harm, ranging from renal and cardiac injury to increased mortality. A systolic blood pressure <90 mmHg[5] and a mean arterial pressure <65 mmHg are found to be associated with similar adverse outcomes.[2,6] Each of these outcomes appears to exhibit a dose-response relationship with greater harms associated with prolonged and more profound episodes of hypotension. It should be noted that in patients with preexisting hypertension, harm may occur even at blood pressures above these thresholds.[2] If in doubt, clinical evidence of adequate end-organ perfusion should be sought.

Just as in hypertension, the underlying etiology is vital in defining the appropriate treatment. Table 36-3 provides common examples. Once again, all clinicians should familiarize themselves with the intraoperative course as blood loss, fluid therapy, or neuraxial

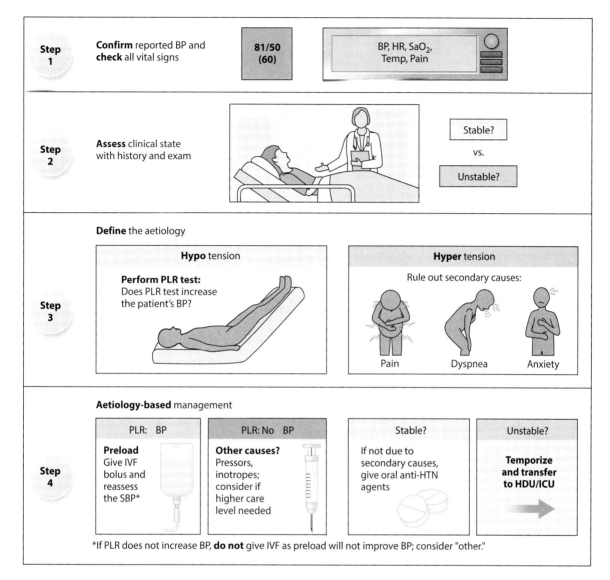

FIGURE 36-1. A rational approach to postoperative BP assessment.
Reproduced with permission from McEvoy MD, Gupta R, Koepke EJ, et al. Perioperative quality initiative consensus statement on postoperative blood pressure, risk and outcomes for elective surgery. *Br J Anaesth.* 2019;122(5):575-586.

blockade during surgery can all have profound effects on cardiovascular status in the postoperative period.

A number of tools for evaluating the cause of hemodynamic instability exist (see Figure 36-1). These include simple bedside examination, examining perfusion, and volume status. This may be supplemented by specific tests such as the passive leg raise (PLR), which strongly predicts fluid responsiveness.

Continuous advanced hemodynamic monitoring, which can be performed using noninvasive technologies, may also help to define the nature of hypotension and guide therapy.[7] Finally, the use of point of care ultrasound, including echocardiography, is becoming more widespread and can be used to diagnose the probable cause of hypotension.[1]

TABLE 36-2. Commonly Used IV Antihypertensive Agents for Treatment of Acute Postoperative Hypertension (APH)

AGENT	DOSE	ONSET/DURATION	SIDE EFFECTS/USE WITH CAUTION	NOTES
Labetalol	**Initial bolus:** 20 mg May repeat 20–80 mg every 10 mins **Max dose:** 300 mg **Continuous infusion:** 1–2 mg/min	**Onset:** 2–5 mins **Duration:** 6 hours	**Side effects:** Hypotension, dizziness, N/V, paresthesias, scalp tingling, bronchospasm **Use with caution:** HF, bradycardia, heart block, bronchospasm	• Alpha:beta blocking activity is 1:7. • Reduces SVR at mildly reduced heart rate. • Studied in multiple surgery types and found to be safe and effective.[2]
Esmolol	**Initial bolus:** 500 ug/kg **Continuous infusion:** 50 ug/kg **Increase infusion:** Q10–20 mins **Max dose:** 300 ug/kg/min	**Onset:** <1 min **Duration:** 10–20 mins	**Side effects:** 1° heart block, pain at infusion site, nausea, flushing **Use with caution:** COPD/asthma, bradycardia, heart block, HF, anemia	• Very short-acting agent with abrupt onset and duration. • Attractive for situations whereby both pulse and blood pressure are elevated. • Not dependent on renal or hepatic metabolism.[2]
Nitroglycerin	**Infusion:** 5 ug/min, increase by 5 ug/min every 5 mins **Max dose:** 60 ug/min	**Onset:** 2–5 mins **Duration:** 3–5 mins	**Side effects:** Headaches, dizziness, hypotension, reflex tachycardia, tachyphylaxis **Use with caution:** Volume depletion	• Potent venodilator in volume-depleted patients, may cause severe hypotension and reflex tachycardia since it reduces preload and cardiac output. • Can worsen adrenergic response of APH. • If coronary insufficiency and APH are present, nitroglycerin is a potent coronary vasodilator; may be useful in combination with other agents.[6]
Nitroprusside	**Infusion:** 0.5 ug/kg/min **Max dose:** 2 ug/kg/min	**Onset:** Immediate **Duration:** 1–2 mins	**Side effects:** Thiocyanate and cyanide toxicity, headache, N/V, muscle spasms, flushing **Use with caution:** Myocardial ischemia, liver/renal disease, cerebrovascular disease, increased ICP	• Potent arterial and venous vasodilator. • Avoid in setting of acute MI given coronary steal and increased mortality. • Not a first-line agent.[2,6]

(Continued)

TABLE 36-2. Commonly Used IV Antihypertensive Agents for Treatment of Acute Postoperative Hypertension (APH)

AGENT	DOSE	ONSET/DURATION	SIDE EFFECTS/USE WITH CAUTION	NOTES
Enalaprilat	**Bolus:** 1.25 mg over 5 mins Q6 hrs **Titrate:** by 1.25 mg **Max dose:** 5 mg Q6 hrs	**Onset:** 15 mins **Duration:** 12–24 hrs	**Side effects:** Variable response, headache, dizziness, hypotension with anesthetics **Use with caution:** Renal dysfunction, hyperkalemia, hypovolemia	• Not recommended for hypertensive emergencies due to prolonged half-life. • Recommended to use in combination with short-acting agents that can be titrated in the setting of the long-acting enalaprilat. • Can cause AKI by reducing MAP that results in insufficient renal perfusion. • Attractive to use in neurosurgical procedures because it does not affect intracranial pressure.[6]
Hydralazine	**Bolus:** 10–20 mg Q6 hrs	**Onset:** 5–15 mins **Duration:** up to 12 hrs	**Side effects:** Reflex tachycardia, headache, flushing, vomiting **Use with caution:** Increased ICP, aortic dissection, myocardial ischemia	• Rapid acting arterial vasodilator lasting up to 12 hrs, so r ot ideal for titration. • Drops diastolic blood pressure, resulting in reflex tachycardia, increased cardiac output, and sympathetic activity. • Avoid in myocardial ischemia, aortic dissection, or increased ICP. • May reduce blood pressure in a manner that is difficult to correct.[6]
Fenoldopam	**Infusion:** 0.1 mg/kg **Titrate:** 0.1 ug/kg/min every 15 mins **Max dose:** 1.6 ug/kg/min	**Onset:** 5 mins **Duration:** 30–60 mins	**Side effects:** Headache, flushing, nausea, increased IOP, tachycardia **Use with caution:** Avoid in glaucoma, increased ICP or myocardial ischemia	• A dopamine-1 receptor agonist. • Works as an arteriolar vasodilator. • Rapidly drops blood pressure resulting in reflex tachycardia. • Good choice in patients with renal dysfunction because it improves creatinine clearance, urine flow rates, and sodium excretion.[2,6]

(Continued)

TABLE 36-2. Commonly Used IV Antihypertensive Agents for Treatment of Acute Postoperative Hypertension (APH) *(Continued)*

AGENT	DOSE	ONSET/DURATION	SIDE EFFECTS/USE WITH CAUTION	NOTES
Nicardipine	**Infusion:** 5 mg/hr **Titrate:** 2.5 mg/hr every 5 mins **Max dose:** 15 mg/hr	**Onset:** 5–15 mins **Duration:** 4–6 hrs	**Side effects:** Headache, flushing, dizziness, nausea, edema, tachycardia **Use with caution:** Elevated ICP	• Second-generation dihydropyridine type calcium channel blocker. • Dilates cerebral and coronary vascular beds, reducing cardiac ischemia and improving cardiac output. • Easily titratable with a rapid onset but duration of 4–6 hrs. • Very effective in the management of APH. • Avoid in patients with elevated ICP.[6]
Clevidipine	**Infusion:** 2 mg/hr **Titrate:** Double dose every 3 mins **Max dose:** 132 mg/hr	**Onset:** 2–4 mins **Duration:** 5–15 mins	**Side effects:** N/V, anxiety, tachycardia **Use with caution:** Anemia	• Ultra-short-acting third-generation calcium channel blocker targeting arteriolar beds. • Reduces blood flow without reflex tachycardia. • Safe in patients with end-stage renal disease and hepatic dysfunction and is a direct coronary vasodilator. • Excellent agent for management of APH.[2,6]

TABLE 36-3. Etiologies of Intraoperative/Postoperative Hypotension

INTRAOP	POSTOP
Anesthetic drugs	Hypovolemia (dehydration/blood loss)
Neuraxial blockade	Perioperative myocardial ischemia
Patient positioning	Sepsis
Fluid shifts	BP medications administered perioperatively
Blood loss	Heart failure
Preoperative treatment with ACEIs/ARBs	Arrhythmias
Myocardial ischemia/infarction	Pulmonary embolism
Heart failure	
Arrhythmias	

Treatment is based on the identified cause. In cases of hypovolemia, additional intravenous fluid may be administered, including in the form of blood products where indicated. For vasodilatory shock, vasopressors may be titrated to achieve an adequate blood pressure. The choice of agent will vary between settings and institutions, but common examples include phenylephrine and norepinephrine. Where clinicians are unfamiliar with these drugs, specialist help should be sought, and early referral to critical care is advised. The same holds true where contractility is impaired and inotropy is required, and specialist advice is recommended.

Clinical pearls

- Confirm the accuracy of reported readings. Repeat where necessary and consider more regular or invasive monitoring.
- Consider the intraoperative course, particularly in the early postoperative phase, which can have direct effects beyond the operating room.

- For both hypo- and hypertension, the etiology is vital. Many cases can be resolved without vasoactive drugs through the management of related factors like pain in hypertension or fluid status in hypotension.
- Although cut-off values for high and low blood pressure for the avoidance of harm have been suggested, none are perfect, and they should always be placed in the clinical context of the patient.

REFERENCES

1. Ludbrook G, Grocott MPW, Heyman K, et al. Outcomes of postoperative overnight high-acuity care in medium-risk patients undergoing elective and unplanned noncardiac surgery. *JAMA Surg.* 2023 Jul 1;158(7):701-708. PMID: 37133876
2. McEvoy MD, Gupta R, Koepke EJ, et al. Perioperative quality initiative consensus statement on postoperative blood pressure, risk and outcomes for elective surgery. *Br J Anaesth.* 2019 May;122(5):575-586. PMID: 30916008
3. Marik PE, Varon J. Hypertensive crises: challenges and management. *Chest.* 2007;131:1949-1962. PMID: 17565029
4. Rose DK, Cohen MM, DeBoer DP. Cardiovascular events in the postanesthesia care unit: contribution of risk factors. *Anesthesiology.* 1996;84:772-781. PMID: 8638830
5. Sessler DI, Meyhoff CS, Zimmerman NM, et al. Period-dependent associations between hypotension during and for four days after noncardiac surgery and a composite of myocardial infarction and death: a substudy of the POISE-2 trial. *Anesthesiology.* 2018;128:317-327. PMID: 29189290
6. Salmasi V, Maheshwari K, Yang D, et al. Relationship between intraoperative hypotension, defined by either reduction from baseline or absolute thresholds, and acute kidney and myocardial injury after noncardiac surgery: a retrospective cohort analysis. *Anesthesiology.* 2017;126:47-65. PMID: 27792044
7. Eyeington CT, Lloyd-Donald P, Chan MJ, et al. Non-invasive continuous haemodynamic monitoring and response to intervention in haemodynamically unstable patients during rapid response team review. *Resuscitation.* 2019;143:124-133. PMID: 31446156

## 37

Myocardial Infarction/Injury After Noncardiac Surgery

Steven L. Cohn, MD, MACP, SFHM, FRCP

COMMON CLINICAL QUESTIONS

1. What is perioperative myocardial injury and its clinical significance?
2. What are the risk factors for MINS?
3. How should MINS be managed?

DEFINITION AND CHARACTERISTICS OF MYOCARDIAL INJURY

Troponin elevations can be seen in many conditions (Table 37-1). Myocardial injury is defined as an elevated troponin above the 99th percentile upper reference level and is classified as acute or chronic, ischemic or nonischemic, and injury or infarction (Figure 37-1). In *acute* myocardial injury, there is a rise and fall of troponin with at least one elevated value, whereas *chronic* myocardial injury has an elevated troponin but no rise and fall pattern. Myocardial injury after noncardiac surgery (MINS)[1] is an acute myocardial injury of presumed ischemic etiology (excludes nonischemic conditions such as pulmonary embolism, stroke, sepsis) that may, but does not have to, meet criteria for myocardial infarction (ischemic signs, symptoms, ECG changes, or other cardiac imaging changes) and occurs within 30 days (typically within 72 hours) of surgery. This category also encompasses acute myocardial infarction (MI) which is further defined as Type I with acute plaque rupture (STEMI or NSTEMI) or Type II (NSTEMI)

where there is an oxygen supply-demand mismatch. Acute nonischemic myocardial injury (NIMI) has a rise and fall in troponin but no signs or symptoms of an ischemic etiology.

Definitions vary somewhat among investigators based on troponin used, specific criteria defining an elevated value, and need for absolute change in levels.[2] The incidence of MINS varies based on the specific troponin used, the patient group studied, and whether there was systematic or routine screening as opposed to only testing symptomatic patients.[3,4] It has been reported to be between 10% and 20% but higher with systematic screening, and as high as 65% using fifth-generation hsTnT, depending on variable diagnostic criteria.[5,6] Preoperative risk factors for MINS include older age, emergency surgery, heart disease, hypertension, and chronic kidney disease. Intraoperative risk factors include hypotension and tachycardia.

The CCS guidelines[7] recommend obtaining postoperative troponins in patients with an elevated BNP/NTproBNP. The 2022 ESC guidelines[8] have a Class I recommendation to measure hs-cTn T or hs-cTn I before intermediate- and high-risk NCS, and at 24 and 48 hours afterwards in patients who have known CVD, CV risk factors (including age $\geq$ 65 years), or symptoms suggestive of CVD. The 2023 ESAIC focused guideline[9] suggests that routine measurement of postoperative troponins may be used to evaluate the risk of adverse postoperative outcomes and potentially predict 30-day mortality (weak recommendation; low to moderate evidence), but caution using

TABLE 37-1.   Etiologies of Troponin Elevation*

ISCHEMIC (CORONARY OR MYOCARDIAL)	NONISCHEMIC
ACS—Atherosclerotic plaque rupture (STEMI/NSTEMI)	Sepsis/critical illness
Sustained tachyarrhythmias	Pulmonary embolism
Sustained bradyarrhythmias	Stroke/subarachnoid hemorrhage/head trauma
Coronary artery spasm	Acute kidney injury/chronic kidney disease
Hypotension/shock	Pulmonary hypertension
Severe anemia	Respiratory failure/COPD
Severe hypertension	Extensive burns
Aortic dissection	Extreme exertion
Acute heart failure	Rhabdomyolysis
	Infiltrative disease (amyloidosis, sarcoidosis)
	Cardiomyopathy
	Vasculitis, myocarditis, endocarditis, pericarditis
	Cardiotoxic drugs
	Cardiac procedures

*There may be an overlap between categories.

them to improve outcome (no recommendation; very low-quality evidence). The 2021 AHA Scientific Statement[10] and the 2024 AHA/ACC guidelines[11] state that it may be reasonable to measure troponins 24 and 48 hours postoperatively in essentially the same group of at-risk patients as the ESC (COR 2b/LOE B), but not to measure them in asymptomatic patients undergoing low-risk surgery without signs or symptoms of ischemia (COR 3/LOE B).

The importance of MINS is that it is associated with an increased 30-day risk of mortality, heart failure, and stroke, as well as 1-year mortality, and most patients are asymptomatic. The mortality rate ranges from 8% to 13% and increases with increasing levels of troponin.[12] Specific thresholds have been associated with adverse prognosis—fourth-generation troponin >30 ng/dL, and hsTnT ≥20–<65 ng/L with an absolute change of ≥5 ng/L or any elevation ≥65 ng/L or any absolute change ≥14 ng/L.[13]

MANAGEMENT

Because there are multiple causes for troponin elevation, perioperative myocardial injury (PMI) cannot be treated as a single entity, and treatment needs to be individualized. While there is evidence-based therapy for Type I MI, treating other troponin elevations in a similar fashion with antiplatelet therapy and anticoagulation may result in increased bleeding or unnecessary cardiac catheterization, and starting beta-blockers in the perioperative period may be harmful.

In POISE, patients with postoperative myocardial infarctions who were given aspirin and a statin did better,[14] and there was also a suggestion from a smaller study that intensification of medical therapy (aspirin, statin, beta-blocker, ACE-inhibitor) in patients with postoperative troponin elevations was associated with improved outcome at 1 year.[15] Since most patients with MINS will have a history of CAD or risk factors

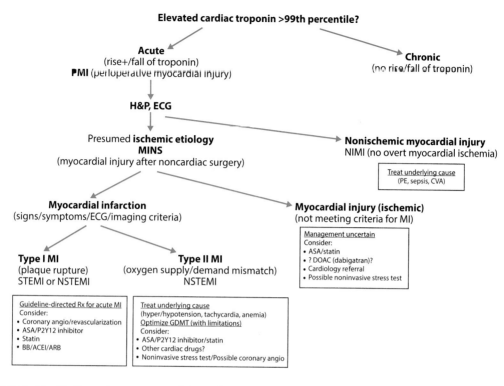

FIGURE 37-1. Classification and management of elevated postoperative troponin.
Adapted from Cohn SL, Rohatgi N, Patel P, Whinney C. Clinical progress note: myocardial injury after noncardiac surgery. *J Hosp Med.* 2020;15(7):412-415.

for it, starting aspirin and a statin may be reasonable assuming the risk of postoperative bleeding is not high. However, many patients do not receive these medications. Referral for further cardiac evaluation, such as echocardiography, stress testing, and possibly coronary angiography should be individualized, and the patient should be made aware of the diagnosis and prognostic importance.

MANAGE, the only randomized control trial to evaluate the treatment of MINS, reported that dabigatran improved the primary efficacy outcome, a composite of vascular mortality and nonfatal myocardial infarction, nonhemorrhagic stroke, peripheral arterial thrombosis, amputation, and symptomatic venous thromboembolism, with no increase in the primary safety outcome, a composite of life-threatening, major, and critical organ bleeding.[16] However, there were many criticisms of the study including lower patient enrollment than planned, changing outcomes during the trial, definition of bleeding, and significant

premature discontinuation of the drug. Additionally, subgroup analysis showed differences in outcomes based on early versus late enrollment and between patients with confirmed MI versus isolated troponin elevation. An accompanying editorial suggested that the benefit of dabigatran may have been driven by a reduction in nonhemorrhagic stroke (the only individual outcome that was statistically significant) with some of the troponin elevations related to paroxysmal asymptomatic atrial fibrillation. The INTREPID study, designed to see if aspirin or ticagrelor would reduce postoperative complications in patients with elevated troponin after noncardiac surgery, was terminated due to enrollment difficulties.

SUMMARY

Unfortunately, MINS predicts mortality but currently lacks a clear treatment algorithm other than for myocardial infarction. While aspirin, statins, and dabigatran may help some patients, there is no consensus on the treatment of patients with troponin elevations not meeting the criteria for myocardial infarction. Several randomized trials are underway to assess the benefit of ivabradine, esmolol, and colchicine in preventing MINS, and additional trials are needed to investigate the treatment of MINS. In patients currently on appropriate GDMT, it is unclear how a diagnosis of MINS would change management. Although guidelines have made recommendations, until we have better evidence, we can only speculate as to whether it is beneficial to screen these patients with postoperative troponins and what the best treatment should be to improve outcomes.

Clinical pearls

- MINS is associated with an elevated 30-day mortality that increases with increasing levels of troponin.

- Most patients with MINS are asymptomatic, and only about 20% meet the criteria for acute myocardial infarction.

- Because there are multiple causes for troponin elevation, PMI/MINS cannot be treated as a single entity, and therapy should be tailored to the specific etiology and clinical setting.

REFERENCES

1. Botto F, Alonso-Coello P, Chan MT, et al. Myocardial injury after noncardiac surgery: a large, international, prospective cohort study establishing diagnostic criteria, characteristics, predictors, and 30-day outcomes. *Anesthesiology.* 2014;120(3):564-578. PMID: 24534856

2. Puelacher C, Lurati Buse G, Seeberger D, et al.; BASEL-PMI Investigators. Perioperative myocardial injury after noncardiac surgery: incidence, mortality, and characterization. *Circulation.* 2018;137(12):1221-1232. PMID: 29203498

3. Beattie WS, Karkouti K, Tait G, et al. Use of clinically based troponin underestimates the cardiac injury in non-cardiac surgery: a single-centre cohort study in 51,701 consecutive patients. *Can J Anaesth.* 2012;59(11):1013-1022. PMID: 22961610

4. Smilowitz NR, Redel-Traub G, Hausvater A, et al. Myocardial injury after noncardiac surgery: a systematic review and meta-analysis. *Cardiol Rev.* 2019;27:267-273. PMID: 30985328

5. Writing Committee for the VISION Study Investigators; Devereaux PJ, Biccard BM, Sigamani A, et al. Association of postoperative high-sensitivity troponin levels with myocardial injury and 30-day mortality among patients undergoing noncardiac surgery. *JAMA.* 2017;317(16):1642-1651. PMID: 28444280

6. Brown JC, Samaha E, Rao S, et al. High-sensitivity cardiac troponin T improves the diagnosis of perioperative MI. *Anesth Analg.* 2017;125(5):1455-1462. PMID: 28719430

7. Duceppe E, Parlow J, MacDonald P, et al. Canadian Cardiovascular Society guidelines on perioperative cardiac risk assessment and management for patients who undergo noncardiac surgery. *Can J Cardiol.* 2017;33(1):17-32. PMID: 27865641

8. Halvorsen S, Mehilli J, Cassese S, et al.; ESC Scientific Document Group. 2022 ESC guidelines on cardiovascular assessment and management of patients undergoing non-cardiac surgery. *Eur Heart J.* 2022;43(39):3826-3924. PMID: 36017553

9. Lurati Buse G, Bollen Pinto B, Abelha F, et al. ESAIC focused guideline for the use of cardiac biomarkers in perioperative risk evaluation. *Eur J Anaesthesiol.* 2023;40(12):888-927. PMID: 37265332

10. Ruetzler K, Smilowitz NR, Berger JS, et al. Diagnosis and management of patients with myocardial injury after noncardiac surgery: a Scientific Statement From the American Heart Association. *Circulation.* 2021;144(19):e287-e305. PMID: 34601955

11. Thompson A, Fleischmann KE, Smilowitz NR, et al. 2024 AHA/ACC/ACS/ASNC/HRS/SCA/SCCT/SCMR/SVM guideline for perioperative cardiovascular management for noncardiac surgery: a report of the American College of Cardiology/American Heart Association Joint Committee on Clinical Practice Guidelines. *J Am Coll Cardiol.* 2024;84(19):1869-1969. doi:10.1016/j.jacc.2024.06.013. PMID: 39320289

12. Vascular Events in Noncardiac Surgery Patients Cohort Evaluation (VISION) Study Investigators; Devereaux PJ, Chan MT, Alonso-Coello P, et al. Association between postoperative troponin levels and 30-day mortality among patients undergoing noncardiac surgery. *JAMA.* 2012;307(21):2295-304. PMID: 22706835

13. Devereaux PJ, Biccard BM, Sigamani A, et al; Writing Committee for the VISION Study Investigators. Association of postoperative high-sensitivity troponin levels with myocardial injury and 30-day mortality among patients undergoing noncardiac surgery. *JAMA.* 2017;317:1642-1651. PMID: 28444280

14. Devereaux PJ, Xavier D, Pogue J, et al. Characteristics and short-term prognosis of perioperative myocardial infarction in patients undergoing noncardiac surgery:

a cohort study. *Ann Intern Med.* 2011;154(8):523-528. PMID: 21502650

15. Foucrier A, Rodseth R, Aissaoui M, et al. The long-term impact of early cardiovascular therapy intensification for postoperative troponin elevation after major vascular surgery. *Anesth Analg.* 2014;119(5):1053-1063. PMID: 24937347

16. Devereaux PJ, Duceppe E, Guyatt G, et al.; MANAGE Investigators. Dabigatran in patients with myocardial injury after non-cardiac surgery (MANAGE): an international, randomised, placebo controlled trial. *Lancet.* 2018;391(10137):2325-2334. PMID: 29900874

## 38

Atrial Fibrillation

Nidhi Rohatgi, MD, MS, SFHM and Paul J. Wang, MD, FAHA, FACC, FHRS, FESC

COMMON CLINICAL QUESTIONS

1. What is the risk of stroke and systemic embolism with postoperative atrial fibrillation after noncardiothoracic surgery?
2. What are the management strategies for postoperative atrial fibrillation after noncardiothoracic surgery?

INTRODUCTION

Postoperative atrial fibrillation (POAF) is the most common sustained arrhythmia after cardiothoracic surgeries and noncardiothoracic surgeries (most commonly abdominal and orthopedic surgery). Although most literature on atrial fibrillation (AF) has focused on nonsurgical settings or postcardiothoracic surgeries, this chapter will focus on POAF after noncardiothoracic surgeries.

CLINICAL PRESENTATION

AF has conventionally been described using the duration of the episode, symptoms, or presence of valvular disease (Table 38-1).[1]

Episodes of POAF are most common on postoperative days 2–4 and are often self-terminating.[2] Patients with AF may be asymptomatic or have symptoms ranging from fatigue, palpitations, dizziness, syncope, or acute heart failure. Episodes of asymptomatic

POAF may often go undetected after noncardiothoracic surgeries as continuous cardiac monitoring seldom extends beyond the postoperative acute care units. In patients with a new diagnosis of AF in the postoperative setting, recurrence within 2 years has been reported in 16.8% of the patients. Risk factors for recurrence of AF include moderate to severe left atrial enlargement, uncontrolled hypertension, left ventricular hypertrophy, reduced left ventricular ejection fraction, and valvular heart disease.[3] The exact etiology of POAF is not established. Although transient factors related to the surgery (e.g., anatomical location of the procedure, duration of surgery, surgical complications, amount of blood loss) play an important role in the development of POAF, the majority of episodes of POAF occur in patients with preexisting risk factors (Table 38-2).[1,4]

In patients with no history of AF, it is often difficult to discern if the episode of POAF is the first true occurrence of AF in that patient or if it is the first detection of a previously undiagnosed AF, especially if they have preexisting risk factors for AF.

PREVENTION OF POAF

In contrast to cardiothoracic surgery, there are no guideline-directed pharmacological strategies for prevention of POAF for noncardiothoracic surgeries, except that patients who are on beta-blockers or nondihydropyridine calcium channel blockers should continue these medications in the perioperative

TABLE 38-1. Definitions of Atrial Fibrillation Based on Duration, Symptoms, and Presence of Valvular Disease

Acute or chronic AF	These terms are no longer recommended
Subclinical or silent AF	Asymptomatic AF
Paroxysmal AF	Terminates within 7 days of onset but may recur
Persistent AF	AF sustains for >7 days
Long-standing persistent AF	AF sustains for >12 months
Permanent AF	AF sustains and the decision is made to not pursue rhythm control strategies anymore
Valvular AF	Mechanical valve or moderate to severe mitral stenosis
Nonvalvular AF	Does not imply no valvular disease (it excludes mechanical valve and moderate to severe mitral stenosis)
MARM AF	Mechanical and rheumatic mitral AF

AF, Atrial fibrillation.

period if the blood pressure and heart rate allow. Hypervolemia, severe anemia, hypoxia, electrolyte imbalance, and alcohol withdrawal should be avoided or promptly managed, and compliance with continuous or bi-level positive airway pressure (CPAP/BiPAP) in patients with obstructive sleep apnea should be maintained whenever possible. To reduce the risk of recurrence of AF, patient-related factors should be optimized in the long term (Table 38-2).

EVALUATION OF POAF

The first step in evaluation of postoperative AF is establishing hemodynamic stability and confirmation of the rhythm. A 12-lead electrocardiogram should be obtained and cardiac monitoring (telemetry) should be considered until rate or rhythm control is achieved.[5] Careful history and physical examination should be performed to identify the potential risk factors and triggers of POAF in that patient (Table 38-2). Important diagnoses such as sepsis, bleeding, or pulmonary embolism should be excluded, if there is a clinical suspicion. Caffeine abstention is of no benefit, unless it is known to be a trigger for AF for that patient.[1] All patients should have a complete blood count and chemistry panel. Thyroid function studies should be obtained but interpreted with caution as the results may be inaccurate in the postoperative setting. Obtaining cardiac biomarkers (e.g., troponin, B-type

TABLE 38-2. Risk Factors and Triggers for Atrial Fibrillation

PATIENT-RELATED FACTORS		SURGICAL FACTORS	BIOMARKERS AND ECHOCARDIOGRAPHIC FEATURES
Age	Prior atrial fibrillation	Increased sympathetic response	Increased C-reactive protein
Obesity	Premature atrial beats	Inflammation and oxidative stress	Increased B-type natriuretic peptide
Sleep apnea	Diabetes mellitus	Mitral valve surgery	Increased lipoprotein(a)
Alcohol use	Smoking	Hypovolemia	Left atrial enlargement
Hypertension	Exercise	Hypervolemia	Increased left ventricular wall thickness
Coronary artery disease	Family history	Anemia	Decreased left ventricular fractional shortening
Valvular heart disease	Pneumonia/sepsis	Pain	
Heart failure	Renal failure	Hypokalemia	
Discontinuation of home beta-blockers	Chronic obstructive lung disease	Hypomagnesemia	
	Hyperthyroidism		

natriuretic peptide) is not routinely recommended unless there is a clinical suspicion of ischemia or heart failure. All patients with POAF should have a transthoracic echocardiogram as an inpatient or outpatient based on the AF burden and duration, and ideally when rate or rhythm control has been achieved.[1,5] At the time of discharge from the hospital, ambulatory rhythm monitoring should be considered for 2–4 weeks to assess for recurrence of AF and the AF burden, although the optimal duration and frequency of monitoring remains unclear.[1] A strategy for assessment, evaluation, and management of POAF is presented in Figure 38-1.

MANAGEMENT OF POAF

The first step in management of POAF should be to correct the potential trigger for AF because this can often terminate AF (e.g., correcting fluid overload or hypovolemia, managing pain to reduce the sympathetic tone). In hemodynamically unstable patients, cardioversion is indicated. Early cardioversion prior to

48 hours is often a consideration to increase the likelihood of maintaining sinus rhythm and potentially reducing the risk of thromboembolic risk, particularly when anticoagulation is subtherapeutic. In the nonsurgical setting, transesophageal echocardiography (TEE) and therapeutic anticoagulation should be considered prior to cardioversion in patients with AF of unknown or ≥48 hours duration and then for at least 4 weeks after cardioversion; however, anticoagulation recommendations require an even more careful and individualized discussion about the bleeding risk and thromboembolic risk in the postoperative setting.[1]

Rate and Rhythm Control

Common pharmacological strategies for rate or rhythm control of POAF include beta-blockers, nondihydropyridine calcium channel blockers, digoxin, and amiodarone (Table 38-3).

In most patients with POAF, a rate control strategy will suffice except in those who are either hemodynamically unstable, difficult to rate control, or are

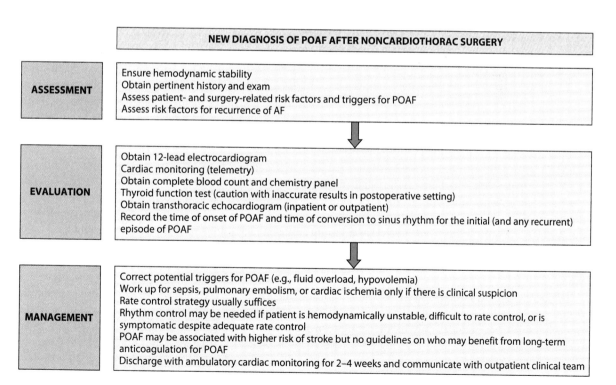

FIGURE 38-1. Assessment, evaluation, and management of postoperative atrial fibrillation after noncardiothoracic surgery. POAF, postoperative atrial fibrillation; AF, atrial fibrillation.

TABLE 38-3. Medications for Rate Control

DRUG	INDICATIONS/PRECAUTIONS
Beta-blocker	• Effective for rate control • First-line therapy
Nondihydropyridine calcium channel blocker	• Given if poor candidate for or inadequate control after beta-blocker • Avoid with left ventricular ejection fraction <40%
Digoxin	• Should not be used as the sole or first-line agent—limited effectiveness if high sympathetic tone • Avoid with significant renal dysfunction
Amiodarone	• Primarily for rhythm control but may also provide rate control • Used when other drugs are contraindicated or ineffective • Risk of chemical cardioversion, so consider transesophageal echocardiogram and anticoagulation prior to administration if onset of atrial fibrillation >48 hours ago and higher CHA_2DS_2-VASc score

symptomatic despite adequate rate control. The target heart rate depends on the patient's symptoms, blood pressure, and left ventricular systolic function. In general, a target heart rate of 80–110 bpm at rest and <110 bpm with moderate exertion (e.g., 6-minute-walk test) is acceptable.[1] In the postoperative setting, a more liberal target heart rate of 100–120 bpm at rest with minimal symptoms with exertion may be acceptable to avoid hypotension.

Thromboembolic Risk

The new diagnosis of POAF was previously considered to be a transient and benign rhythm. However, at least two large meta-analyses showed a higher risk of stroke in patients with POAF after noncardiac surgery compared to patients who did not have POAF.[6,7] In the nonsurgical setting, primarily in patients with cardiovascular implantable electronic devices, AF lasting even few minutes has been associated with a higher rate of stroke. However, there are no similar studies for POAF after noncardiothoracic surgery.

In the nonsurgical setting, CHA_2DS_2-VASc score is recommended to assess the annual thromboembolic risk with AF, but it provides only moderate discrimination between patients at low or high risk and is not validated for POAF.[1] Long-term anticoagulation is *not recommended* for patients with AF who have CHA_2DS_2-VASc score of 0 for men or 1 for women unless conversion to sinus rhythm is planned, in

which case all patients with AF ≥48 hours in duration should be anticoagulated for at least 1 month.[1,5] Long-term anticoagulation is *reasonable* for patients with AF who have CHA_2DS_2-VASc score of 1 for men or 2 for women, and anticoagulation is *recommended* for those at higher CHA_2DS_2-VASc score.[1] Bleeding risk scores such as HAS-BLED should not be used in isolation to determine eligibility for anticoagulation in patients with POAF at high risk of stroke as they provide poor discrimination even in the nonsurgical setting and have not been validated in the surgical setting. They can, however, supplement medical-decision making.[1]

For AF in the nonsurgical setting: (a) direct oral anticoagulants (DOACs) are recommended over vitamin K antagonists (VKA) in DOAC-eligible patients (excluding patients with moderate to severe mitral stenosis or mechanical heart valve), and (b) if the patient is at increased risk of stroke but has a contraindication to long-term anticoagulation, percutaneous left atrial appendage occlusion may be considered.[1] This has not been evaluated for POAF and the major clinical trials comparing DOAC to VKA excluded patients within 30 days of major surgery. Aspirin alone or with clopidogrel is not recommended to reduce the risk of stroke.[1] If DOACs are prescribed, concomitant drug interactions with CYP3A4 and P-glycoprotein inhibitors or inducers should be addressed.

Data from a meta-analysis showed that anticoagulation use for POAF after noncardiac surgery was associated with a lower risk of stroke and mortality but a higher risk of bleeding, though the quality of evidence is poor.[8] It remains unclear which patients with a new diagnosis of POAF after noncardiothoracic surgery should be anticoagulated. A randomized clinical trial (ASPIRE-AF) is underway to evaluate this.[9]

Clinical pearls

- Optimize and treat the risk factors and triggers for POAF.

- Although previously thought to be transient and benign, newly diagnosed POAF may be associated with an increased risk of stroke and systemic embolism.

- It remains unclear which patients with POAF after noncardiothoracic surgery should be anticoagulated.

REFERENCES

1. Joglar JA, Chung MK, Armbruster AL, et al. 2023 ACC/AHA/ACCP/HRS guideline for the diagnosis and management of atrial fibrillation: a report of the American College of Cardiology/American Heart Association Joint Committee on Clinical Practice Guidelines. *Circulation.* 2024;149:e1-e156. PMID: 38033089

2. Gaudino M, Di Franco A, Rong LQ, et al. Postoperative atrial fibrillation: from mechanisms to treatment. *Eur Heart J.* 2023;44:1020–1039. PMID: 36721960

3. Hyun J, Cho MS, Nam G, et al. Natural course of new-onset postoperative atrial fibrillation after noncardiac surgery. *J Am Heart Assoc.* 2021;10:e018548. PMID: 33739130

4. Karamchandani K, Khanna AK, Bose S, et al. Atrial fibrillation: current evidence and management strategies during the perioperative period. *Anesth Analg.* 2020;130:2–13. PMID: 31569164

5. Hindricks G, Potpara T, Dagres N, et al, ESC Scientific Document Group. 2020 ESC guidelines for the diagnosis and management of atrial fibrillation developed in collaboration with the European Association for Cardio-Thoracic Surgery (EACTS): the task force for the diagnosis and management of atrial fibrillation of the Europea. *Eur Heart J.* 2021;42:373–498. PMID: 32860505

6. Lin M-H, Kamel H, Singer DE, et al. Perioperative/postoperative atrial fibrillation and risk of subsequent stroke and/or mortality. *Stroke.* 2019;50:1364–1371. PMID: 31043148

7. AlTurki A, Marafi M, Proietti R, et al. Major adverse cardiovascular events associated with postoperative atrial fibrillation after noncardiac surgery: a systematic review and meta-analysis. *Circ Arrhythm Electrophysiol.* 2020;13:e007437. PMID: 31944855

8. Ke Wang M, Heo R, Meyre PB, et al. Anticoagulation use in perioperative atrial fibrillation after noncardiac surgery: a systematic review and meta-analysis. *Swiss Med Wkly.* 2023;153:40056. PMID: 37080190

9. Anticoagulation for stroke prevention in patients with recent episodes of perioperative atrial fibrillation after noncardiac surgery (ASPIRE-AF)—NCT03968393. Accessed September 17, 2022. https://clinicaltrials.gov/ct2/show/NCT03968393.

## 39

Pulmonary Complications

J. Njeri Wainaina, MD, FACP, FHM, FIDSA

COMMON CLINICAL QUESTIONS

1. What respiratory complications can occur after surgery?
2. What physiological mechanisms underlie postoperative respiratory failure?
3. What can be done during or after surgery to mitigate pulmonary complications?

BACKGROUND

The term postoperative pulmonary complications (PPCs) refers to any adverse event involving the respiratory system that occurs after surgery.[1] Incidence ranges from 5% to 80% depending on definitions used, surgery type, and population referenced.[2] For instance, the European Perioperative Clinical Outcome (EPCO) definition[3] encompasses respiratory failure, pneumonia/respiratory infection, pleural effusion, atelectasis, pneumothorax, bronchospasm, aspiration pneumonitis, acute respiratory distress syndrome (ARDS), tracheobronchitis, pulmonary edema, and exacerbation of preexisting lung disease while the American College of Surgery's (ACS) National Surgical Quality Improvement Program (NSQIP) includes only pneumonia and respiratory failure which comprises unplanned intubation and failure to wean from mechanical ventilation within 48 hours of surgery. Table 39-1 outlines accepted definitions of respiratory failure and pneumonia which comprise the largest slice of PPCs.

TABLE 39-1. Definitions of Complications

RESPIRATORY FAILURE	PNEUMONIA (CDC DEFINITION)

• Postoperative PaO_2 < 60 mmHg on room air
• O_2 sat < 90% and requiring oxygen
• Ventilator dependence for >1 postoperative day or reintubation
• Need for postoperative mechanical ventilation >48 hours
• Unplanned reintubation because of respiratory distress, hypoxia, hypercarbia, or respiratory acidosis within 30 days of surgery
• Postoperative acute lung injury
• ARDS
• Requiring mechanical ventilation within 7 days of surgery
• Requiring noninvasive ventilation
	• CXR with at least one of the following: infiltrate, consolidation, cavitation; *plus* at least one of the following:
	  • Fever > 38°C with no other cause
	  • WBC < 4000 or > 12,000
	• For adults > 70 years of age, altered mental status with no other cause; *plus* at least two of the following:
	• New purulent/changed sputum, increased secretions/suctioning requirements
	• New/worsening cough/dyspnea/tachypnea
	• Rales/bronchial breath sounds
	• Worsening gas exchange

While there is a disparity in reported occurrence rates, there is no disagreement on the increase in morbidity, morbidity, and cost that ensues. The impact of PPCs was starkly demonstrated when a landmark study showed 51.8% of patients who contracted COVID-19 perioperatively early in the pandemic developed pulmonary complications and 23.8% died within 30 days of surgery. The 30-day mortality in patients who developed PPCs was 38% and pulmonary complications accounted for 81.7% of all deaths.[4] Pre-pandemic data shows 14–30% of patients who experience a PPC within 30 days of major surgery will die compared to 0.2–3% in those without a PPC, and 90-day mortality goes up from 1.2% to 24.4% with 30% excess mortality at 5 years. PPCs also prolong the length of stay 13–17 days, inflating costs to patients and the healthcare system by up to 50%.[1]

Patient- and surgery-specific risk factors, risk calculators to quantify the hazard of PPCs, and preoperative mitigation and optimization strategies are discussed in Chapter 16.

APPROACH TO POSTOPERATIVE RESPIRATORY FAILURE: DIAGNOSIS AND TREATMENT

Respiratory failure, the most severe postoperative pulmonary complication, typically occurs early—either immediately after the procedure or within the first week. Physiologically, respiratory failure is the result of impaired lung perfusion, alveolar airflow and/or pulmonary interstitial gas exchange arising from hypoventilation, ventilation-perfusion (V/Q) mismatch, right to left shunt, and impaired oxygen diffusion. An anatomical approach that localizes the primary pathology to the cardiopulmonary vasculature, interstitium, alveolus, airways, and pleura can guide a structured approach to clinical evaluation. Nonpulmonary causes including sedating medications, such as anesthetics and opioid analgesics, neuromuscular blockade and disorders, central nervous system (CNS) disorders, electrolyte derangements, and metabolic disorders should also be kept in mind. Etiologies of respiratory failure are categorized in Table 39-2.

The diagnosis of respiratory failure requires an assessment of gas exchange effectiveness. Pulse oximetry is the quickest and easiest method, though is

TABLE 39-2. Causes of Postoperative Respiratory Failure

HYPOVENTILATION	
Airway obstruction	Laryngeal edema, OSA, COPD
Impaired respiratory drive	Residual general anesthetics, other CNS suppressants—opioids, gabapentinoids
Pump failure	Pleural effusions, obesity hypoventilation syndrome
Neuromuscular	Prolonged neuromuscular blockade, preexisting neuromuscular disease
V/Q MISMATCH	
Decreased V/Q ratio	Pulmonary edema, mucus plugs, chronic obstructive airway disease
Increased V/Q ratio	Pulmonary embolism, Emphysema
RIGHT TO LEFT SHUNT	
Anatomic	Intracardiac, pulmonary arteriovenous malformations, hepatopulmonary syndrome
Physiologic	Atelectasis, pneumonia, chemical pneumonitis, ARDS
IMPAIRED OXYGEN DIFFUSION	Pulmonary edema, underlying interstitial lung disease

limited to identifying hypoxia. Arterial blood gas analysis carries the drawback of a painful blood draw but adds the ability to detect hypercapnia which pulse oximetry cannot capture. Assessment of airway patency and ventilation via physical examination should occur concurrently. Consider additional testing, such as imaging, to determine the cause and extent of involvement.

Treatment starts with correcting the impaired process—hypoventilation, ventilation-perfusion (V/Q) mismatch, right to left shunt, and impaired oxygen diffusion by ensuring airways are patent, providing supplemental oxygen, ideally noninvasively whenever possible, and improving interstitial oxygen diffusion. Diagnosing and addressing the cause of impairment is necessary for complete resolution.

APPROACH TO POSTOPERATIVE PNEUMONIA: DIAGNOSIS AND TREATMENT

Postoperative pneumonia usually occurs within the first week of surgery, and should be considered hospital-acquired regardless of patient location at the time symptoms manifest. Patients classically present with fever, new or increased cough, and new or increased purulent respiratory secretions. This could be accompanied by new hypoxic respiratory failure, hypotension, or septic shock. Less typical symptoms should prompt consideration of other postoperative pulmonary complications such as atelectasis, pulmonary embolism, aspiration pneumonitis, pleural effusion, medication or blood product-induced acute lung injury, and exacerbations of chronic lung disease. Nonpulmonary conditions such as decompensated heart failure, acute kidney injury, and decompensated cirrhosis causing pulmonary edema should also be kept in mind.

Management includes obtaining a chest x-ray which would be expected to reveal new infiltrates, sampling respiratory secretions for bacterial culture, and initiation of empiric antibiotics that cover hospital-acquired organisms including but not limited to *Pseudomonas aeruginosa* and Methicillin-resistant *Staphylococcus aureus* based on the institution's epidemiology and antibiogram as well as individual patient risk factors for multidrug resistant organisms. Table 39-3 catalogs additional common pathogens with surgical and medical predisposing factors. Once a microbiological diagnosis is made, antibiotics should be de-escalated to target the culprits. Both American[5] and European[6] guidelines recommend a 7-day duration for patients that respond adequately regardless of whether they are mechanically ventilated or not. Longer courses may be appropriate in patients with complicated or metastatic infections, structural lung disease, and/or immunosuppression.

PREVENTION

To prevent postoperative respiratory failure and pneumonia, it is important to address any modifiable risk factors as comprehensively as possible before surgery. I-COUGH, a multidisciplinary, standardized patient care program that includes pulmonary interventions, early mobilization, and patient education, was associated with a reduction in the incidence of postoperative pneumonia and unplanned intubation,[7] but it requires a coordinated, ongoing institutional commitment.

TABLE 39-3. Common Pathogens and Association with Medical and Surgical Factors

	SURGICAL PREDISPOSITION	MEDICAL PREDISPOSITION
Hemophilus influenzae	Trauma	
Streptococcus pneumoniae	Trauma	
Staphylococcus aureus	Neurosurgery Trauma	CKD, DM, injection drug use, recent influenza
MRSA	Long surgery Emergency surgery	Positive nasal screen
Pseudomonas aeruginosa	Nonspecific	Long intubation, bronchiectasis, cystic fibrosis, COPD, treatment with steroids, malnutrition, prolonged exposure to antibiotics
Acinetobacter species	Nonspecific	Mechanical ventilation
Anaerobes—uncommon	Abdominal surgery	

TABLE 39-4. Postoperative Measures to Prevent PPCs[7] (Including I-COUGH)

- **I**ncentive spirometry (10 times/hr with 3–5 efforts each set)
- **C**oughing and deep breathing
- **O**ral hygiene with twice daily teeth brushing and mouthwash
- **U**nderstanding (patient and family education)
- **G**etting out of bed >3 times daily—standing/walking within the first 24 hours after surgery
- **H**ead of the bed elevated >30 degrees and sitting in a chair
- Addition of epidural analgesia when general anesthesia is used
- Reducing dose of opioids in patients who have or are at risk for OSA
- Pulse oximetry/capnography with central station monitoring in high-risk patients

Its components and other postoperative strategies to decrease risk are listed in Table 39-4.

Clinical pearls

- Postoperative pulmonary complications (PPCs) are common, and confer significant morbidity, mortality, and cost.
- Evaluation and treatment of postoperative pneumonia is like that in a hospitalized nonsurgical patient. While gram negative bacilli and *Staphylococcus aureus* are common pathogens, consider other organisms that the antecedent surgery may predispose.
- Using the I-COUGH bundle may prevent PPCs.

REFERENCES

1. Miskovic A, Lumb AB. Postoperative pulmonary complications. *Br J Anaesth*. 2017:118(3):317-334. PMID: 28186222
2. Shander A, Fleisher LA, Barie PS, et al. Clinical and economic burden of postoperative pulmonary complications: patient safety summit on definition, risk-reducing interventions, and preventive strategies. *Crit Care Med*. 2011;39(9):2163-2172. PMID: 21572323
3. Jammer I, Wickboldt N, Sander M, et al. Standards for definitions and use of outcome measures for clinical effectiveness research in perioperative medicine: European Perioperative Clinical Outcomes (EPCO) definitions: a statement from the ESA-ESICM joint taskforce on perioperative outcome measures. *Eur J Anaesthesiol*. 2015;32:88-105. PMID: 25058504
4. Nepogodiev D, Glasbey JC, Li E, et al. Mortality and pulmonary complications in patients undergoing surgery with perioperative SARS-CoV-2 infection: an international cohort study. *Lancet*. 2020;396:27-38. PMID: 32531186
5. Kalil AC, Metersky ML, Klompas M, et al. Management of adults with hospital-acquired and ventilator-associated pneumonia: 2016 clinical practice guidelines by the Infectious Diseases Society of America and the American Thoracic Society. *Clin Infect Dis*. 2016;63(5):e61. PMID: 27418577
6. Torres A, Niederman MS, Chastre J, et al. International ERS/ESICM/ESCMID/ALAT guidelines for the management of hospital-acquired pneumonia and ventilator-associated pneumonia: guidelines for the management of hospital-acquired pneumonia (HAP)/ventilator-associated pneumonia (VAP) of the European Respiratory Society (ERS), European Society of Intensive Care Medicine (ESICM), European Society of Clinical Microbiology and Infectious Diseases (ESCMID) and Asociación Latinoamericana del Tórax (ALAT). *Eur Respir J*. 2017;50(3):1700582. PMID: 28890434
7. Cassidy MR, Rosenkranz P, McCabe K, et al. I COUGH: reducing postoperative pulmonary complications with a multidisciplinary patient care program. *JAMA Surg*. 2013;148:740-745. PMID: 23740240

## 40

Deep Venous Thrombosis and Pulmonary Embolism

Scott Kaatz, DO, MSc, FACP, SFHM and James D. Douketis, MD, FRCP(C)

COMMON CLINICAL QUESTIONS

1. Is d-dimer recommended for the diagnosis of postoperative DVT/PE?
2. What is the preferred treatment for postoperative DVT/PE and for what duration?
3. When is an inferior vena cava filter indicated?

VTE DIAGNOSIS

Postoperative venous thromboembolic disease (VTE) accounts for approximately 25% of all VTE despite prophylaxis.[1] Common signs and symptoms of deep vein thrombosis (DVT) include swelling, edema, pain, and increased warmth, and these findings are somewhat sensitive but not specific. Pulmonary embolism (PE) can present with signs of DVT as well as dyspnea, pleuritic pain, cough, orthopnea, wheezing, hemoptysis, tachycardia, tachypnea, and hypotension. Validated pretest probability prediction rules should be used when evaluating patients with suspected VTE. Most postoperative patients will have an intermediate or high pretest probability of VTE. D-dimer testing in the postoperative patient has limited utility because of the high frequency of elevated results, and the American Society of Hematology (ASH) guidelines recommend against using d-dimer for the diagnosis of VTE.[2] Computed tomographic pulmonary angiography and compression venous ultrasound are suggested as initial studies to assess for PE and DVT, respectively, and serial venous ultrasound should be used in patients with high suspicion of DVT and an initial negative study.[2]

VTE TREATMENT

Key aspects to treatment include choice of anticoagulants, use of inferior vena cava (IVC) filters, and length of treatment. If surgical site hemostasis is uncertain or not secured, an anticoagulant that can be titrated and easily reversed, like unfractionated heparin, or placement of a temporary IVC filter should be used until hemostasis is secured (Figure 40-1).

Choice of Anticoagulants

The American College of Chest Physicians (ACCP) guidelines suggest using direct oral anticoagulants (DOACs) over vitamin K antagonists like warfarin for the treatment of VTE.[3] Oral apixaban and rivaroxaban are initiated at higher doses for 1 and 3 weeks, respectively, whereas dabigatran and edoxaban require at least 5 days of parenteral anticoagulant lead-in (not overlap) (Table 40-1). The ACCP recommends apixaban, edoxaban, or rivaroxaban over low-molecular weight heparin (LMWH) for patients with cancer-associated VTE.[3] Common concerns with DOACs include use in patients with severe renal insufficiency (i.e., creatinine clearance [CrCl] < 30 mL/min) and potential DOAC-drug interactions (e.g., anticonvulsants, antimicrobials).

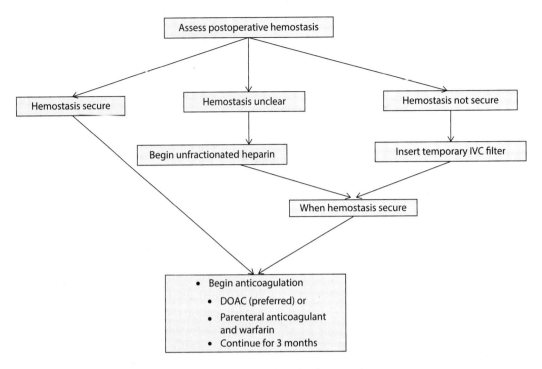

FIGURE 40-1. Postoperative venous thromboembolism treatment based on hemostasis. DOAC, direct oral anticoagulant.

DOAC Use with Renal Impairment. CrCl differs slightly from the estimated glomerular filtration rate and should be calculated with the Cockcroft-Gault formula using actual body weight when making DOAC decisions. The U.S. Food and Drug Administration (FDA) provides recommendations regarding use and dose adjustment for each DOAC based on CrCl and potentially interacting drugs that inhibit the P-glycoprotein transport system and/or CYP3A metabolism (Table 40-1). Their recommendations for apixaban are based on pharmacokinetic and pharmacodynamic (anti-FXa activity) data, noting patients with CrCl < 15 mL/min were not enrolled in trials, and state that no dose adjustment is recommended for patients with renal impairment including those on dialysis. For rivaroxaban, the FDA states to avoid use with CrCl < 15 mL/min.

DOACs and Obesity. Guidance from the International Society on Thrombosis and Haemostasis (ISTH) suggests use of apixaban or rivaroxaban regardless of high body mass index (BMI) or weight,[4] and there are limited data for the use of DOAC for the treatment of acute VTE in such patients.[5]

DOAC Reversal. Idarucizumab is approved by the FDA for dabigatran reversal based on the REVERSE-AD nonrandomized trial, which included 301 patients with uncontrolled bleeding and 202 needing an urgent procedure or surgery.[6] Cessation of bleeding in those that could be assessed occurred in 67.7% at 24 hours, and hemostasis was judged as normal in 93.4% of the procedural/surgical group. Three patients in the surgery group had postoperative bleeding and were re-dosed.

Andexanet alfa is FDA-approved for reversal of apixaban and rivaroxaban based on the ANNEXA-4 nonrandomized trial, which included 352 patients with acute major bleeding.[7] Excellent or good hemostasis was achieved within 12 hours in 82%. If a specific reversal agent is not available, use of four-factor nonactivated prothrombin complex concentrate has been suggested.[8]

Inferior Vena Cava (IVC) Filters

IVC filters, particularly temporary filters that are retrievable, are widely used when therapeutic (full)–dose anticoagulation is contraindicated due to active

TABLE 40-1. Standard Treatment Dosing and Renal Adjustment for Direct Oral Anticoagulants

	APIXABAN	DABIGATRAN	EDOXABAN	RIVAROXABAN
Renal elimination	27%	80%	50%	33%
CrCl for exclusion in trials	<25 mL/min	<30 mL/min	<30 mL/min	<30 mL/min
FDA recommendations				
Initial treatment	10 mg twice daily for the first 7 days	Parenteral anticoagulant for 5–10 days	Parenteral anticoagulant for 5–10 days	15 mg twice daily for the first 21 days
Subsequent dosing	5 mg twice daily	150 mg twice daily following (not overlap) parenteral anticoagulant	60 mg once daily following (not overlap) parenteral anticoagulant	20 mg once daily
CrCl < 15 mL/min or dialysis	No dose adjustment is recommended	Dosing recommendation cannot be provided	Not recommended	Avoid use
CrCl 15 to < 30 mL/min	No dose adjustment is recommended	Dosing recommendation cannot be provided	Reduce dose	Observe closely
P-gp inhibitor	Not applicable	Avoid with CrCl < 50 mL/min	Not applicable	Not applicable
Combined P-gp and moderate CYP3A inhibitors with CrCl 15 to < 80 mL/min	Not applicable	Not applicable	Not applicable	Should not be used unless the potential benefit justifies the potential risk

CrCl, creatinine clearance; P-gp, P-glycoprotein.

bleeding or in the immediate perioperative period. Ideally, once the bleeding risk subsides and anticoagulant therapy can be resumed, we suggest IVC filter removal within 2–4 weeks, as with the increased duration of filter placement, the risk of filter-associated tilting, thrombosis, migration, and strut fracture also increases.[9]

Length of Treatment

In patients with VTE provoked by surgery, the ACCP guidelines recommend treatment of proximal DVT or PE for 3 months and suggest a similar length of treatment for isolated distal DVT.[3]

Clinical pearls

- D-dimer testing has very limited utility in diagnosing postoperative VTE.
- Assuming adequate hemostasis, anticoagulation is the treatment of choice for VTE, with DOACs preferred over warfarin.
- IVC filters (temporary) should only be used if anticoagulation is contraindicated, and they should be removed when anticoagulation can be started.
- The recommended treatment duration for a VTE provoked by surgery is 3 months.

REFERENCES

1. Anderson DR, Morgano GP, Bennett C, et al. American Society of Hematology 2019 guidelines for management of venous thromboembolism: prevention of venous thromboembolism in surgical hospitalized patients. *Blood Adv*. 2019;3(23):3898-3944. PMID: 31794602

2. Lim W, Le Gal G, Bates SM, et al. American Society of Hematology 2018 guidelines for management of venous thromboembolism: diagnosis of venous thromboembolism. *Blood Adv*. 2018;2(22):3226-3256. PMID: 30482764

3. Stevens SM, Woller SC, Kreuziger LB, et al. Antithrombotic therapy for VTE disease: second update of the CHEST guideline and expert panel report. *Chest*. 2021;160(6):e545-e608. PMID: 34352278

4. Martin KA, Beyer-Westendorf J, Davidson BL, et al. Use of direct oral anticoagulants in patients with obesity for treatment and prevention of venous thromboembolism: updated communication from the ISTH SSC subcommittee on control of anticoagulation. *J Thromb Haemost*. 2021;19(8):1874-1882. PMID: 34259389

5. Sebaaly J, Kelley D. Direct oral anticoagulants in obesity: an updated literature review. *Ann Pharmacother*. 2020;54(11):1144-1158. PMID: 32443941

6. Pollack CV Jr, Reilly PA, van Ryn J, et al. Idarucizumab for dabigatran reversal: full cohort analysis. *N Engl J Med*. 2017;377(5):431-441. PMID: 28693366

7. Connolly SJ, Crowther M, Eikelboom JW, et al. Full study report of Andexanet Alfa for bleeding associated with factor Xa inhibitors. *N Engl J Med*. 2019;380(14): 1326-1335. PMID: 30730782

8. Cuker A, Burnett A, Triller D, et al. Reversal of direct oral anticoagulants: guidance from the Anticoagulation Forum. *Am J Hematol*. 2019;94(6):697-709. PMID: 30916798

9. Duffett L, Carrier M. Inferior vena cava filters. *J Thromb Haemost*. 2017;15(1):3-12. PMID: 28019712

## 41

Acute Kidney Injury

Barbara Slawski, MD, MS, SFHM

COMMON CLINICAL QUESTIONS

1. What are the risk factors and etiologies for post-operative acute kidney injury (AKI)?
2. How do you diagnose postoperative AKI?
3. How is postop AKI treated?

INTRODUCTION

Acute kidney injury (AKI) is a potentially reversible decline in kidney function/glomerular filtration rate (GFR) that occurs over hours to days, ranging from mild to severe injury requiring renal replacement therapy (RRT). The Kidney Disease: Improving Global Outcomes (KDIGO) criteria are to define AKI (Table 41-1).[1] While AKI can occur in patients with normal kidney function, chronic kidney disease (CKD) increases perioperative risk. Although AKI is more common after cardiac surgery, its incidence after noncardiac surgery is high as well. Even small postoperative increases in creatinine are associated with adverse outcomes including higher rates of cardiovascular events, longer lengths of stay, cost, poor surgical outcomes, and mortality.

EPIDEMIOLOGY

The incidence of AKI varies depending on the population studied and definition used. Approximately 12% of postoperative patients develop AKI.[2] Cardiac and noncardiac surgeries differ in patient demographics and procedural risks, so their AKI risk also differs at 19% and 4–8% respectively.[3] Age, African American race, CKD, hypertension, and diabetes pose the greatest risk for postoperative AKI.[2]

DIAGNOSIS OF POSTOPERATIVE AKI

Serum creatinine is most commonly used to assess renal function. Small changes at low creatinine numbers reflect large changes in GFR. Creatinine levels can be misleading in patients with abnormal body habitus (amputations, paralysis, etc.), and extremes of age. GFR formulas are based on steady-state creatinine concentrations and are not reliable in extreme states. A drawback of using creatinine as an AKI indicator is that the rise in creatinine lags behind the development of AKI, delaying detection. Oliguria may also portend AKI. The Acute Disease Quality Initiative and Perioperative Quality Initiative suggested that postoperative AKI occurs when KDIGO criteria, which use a combination of the rise in creatinine and urine output, have been met within 7 days of surgery. Novel biomarkers such as neutrophil gelatinase–associated lipocalin (NGAL), IGFBP7, Cystatin C, tissue inhibitor of matrix metalloproteinase-2 (TIMP-2), and soluble urokinase plasminogen activator receptor (suPAR) show promise in detecting early AKI, particularly in cardiac surgery.[4–6] They are not widely available for clinical use, and a standard definition of AKI using these biomarkers is not available.[5]

TABLE 41-1. 2012—KDIGO Criteria for Diagnosing Acute Kidney Injury

AKI STAGE	CREATININE CHANGE	URINE OUTPUT	OTHER
1	Increased 1.5–1.9 times baseline or absolute increase of >0.3 mg/dL	<0.5 mL/kg/hr for 6–12 hours	
2	Increased 2.0–2.9 times baseline	<0.5 mL/kg/hr for >12 hours	
3	Increased >3 times baseline or absolute increase of >4 mg/dL	<0.3 mL/kg/hr for >24 hours or anuria for >12 hours	Initiation of renal replacement therapy

CAUSES AND MANAGEMENT OF POSTOPERATIVE AKI

Postoperative AKI can be multifactorial.[2] Risk factors associated with AKI are listed in Table 41-2 and are discussed below.[7] Common injury pathways affect the kidney microcirculation resulting in decreased blood flow, increased oxygen demand, and release of inflammatory mediators. Once urinary obstruction

TABLE 41-2. Perioperative Risk Factors/Etiologies for AKI

PREOPERATIVE	INTRA/POSTOPERATIVE
• Preexisting kidney dysfunction • Diabetes • Cardiac dysfunction • Age > 50 years • Sepsis • Volume depletion • Hepatic failure • Crush injury • Exposure to nephrotoxins	• Hypovolemia (due to bleeding and insensible fluid losses) • Kidney ischemia • Inflammation • Increased intra-abdominal pressure • Decreased cardiac output (anesthetic-related) • Vasodilatation (anesthetic-related) • Exposure to nephrotoxins • Urinary obstruction • Embolism • Acute lung injury • Mechanical ventilation

Source: Reproduced from Prowle JR, Forni LG, Bell M, et al. Postoperative acute kidney injury in adult non-cardiac surgery: joint consensus report of the Acute Disease Quality Initiative and PeriOperative Quality Initiative. *Nat Rev Nephrol.* 2021;17(9):605-618.

has been ruled out, the KDIGO bundle consisting of supportive measures, including volume replacement, maintenance of adequate BP targets, and avoidance of nephrotoxic agents, can be used to treat postoperative AKI.

- *Procedural risks*—cardiac surgery carries more risk than noncardiac surgery. Abdominal surgeries with high intra-abdominal venous pressure may compromise kidney blood flow and cause AKI. Enhanced recovery after surgery (ERAS) protocols do not reduce the incidence of postoperative AKI.[8]

- *Anesthesia* can result in hemodynamic changes including vasodilation that decreases blood pressure, and positive pressure ventilation that may impair cardiac venous return, resulting in lower kidney perfusion and AKI. There is growing evidence that dexmedetomidine may have postoperative renoprotective effects.[9] Recent data also demonstrate some evidence that atrial natriuretic peptides and inodilators may reduce AKI risk, mostly in the cardiac surgery population. There is no good evidence that nitric oxide donors, alpha-2-agonists, calcium channel blockers, steroids, N-acetylcysteine, or sodium bicarbonate have renoprotective effects.[10]

- *Inflammatory mediators* are released due to tissue hypoperfusion, sepsis, or cardiopulmonary bypass and can contribute to AKI.

- *Intraoperative hypotension and hypertension* have been linked to postoperative AKI, but despite multiple studies, a recommendation for a specific intraoperative mean arterial pressure is not available. Patients with older age, renal artery stenosis, diabetes, hypertension, CKD, sepsis, and hepatorenal syndrome and patients on nonsteroidal anti-inflammatory drugs (NSAIDs), angiotensin-converting enzyme inhibitors/angiotensin II receptor blockers (ACEI/ARBs), cyclosporine, and tacrolimus are at higher risk for developing normotensive ischemic acute renal failure.[11]

- *Volume status* Hypovolemia can be caused by preoperative fasting and blood loss. Hypervolemia due to fluid administration or decompensated heart failure is associated with increased AKI risk. Maintaining adequate volume status in the perioperative period is crucial.

- *Nephrotoxins* given perioperatively period increase AKI risk. NSAIDs, radiocontrast agents, and nephrotoxic antibiotics should be avoided or minimized. There is no definitive evidence that hydroxyethyl starch is associated with AKI.

- *Urinary tract obstruction related to mechanical obstruction or surgical trauma* can cause AKI. Medications can also cause urinary retention, such as anticholinergic agents, opioids, some anesthetics, alpha-adrenoceptor agonists, and benzodiazepines. Ultrasound can detect obstruction and early relief of obstruction can reverse AKI.

SUMMARY

Postoperative AKI is associated with several adverse outcomes. Aggressive preventive measures to avoid both normotensive and hypotensive ischemic acute kidney injury, avoidance of nephrotoxins, early detection and determination of AKI etiology, intervention based on etiology, and early consultation from nephrology can help prevent or improve outcomes of AKI.

Clinical pearls

- Postoperative AKI is usually diagnosed using the KDIGO criteria.

- Risk factors for AKI include type of surgical procedure, anesthesia, intraoperative hypotension, hyper/hypovolemia, nephrotoxic agents, and urinary tract obstruction.

- Treatment is directed toward the specific etiology, and nephrology consultation may be helpful.

REFERENCES

1. Kellum JA, Lameire N, Aspelin P, et al. Kidney Disease: Improving Global Outcomes Acute Kidney Injury Work Group. KDIGO clinical practice guideline for acute kidney injury. *Kidney Int Suppl.* 2012;2:1-138. PMID: 2349904

2. Gelman S. Acute kidney injury after surgery. *Anesthesiology.* 2020;132(3):5-7. PMID: 31687985

3. Grams ME, Sang Y, Coresh J, et al. Acute kidney injury after major surgery: a retrospective analysis of VHA Data. *Am J Kidney Dis.* 2016;67(6):872-880. PMID: 26337133

4. Prowle JR, Forni LG, Bell M, et al. Postoperative acute kidney injury in adult non-cardiac surgery: joint consensus report of the Acute Disease Quality Initiative and PeriOperative Quality Initiative. *Nat Rev Nephrol.* 2021;17(9):605-618. PMID: 33976395

5. Hussain ML, Hamid PF, Chakane N. Will urinary biomarkers provide a breakthrough in diagnosing cardiac surgery associated AKI?—A systematic review. *Biomarkers.* 2020;25(5):375-383. PMID: 32479185

6. Antonelli A, Allinovi M, Cocci A, et al. The predictive role of biomarkers for the detection of acute kidney injury after partial or radical nephrectomy: a systematic review of the literature. *Eur Urol Focus.* 2020;6(2):344-353. PMID: 30309817

7. Zarbock A, Koyner JL, Hoste EA, Kellum JA. Update on perioperative acute kidney injury. *Anesth Analg.* 2018;127(5):1236-1245. PMID: 30138176

8. Shen W, Wu Z, Wang Y, et al. Impact of enhanced recovery after surgery (ERAS) protocol versus standard of care on postoperative acute kidney injury (AKI): a meta-analysis. *PLoS One.* 2021;16(5):e0.251476. PMID: 34015002

9. Loomba R, Villarreal E, Dhargalker J, et al. The effect of dexmedetomidine of renal function after surgery: a systematic review and meta-analysis. *J Clin Ther.* 2022;47(3):287-297. PMID: 34510502

10. Pathal S, Olivieri G, Mohamed W, et al. Pharmacologic interventions for the prevention of renal injury in surgical patients: a systematic literature review and meta-analysis. *Br J Anes.* 2021;126(1):131-138. PMID: 32828488

11. Abuelo G. Normotensive ischemic acute renal failure. *N Engl J Med.* 2007;357:797-805. PMID: 17715412

## 42

Urinary Retention (POUR)

Paul J. Grant, MD, SFHM, FACP

COMMON CLINICAL QUESTIONS

1. What are the risk factors for POUR?
2. What are the available strategies to decrease the risk of POUR?
3. When is urinary catheterization recommended for managing POUR?

INTRODUCTION

Postoperative urinary retention (POUR) is a common postprocedural complication with a widely ranging incidence of 5–70%.[1] POUR can be defined as the inability to void after surgery despite having a full bladder. Although clinical evaluation may be suggestive of the diagnosis of POUR, it has been shown to lack sensitivity.[2] Portable ultrasound is the preferred method to diagnose POUR as urinary volumes on scan have shown a good correlation with volumes obtained from urinary catheterization. Occasionally, the diagnosis of POUR is made via urinary catheterization (which may also be therapeutic). Complications of POUR can include:

- Pain, discomfort
- Urinary infection
- Autonomic dysregulation (i.e., vomiting, bradycardia, hypo- or hypertension, cardiac arrhythmias)
- Acute kidney injury
- Bladder overdistention injury (causing adverse effects on urodynamics)
- Prolonged hospital length of stay

RISK FACTORS

Perioperative risk factors for POUR can be categorized into patient-related, procedural, and anesthetic/analgesic factors[1,2] (see Table 42-1).

PREVENTION STRATEGIES

Although limited, measures exist that may decrease the risk of POUR. If a urinary catheter is used intraoperatively, early removal is strongly advised (i.e., within 24 hours of surgery). Multimodal analgesia is an important strategy to limit the use of opioids which are a known risk factor for POUR. Early ambulation has also shown to reduce the risk of POUR.[3]

Alpha-blockers appear to be effective in reducing the risk of POUR.[4] A recent meta-analysis of randomized-controlled trials demonstrated that prophylactic use of tamsulosin (a uroselective alpha-1 blocker) was effective in reducing the risk of POUR.[5] However, tamsulosin was associated with more side effects, primarily dizziness.

TABLE 42-1. Perioperative Risk Factors for Postoperative Urinary Retention (POUR)		
PATIENT CHARACTERISTICS	**PROCEDURE-RELATED**	**ANESTHETIC/ANALGESIA FACTORS**

• Advanced age
• Men
• Benign prostatic hyperplasia
• Personal history of voiding dysfunction
• Medications:
  • Anticholinergic
  • Beta-blockers
  • Sympathomimetics
• Neurologic comorbidities:
  • Prior stroke
  • Cerebral palsy
  • Multiple sclerosis
  • Spinal lesion
  • Diabetic or alcohol-related neuropathy
	• Prolonged surgery
	• Excessive IV fluids
	• Type of surgery:
	  • Hernia
	  • Anorectal
	  • Incontinence surgery
	  • Joint arthroplasty
	• Postoperative pain
		• Spinal anesthesia
		• Epidural anesthesia
		• Perioperative opioids

MANAGEMENT

The management options for POUR consist of pharmacologic therapies and urinary catheterization. Medications can increase detrusor muscle contractility, decrease bladder outlet resistance, and facilitate micturition. Despite limited data, peripherally acting alpha-blockers (i.e., tamsulosin, alfuzosin, silodosin) quickly achieve peak serum concentrations and are reasonable options for the treatment of POUR.[1,2]

Urinary catheterization may be necessary for treating POUR and is indicated when bladder volumes exceed 600 mL on portable ultrasound. The decision to use intermittent catheterization versus an indwelling catheter is controversial. Intermittent catheterization is associated with a lower risk of urinary infection and is the preferred approach for patients who develop POUR after ambulatory surgery. If an indwelling catheter is used (i.e., after multiple intermittent catheterizations, for patient comfort or preference), removal is advised within 24 hours. If this fails, the catheter can be reinserted for prolonged bladder decompression with the goal of return to normal urinary function.[1,2] The addition of an alpha-blocker may increase the success of catheter removal.[6]

See Table 42-2 for preventive and management strategies for POUR.

TABLE 42-2. Prevention and Treatment Strategies for POUR	
Prevention	• Preoperative voiding (empty bladder) • Judicious use of IV fluids (excessive IV fluids may increase the risk of POUR) • Early removal of indwelling urinary catheter • Multimodal analgesia • Early ambulation • Consideration of alpha-blockers* (off-label use)
Treatment	• Bladder catheterization (particularly if bladder scan with >600 mL) • Consideration of alpha-blockers* (off-label use)

*Examples include tamsulosin, alfuzosin, and silodosin.

Clinical Pearls

- Prevention strategies include early removal of urinary catheters, multimodal anesthesia, early ambulation after surgery, and off-label use of alpha-blockers (i.e., tamsulosin) for high-risk patients.

- Treatment of POUR includes bladder decompression, with intermittent urinary catheterization generally preferred over an indwelling catheter, and off-label use of alpha-blockers (i.e., tamsulosin).

REFERENCES

1. Baldini G, Bagry H, Aprikian A, Carli F. Postoperative urinary retention: anesthetic and perioperative considerations. *Anesthesiology*. 2009;110:1139-1157. PMID: 19352147

2. Darrah DM, Griebling TL, Silverstein JH. Postoperative urinary retention. *Anesthesiology Clin*. 2009;27(3): 465-484. PMID: 19825487

3. Jackson J, Davies P, Leggett N, et al. Systematic review of interventions for the prevention and treatment of postoperative urinary retention. *BJS Open*. 2018;3(1):11-23. PMID: 30734011

4. Ghuman A, de Jonge SW, Dryden SD, et al. Prophylactic use of alpha-1 adrenergic blocking agents for prevention of postoperative urinary retention: a review & meta-analysis of randomized clinical trials. *Am J Surg*. 2018;215(5):973-979. PMID: 29397894

5. Zhou Z, Gan W, Li Z, et al. Can prophylactic tamsulosin reduce the risk of urinary retention after surgery? A systematic review and meta-analysis of randomized control trials. *Int J Surg*. 2023;109(3):438-448. PMID: 36912745

6. Fisher E, Subramonian K, Omar MI. The role of alpha blockers prior to removal of urethral catheter for acute urinary retention in men. *Cochrane Database Syst Rev*. 2014;(6):CD006744. PMID: 24913721

Nausea and Vomiting (PONV)

Deborah C. Richman, MBChB, FFA(SA) and Tong J. Gan, MD, MBA, MHS, FASA, FRCA

COMMON CLINICAL QUESTIONS

1. Who is at risk of PONV?
2. What is the best management approach to the patient with resistant recurrent PONV?
3. What is recommended for rescue therapy after failed PONV prophylaxis?

INTRODUCTION

Postoperative nausea and vomiting (PONV) is one of the commonest and most dreaded postoperative complications, often worse than operative pain. Up to 80% of patients will have PONV if not given prophylaxis. Modern anesthetic agents and the standard use of multimodal prophylactic antiemetic agents have reduced both the occurrence and the severity and duration of PONV. PONV usually occurs in the first 24 hours after surgery. It includes early (in the postanesthesia care unit [PACU]) and late symptoms—either in the hospital or postdischarge nausea and vomiting (PDNV) following ambulatory surgery. PONV is associated with a number of complications including low patient satisfaction scores, wound disruption, esophageal injury, pulmonary aspiration, dehydration, and increased length of stay—all associated with additional costs to the healthcare system.

PATHOPHYSIOLOGY

The pathophysiology of PONV is multifactorial, involving multiple sites: supratentorial, nausea, and vomiting center—a central pattern generator and the chemoreceptor trigger zone (CTZ)—both in the medulla, peripheral nervous system, vestibular system, and the gastrointestinal (GI) tract that have different receptors that can all trigger PONV. These sites interact and can be additive. The primary receptors involved are dopamine 2 (DA_2), histamine 1 (H_1), muscarinic 1 (M_1), neurokinin 1—substance P (NK_1), and 5 hydroxytryptamine—3 ($5HT_3$) or serotonin.

RISKS

Risk factors and triggers for PONV include surgical, anesthesia, and patient factors (Table 43-1).

A validated, easy to implement clinical risk score (Apfel score)[1] assigns one point for each of four risk factors—female sex, history of PONV or motion sickness, nonsmoker, postoperative opioid use. PONV incidence increases with each additional point.

PROPHYLAXIS (TABLE 43-2)

General measures to avoid the above risk factors, dehydration, ketosis, and GI instrumentation are all important adjuvants to pharmacological prophylaxis. Standard chemoprophylaxis is intravenous

TABLE 43-1. Risk factors for PONV[1,2]

APFEL RISK SCORE—4 FACTORS *RISK INCREASES WITH EACH ADDITIONAL FACTOR*	GENERAL	PATIENT	SURGICAL (TYPE/ SITE/DURATION)	ANESTHESIA AGENTS
1. Female sex	Pain	Female sex	Otorhinolaryngology	Opioids
2. Nonsmoker	Movement Rapid/jolting transport to PACU	Younger age	Ophthalmology	Nitrous oxide
3. History of: • PONV and/or • Motion sickness	Gagging on airway devices		Gynecology	Volatile inhalational agents
4. Postoperative opioid usage	GI tract: • Stimulation • Hypoperfusion		Plastic surgery	Ketamine
	Preexisting nausea and vomiting • GI pathology • Chemotherapy		Laparoscopic procedure	Etomidate
			Increased duration of procedure	

PONV, postoperative nausea and vomiting; PACU, postanesthesia care unit; GI, gastrointestinal.

ondansetron and dexamethasone for patients with an Apfel score of 2, with the addition of 3rd and 4th agents for those at higher risk.[3-5] Choice of anesthesia agents includes avoidance of inhaled agents by using total intravenous anesthesia (TIVA) with propofol, and multimodal analgesia including the use of local or regional anesthesia to minimize opioid use.

The nonpharmacological option of acupuncture is efficacious in reducing PONV.[1] Cannabinoids, although effective in preventing chemotherapy nausea and vomiting, have not been shown to decrease PONV.[6]

Patients with a history of refractory PONV need special attention and reassurance. They often delay needed procedures out of fear of PONV. One should never promise that their symptoms won't recur. Involve the patient in the process and provide reassurance that there are always additional options that can be used, and that they "should not give up" on us.

RESCUE TREATMENT

First-line treatment in the PACU should be a drug that works at a different site than those given initially for prophylaxis. Amisulpride, diphenhydramine, droperidol, and propofol can be considered.[7] All antiemetics have adverse effects, and these should be considered in treatment decisions.[4,8]

PONV with its attendant complications is the ongoing focus of research and best practice recommendation. The importance of prevention is obvious in the era of ambulatory surgery. Return of normal GI function is a key driver in the success of enhanced recovery after surgery (ERAS) programs, consequently PONV prevention is bundled into comprehensive ERAS protocols.

The 2020 PONV consensus guidelines from Society of Ambulatory Anesthesia (SAMBA) and American Society for Enhanced Recovery (ASER)[2,9] provide a more comprehensive discussion of the topic. Their approach to risk assessment and management is summarized in Figure 43-1. Updates are expected in 2025.

TABLE 43-2. Apfel Score, PONV Risk, and Prophylaxis Recommendations

APFEL SCORE	RISK/% PONV WITHOUT PROPHYLAXIS	PROPHYLAXIS	MEDICATION	RECEPTOR— SITE OF ACTION	SIDE EFFECTS	COMMENTS
0	Low/10	General measures				
1	Low/20	General measures Consider 1–2 agents if PONV poses specific risk (e.g., raised intracranial pressure)	Ondansetron 4 mg IV at end of procedure or:	Serotonin 5HT$_3$	• QT prolongation • Constipation • Headache	
			Palonosetron 0.075 mg IV			2nd generation— higher affinity/longer duration of action
			Corticosteroids dexamethasone 4–8 mg IV on induction		Hyperglycemia	
2	Moderate/40	2 agents:	As above			
3	Moderate/60	3 agents:	As above + other: Aprepitant 40 mg IV or po preoperatively prior to induction	NK$_1$	• Constipation ➡ Efficacy hormonal contraception	Duration—24 hours
			Butyrophenone Droperidol 0.625 mg IV at end of surgery	DA$_2$	• QT prolongation • Extrapyramidal effects	• Avoid in Parkinson's disease • Avoid in patient with hyper-prolactinemia
			Amisulpride 5 mg IV on induction	DA$_2$ (and serotonin)	• Minimal CNS side effects	• Avoid in Parkinson's disease • Avoid in patient with hyper-prolactinemia • **Rescue option** • 24-hour effect

(Continued)

TABLE 43-2. Apfel Score, PONV Risk, and Prophylaxis Recommendations *(Continued)*

APFEL SCORE	RISK/% PONV WITHOUT PROPHYLAXIS	PROPHYLAXIS	MEDICATION	RECEPTOR— SITE OF ACTION	SIDE EFFECTS	COMMENTS
			Anticholinergic Scopolamine patch (1.5 mg placed 4 hours earlier)	M_1	• Sedation/dizziness • Dry mouth • Visual disturbances • Urinary retention	*Beers criteria medication—avoid in elderly Patch releases 0.5 mg/24 hours for 72 hours
			Antihistamine Diphenhydramine 12.5 mg IV Promethazine 6.25 mg IV	H_1	• Sedation	Beers criteria medication—avoid in elderly **Rescue option**
			Olanzapine 10 mg po	$5HT_3$; $DA_{1\&2}$; H_1, M_1	• Sedation	Duration—24 hours
			Opioid sparing techniques			
			Acupuncture prior to induction			
4	High/80	4 agents/ interventions:	• From choice above • TIVA—propofol			
			• Propofol 20 mg IV			**Rescue option**

DA_2, dopamine 2; H_1, histamine 1; IV, intravenous; M_2, muscarinic; NK_1, neurokinin 1; po, per os/orally; PONV, postoperative nausea and vomiting; QT, interval from Q to end of T wave on electrocardiogram; TIVA, total intravenous anesthesia.

*Beers criteria drugs—medications to be avoided in older patients due to increased risk to benefit ratio. First published 1991, current version (7th) American Geriatrics Society 2023 updated AGS Beers Criteria for potentially inappropriate medication use in older adults. *J Am Geriatr Soc.* 2023;71(7):2052-2081.

Adult PONV R̲x Management

1 RISK FACTORS

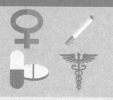

Female sex
Younger age
Nonsmoker
Surgery type

History of
PONV/motion sickness

Opioid analgesia

2 RISK MITIGATION

Minimize use of nitrous oxide, volatile anesthetics, high-dose neostigmine

Consider regional anesthesia

Opioid sparing/ multimodal analgesia (enhanced recovery pathways)

3 RISK STRATIFICATION

Quantify the # of risk factors to determine risk and guide anti-emetic therapy

1–2 Risk Factors

Give 2 agents

>2 Risk Factors

Give 3–4 agents

4 PROPHYLAXIS

5HT₃ receptor antagonists

Antihistamines

Propofol anesthesia

Acupuncture

Corticosteroids

Dopamine antagonists

NK-1 receptor antagonists

Anticholinergics

5 RESCUE TREATMENT

Use antiemetic from different class than prophylactic drug

FIGURE 43-1. Evaluation and management of PONV.
Reproduced with permission from Gan TJ, Belani KG, Bergese S, et al., Fourth Consensus Guidelines for the Management of Postoperative Nausea and Vomiting. *Anesth Analg.* 2020;131(2):411-448.

Clinical Pearls

- Antiemetic prophylaxis is more effective than rescue treatment and is recommended in a stepwise fashion according to risk scores.

- Rescue treatment of PONV in the postanesthesia care unit (PACU) should be with a different agent from those already used for prophylaxis.

- Choice of medication takes into consideration associated interactions/adverse effects.

- There is no guarantee that PONV will not occur/recur with subsequent surgeries, but patients should be reassured that there are many options for PONV prevention and that careful management can be successful.

REFERENCES

1. Apfel CC, Läärä E, Koivuranta M, et al. A simplified risk score for predicting postoperative nausea and vomiting: conclusions from cross-validations between two centers. *Anesthesiology.* 1999;91(3):693-700. PMID: 10485781

2. Gan TJ, Belani KG, Bergese S, et al. Fourth consensus guidelines for the management of postoperative nausea and vomiting. *Anesth Analg.* 2020;131(2):411-448. PMID: 32467512

3. Hyman JB, Park C, Lin HM, et al. Olanzapine for the prevention of postdischarge nausea and vomiting after ambulatory surgery: a randomized controlled trial. *Anesthesiology.* 2020;132(6):1419-1428. PMID: 32229754

4. Huang Q, Wang F, Liang C, et al. Fosaprepitant for postoperative nausea and vomiting in patients undergoing laparoscopic gastrointestinal surgery: a randomised trial. *Br J Anaesth.* 2023;131(4):673-681. PMID: 37423834

5. Kang C, Shirley M. Amisulpride: a review in post-operative nausea and vomiting. *Drugs.* 2021;81(3):367-375. PMID: 33656662

6. Levin DN, Dulberg Z, Chan AW, et al. A randomized-controlled trial of nabilone for the prevention of acute postoperative nausea and vomiting in elective surgery. *Can J Anaesth.* 2017;64(4):385-395. PMID: 28160217

7. Gan TJ, Jin Z, Meyer TA. Rescue treatment of postoperative nausea and vomiting: a systematic review of current clinical evidence. *Anesth Analg.* 2022;135(5):986-1000. PMID: 36048730

8. Weibel S, Rücker G, Eberhart LH, et al. Drugs for preventing postoperative nausea and vomiting in adults after general anaesthesia: an abridged Cochrane network meta-analysis. *Anaesthesia.* 2021;76(7):962-973. PMID: 33075160

9. Scott MJ, Aggarwal G, Aitken RJ, et al. Consensus guidelines for perioperative care for emergency laparotomy enhanced recovery after surgery (ERAS). *World J Surg.* 2023;47(8):1850-1880. PMID: 37277507

## 44

Delirium

Heather E. Nye, MD, PhD, SFHM, FACP and Daniel I. McIsaac, MD, MPH, FRCPC

COMMON CLINICAL QUESTIONS

1. What are the clinical features of delirium?
2. What are risk factors for the development of postoperative delirium?
3. What tools are available to diagnose delirium?
4. What measures can be taken to reduce the risk of developing delirium?

INTRODUCTION

Postoperative delirium is defined as a fluctuating state of confusion marked by impaired cognition, attention, and/or awareness. It occurs with acute onset typically in the first 1–2 days following surgery and is most commonly seen in older adults. Incidence ranges from 5% to 50%, with the highest delirium rates observed following cardiothoracic, major vascular, and emergent orthopedic surgeries.[1] Postoperative delirium is strongly associated with adverse outcomes such as increased risk of prolonged hospitalization, mortality, cognitive and functional decline, and discharge to an institution. Delirium's causal role in adverse outcomes remains unclear; however, given the burden it places on patients, families, and healthcare systems, delirium prevention programs are critical. A three-pronged approach to delirium includes: (1) early delirium risk assessment, (2) evidence-based preventative measures, and (3) prompt diagnosis and treatment of underlying causes (see Figure 44-1).[2]

RISK ASSESSMENT

Preoperative delirium risk assessment is outlined in Chapter 31 and should be performed in all adults over 65 years old undergoing surgery. Though multivariable risk models do exist, none show clear superiority to individual patient-level risk factors. A personal history of delirium, frailty, or preexisting cognitive impairment increases the odds of delirium at least 2.5-fold.[3] Procedural and environmental factors likewise impact risk, with greater delirium incidence seen following emergency, complex or prolonged surgeries, and in patients experiencing immobilization, frequent ward transfers, or disruption of sleep.

DELIRIUM REDUCTION STRATEGIES

Up to 40% of cases of delirium may be prevented through conservative measures. Preoperative interventions include patient and family education, reduction of EtOH intake, and avoiding deliriogenic medications. Studies of cognitive prehabilitation show possible benefit, but additional research is needed.

In hospital, nonpharmacologic multicomponent delirium prevention programs are most likely to reduce delirium incidence (~8% absolute decrease).[4] Such programs can include relatively simple approaches like delirium-friendly preprinted orders, or more resource-intensive nurse-led delirium prevention programs. Orientation, cognitive stimulation, and enhanced sleep hygiene should be prioritized.

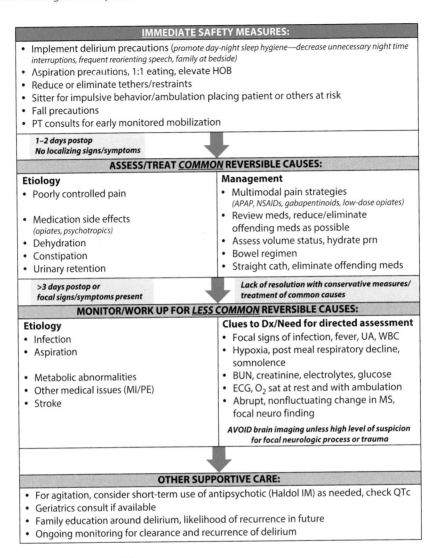

IMMEDIATE SAFETY MEASURES:
- Implement delirium precautions (*promote day-night sleep hygiene—decrease unnecessary night time interruptions, frequent reorienting speech, family at bedside*)
- Aspiration precautions, 1:1 eating, elevate HOB
- Reduce or eliminate tethers/restraints
- Sitter for impulsive behavior/ambulation placing patient or others at risk
- Fall precautions
- PT consults for early monitored mobilization

1–2 days postop
No localizing signs/symptoms

ASSESS/TREAT *COMMON* REVERSIBLE CAUSES:

Etiology	Management
• Poorly controlled pain	• Multimodal pain strategies (*APAP, NSAIDs, gabapentinoids, low-dose opiates*)
• Medication side effects (*opiates, psychotropics*)	• Review meds, reduce/eliminate offending meds as possible
• Dehydration	• Assess volume status, hydrate prn
• Constipation	• Bowel regimen
• Urinary retention	• Straight cath, eliminate offending meds

>3 days postop or focal signs/symptoms present

Lack of resolution with conservative measures/ treatment of common causes

MONITOR/WORK UP FOR *LESS COMMON* REVERSIBLE CAUSES:

Etiology	Clues to Dx/Need for directed assessment
• Infection	• Focal signs of infection, fever, UA, WBC
• Aspiration	• Hypoxia, post meal respiratory decline, somnolence
• Metabolic abnormalities	• BUN, creatinine, electrolytes, glucose
• Other medical issues (MI/PE)	• ECG, O_2 sat at rest and with ambulation
• Stroke	• Abrupt, nonfluctuating change in MS, focal neuro finding

AVOID brain imaging unless high level of suspicion for focal neurologic process or trauma

OTHER SUPPORTIVE CARE:
- For agitation, consider short-term use of antipsychotic (Haldol IM) as needed, check QTc
- Geriatrics consult if available
- Family education around delirium, likelihood of recurrence in future
- Ongoing monitoring for clearance and recurrence of delirium

FIGURE 44-1. Approach to postoperative delirium.

Nutrition, oxygenation, mobilization, medication review, and attention to bowel and bladder care are also likely beneficial.[2,4] Comprehensive risk reduction strategies are outlined in Chapter 31, Table 31-4.

Pharmacologic delirium prevention strategies are also well studied, but most agents, including antipsychotics and cholinesterase inhibitors, do not demonstrate efficacy.[5] Uncertain evidence exists for melatonin, and to a lesser degree, ramelteon.[6] Intraoperatively, several strategies can be considered to reduce delirium risk. Targeting a relatively light plane of general anesthesia reduced delirium risk by 9% in a multicenter trial. Several meta-analyses suggest that use of dexmedetomidine in patients receiving general anesthesia may reduce incidence of delirium. Optimal timing, dosing and duration, and administration remain unclear, and risks of bradycardia and hypotension exist. Some evidence supports the use of propofol-based total intravenous anesthesia (TIVA) instead of volatile anesthesia. Whether use of regional anesthesia reduces delirium remains uncertain; two large multicenter trials in hip fracture showed no benefit from spinal compared to general anesthesia.[7] In hip fracture patients, moderate certainty evidence supports use of peripheral nerve blocks analgesia to reduce delirium.[8]

Diagnosis

Delirium can manifest as either hyperactive, hypo-active, or delirium with mixed features (Table 44-1) and commonly goes underrecognized. Daily screen-ing in high-risk patients is recommended, preferably using validated and feasible tools like the Confusion Assessment Method (CAM, sensitivity 91–97%; speci-ficity 85–94%) and the 4AT (sensitivity 80–93%; spec-ificity 83–93%). Available comparisons suggest that the CAM may have higher specificity and the 4AT higher sensitivity, with clinicians preferring the 4AT (Table 44-2).

Management

Once delirium is diagnosed, supportive measures to prevent subsequent complications should be insti-tuted. Nursing-based protocols may include 1:1 mon-itoring during meals, elevation of the head of the bed, facilitated ambulation (with physical therapy and assist device), and a bedside sitter as necessary.[9] Workup for reversible causes beyond the surgical diagnosis, such as metabolic irregularities, infection, pain, constipa-tion, urinary retention, and myocardial ischemia, can

TABLE 44-1. Features of Postoperative Delirium

HYPERACTIVE	HYPOACTIVE
Agitation	Somnolence
Pacing, restlessness	Social withdrawal
Rapid mood changes	Apathy
Hallucinations	Reduced motor activity
Delusions	Sluggishness

be guided by the clinical scenario. Importantly, both uncontrolled surgical pain due to inadequate analgesia and unnecessarily high doses of opioids may precipi-tate delirium.

Pharmacologic treatment for delirium should be used sparingly and limited to low-dose antipsychotic drugs (APDs) for extreme agitation where patients place themselves or others at risk—and for when behavioral measures have been exhausted.[10] Though current evidence is mixed and of poor quality, APDs may shorten delirium course, but are also associ-ated with increased risk for stroke and sudden death. There is no evidence for delirium treatment with benzodiazepines.

TABLE 44-2. Delirium Screening Tools

CONFUSION ASSESSMENT METHOD (CAM)		
	CLINICAL FEATURE	**EXAMPLES**
1	Acute onset or fluctuating course	Change in behavior over hours to days, worse sometimes than others
2	Inattention	Distractible, poor focus, cannot follow conversation
3	Disorganized thinking	Rambling, tangential, nonsensical speech
4	Altered level of consciousness	Hyperalert, somnolent

Delirium is present when 1 and 2 are BOTH present along with EITHER 3 or 4.
Source: Adapted from Inouye S, van Dyck C, Alessi C. et al. Clarifying confusion: the confusion assessment method. *Ann Intern Med.* 1990;113(12):941-948.

FOUR 'A'S TEST (4AT)			
4AT	**TASK**	**RESULT**	**POINTS**
ALERTNESS	Observe patient, attempt to wake with speech/touch, ask to state name	Alert, no agitation	0
		Mildly sleepy <10 sec	0
		Sleepy	4

(Continued)

FOUR 'A'S TEST (4AT)			
4AT	**TASK**	**RESULT**	**POINTS**
AMT4 *(Abbreviated Mental Test)*	State age, date of birth, place, current year	No mistakes	0
		1 mistake	1
		≥2 mistakes	2
ATTENTION	State months of year backwards	≥7 months correct	0
		<7 months or refuses	1
		Untestable (drowsy, cannot understand)	2
ACUTE CHANGE or FLUCTUATING COURSE		No	0
		Yes	4

SCORING: ≥4 possible delirium +/− cognitive impairment

1–3: possible cognitive impairment

0: delirium or severe cognitive impairment unlikely

Source: Bellelli G, Morandi A, Davis DH, et al. Validation of the 4AT, a new instrument for rapid delirium screening: a study in 234 hospitalised older people. *Age Ageing*. 2014;43:496-502.

Clinical pearls

- In patients at high risk for delirium, nonpharmacologic, multicomponent delirium prevention programs that stress re-orientation, cognitive stimulation and sleep hygiene should be instituted. If delirium develops, take additional measures to prevent complications, such as falls and aspiration and assess and treat reversible causes.

- Optimal approaches to intraoperative analgesia for delirium prevention remain an important target for research, but promising data support use of dexmedetomidine as an adjunct to general anesthesia or as sedation during regional anesthesia.

- For hip fracture patients, a peripheral nerve block is the preferred delirium-sparing analgesic modality.

- Maintain a high index of suspicion for delirium and perform daily screening for those at highest risk using a tool like the confusion assessment method (CAM) or 4AT.

- Pharmacologic treatment for delirium should be used sparingly, limited to low-dose antipsychotic drugs (APDs) such as haloperidol, and reserved for patients with extreme agitation, placing themselves or others at risk, after other behavioral measures have been exhausted.

REFERENCES

1. Jin Z, Hu J, Ma D. Postoperative delirium: perioperative assessment, risk reduction, and management. *Br J Anaesth*. 2020;125(4):492-504. PMID: 32798069
2. American Geriatrics Society Expert Panel on Postoperative Delirium in Older Adults. Postoperative delirium in older adults: best practice statement from the American Geriatrics Society. *J Am Coll Surg*. 2015;220(2):136-148.e1. PMID: 25535170
3. Watt J, Tricco AC, Talbot-Hamon C, et al. Identifying older adults at risk of delirium following elective surgery: a systematic review and meta-analysis. *J Gen Intern Med*. 2018;33(4):500-509. PMID: 29374358
4. Burton JK, Craig LE, Yong SQ, et al. Non-pharmacological interventions for preventing delirium

in hospitalised non-ICU patients. *Cochrane Database Syst Rev.* 2021;7:CD013307. PMID: 34826144

5. Schrijver EJM, de Vries OJ, van de Ven PM, et al. Haloperidol versus placebo for delirium prevention in acutely hospitalised older at risk patients: a multi centre double-blind randomised controlled clinical trial. *Age Ageing.* 2018;47(1):48-55. PMID: 28985255

6. Campbell AM, Axon DR, Martin JR, Slack MK, Mollon L, Lee JK. Melatonin for the prevention of postoperative delirium in older adults: a systematic review and meta-analysis. *BMC Geriatr.* 2019;19(1):272. PMID: 31619178

7. Neuman MD, Feng R, Carson JL, et al. Spinal anesthesia or general anesthesia for hip surgery in older adults. *N Engl J Med.* 2021;385(22):2025-2035. PMID: 34623788

8. Guay J, Kopp S. Peripheral nerve blocks for hip fractures in adults. *Cochrane Database Syst Rev.* 2020;11:CD001159. PMID: 33238043

9. Mohanty S, Rosenthal RA, Russell MM, et al. Optimal perioperative management of the geriatric patient: a best practices guideline from the American College of Surgeons NSQIP and the American Geriatrics Society. *J Am Coll Surg.* 2016;222(5):930-947. PMID: 27049783

10. Scicutella A. The pharmacotherapeutic management of postoperative delirium: an expert update. *Expert Opin Pharmacother.* 2020;21(8):905-916. PMID: 32156151

## 45

Pain Management

Christine E. Boxhorn, MD, DABA

COMMON CLINICAL QUESTIONS

1. What tools are available to assess pain severity?
2. How do you choose and manage opioids?
3. Should buprenorphine be stopped pre-operatively?

INTRODUCTION

It is important to realize the difference between nociception and pain. Nociception is when a noxious stimulus depolarizes sensory nerves, which provide the brain with information about tissue injury. Nociception is neither necessary nor sufficient for pain. Pain is a subjective experience, the consequence of filtering, modulating, and distorting nociception through an individual's affective and cognitive processes.

Pain Management Essentials

Tailoring multimodal approaches (both pharmacologic and nonpharmacologic) to the needs, desires, and circumstances of the patient, as opposed to using a single modality to its "limit," provides better analgesia with the lowest incidence of side effects.[1,2] Use a collaborative plan that includes patient input. Pain management does not end on discharge; coordinating with the outpatient provider is necessary.

ASSESSMENT

Ask the patient which analgesics have either worked or not in the past, as well as the exact doses of any analgesics they were taking prior to admission. The "OPQRST" mnemonic acronym helps ensure a comprehensive pain assessment (Table 45-1).[3]

The most common tools for assessing pain severity are single dimension scales such as the verbal numeric scale where patients state a number between 0 ("no pain") and 10 ("worst pain imaginable").[1] There are also observer-based, behavioral scales for specific patient-populations (e.g., pre-verbal children, sedated ICU patients, and those who are cognitively impaired or have dementia).

Single-dimensional scales are quick and easy; however, one major disadvantage is that they assign a single value to a complex, multidimensional experience, and providers base management decisions on this value. The goals for analgesia should be based on function, not an arbitrary numeric pain value. Therefore, determine the impact of pain on the patient's ability to do the things they need to recover (e.g., coughing, deep breathing, getting out of bed, and ambulating). Using a functional pain scale with subjective and objective components can help with this. The most important part of the assessment is having the patient describe the quality of the pain using adjectives. This provides information on the "mechanism" of the pain and guides the choice of analgesics (Table 45-2).[1]

TABLE 45-1. A Mnemonic Acronym for Pain Assessment

LETTER	ASSESSMENT POINT	QUESTION EXAMPLES
O	Onset	When did the pain start? What was happening at that time?
P	Palliative and provocative factors	What makes the pain better? What makes the pain worse?
Q	Quality	What is the character of the pain? What does it feel like? Describe the pain using adjectives.
R	Region and radiation	Where is the pain? Does it spread to other areas?
S	Severity	How bad is the pain?
T	Timing	When does the pain occur? Has it changed since the onset? If so, how?

TABLE 45-2. Pain Quality Assessment to Determine Mechanism and Treatment Options

MECHANISM	CHARACTERISTICS	EXAMPLES	TREATMENT OPTIONS
Somatic—from musculoskeletal or cutaneous sources	Well localized; constant; sharp, stabbing	Laceration, fracture, burn, abrasion, localized infection or inflammation, muscle spasm	Heat/cold, acetaminophen, NSAIDs, opioids, muscle relaxants, local anesthetics (topical or infiltrate)
Visceral—from internal organs	Not well localized; constant or intermittent; ache, cramp, or pressure, can be sharp	Colic or obstruction (GI or renal), organ infection or inflammation	NSAIDs, opioids, local anesthetics (nerve-blocks)
Neuropathic—from the somatosensory nervous system	Localized or radiating; can also be diffuse; burning, tingling, electric shock, lancinating	Trigeminal, postherpetic, postamputation, peripheral neuropathy, nerve infiltration	Anticonvulsants, antidepressants, NMDA antagonists, neural or neuraxial blockade

PATIENT EDUCATION

Discuss evidence-based options, realistic goals, and reasonable expectations of benefit. Tell patients that they will have pain, but everything will be tried to make them comfortable enough to recover. Promote the benefits of nonpharmacologic and nonopioid options. If opioids are part of the plan, discuss benefits versus risks.

On discharge, explain the likely course of pain over time. Ensure patients understand the characteristics of the analgesics (e.g., dosing, side effect management, precautions). Discuss the medications that must be tapered (e.g., opioids, gabapentin, several muscle relaxants, antidepressants). In addition, if patients are on opioids, describe safe use (e.g., taking as prescribed, no driving, no drinking) and proper storage and disposal. Educate patients on symptoms of neuropathic pain (a potential harbinger of persistent postsurgical pain) and to contact a healthcare provider if they develop, as the analgesic regimen may require adjustment.

ANALGESIC MODALITIES

It is not possible to design "one-size-fits-all" regimens—one must use available modalities, considering patient variability (for analgesia and side effects of medications) and the specific clinical situation.

Nonpharmacologic Measures

Application of cold (for inflammation) or heat (for spasms) is a commonly employed technique but evidence for benefits is mixed.[1,2] Hypnosis has been shown to reduce pain associated with medical procedures. Transcutaneous electrical nerve stimulation (TENS) is associated with less postoperative analgesic use. There is limited evidence of benefit from relaxation and guided imagery in the acute setting. Acupuncture and electroacupuncture improve pain and reduce common opioid side effects. Virtual/augmented reality reduces pain and unpleasantness from certain procedures.

Nonopioid Analgesics

Table 45-3 lists select agents from various classes. These are the most important parts of effective multimodal

TABLE 45-3. Select Nonopioid Analgesics

CLASS	AGENT	COMMENTS
	Acetaminophen	• No anti-inflammatory effect • No incidence of GI complications or antiplatelet effects • Single doses above 1,000 mg do not improve analgesia
NSAIDs	Diclofenac	• Low incidence of GI complications • Possible increased CV and renal complications
	Etodolac	• Low incidence of GI and renal complications • Safest NSAID in liver disease
	Ibuprofen	• Ceiling effect for analgesia at 400 mg • <1500 mg QD has low incidence of GI complications • Possible increased renal complications • Inhibits CV benefits of aspirin when given concomitantly
	Ketorolac	• High incidence of renal and GI complications • Use for no more than 5 days • Doses of 7.5–10 mg as effective as higher doses
	Nabumetone	• Low incidence of GI complications
	Naproxen	• Possible increased liver and renal complications • Probably lowest incidence of CV complications
COX-2 inhibitor	Celecoxib	• Long-term use has serious CV complications
Antiepileptics	Gabapentin, Pregabalin	• Treat neuropathic pain • May not have analgesic and opioid-sparing effects in the perioperative setting, as originally thought • Dizziness and sedation common with high-dose acute administration • Combined with opioids, the risk of overdose death increases 4× through reversal of tolerance and/or an additive effect on respiratory depression, plus sedation is increased • Gabapentin is misused by 40–65% of individuals with prescriptions and between 15% and 22% of people with an opioid use disorder • Do not stop abruptly, must be weaned to avoid possible seizures

(Continued)

TABLE 45-3. Select Nonopioid Analgesics (*Continued*)

CLASS	AGENT	COMMENTS
Antidepressants	Amitriptyline	• Treat neuropathic pain, limited data on effectiveness in acute settings • Anticholinergic symptoms (e.g., dry mouth, confusion), especially in elderly • Sedation common, use at nighttime
	Duloxetine	• Treat neuropathic pain, limited data on effectiveness in acute settings • Anticholinergic symptoms • Possibility of serotonin syndrome if used with similar agents • Can see sedation or insomnia • Sweating common
Skeletal muscle relaxants	Methocarbamol	• Drowsiness, irritability • Avoid in hepatic or renal dysfunction and in elderly
	Tizanidine	• Drowsiness • Sedation and hypotension • Avoid in hepatic or renal dysfunction and in elderly • After long-term use must be weaned to avoid withdrawal
	Orphenadrine	• Drowsiness and anticholinergic symptoms • Avoid in elderly • Caution in CAD, CHF, and cardiac arrythmias • Only muscle relaxant available in an IV formulation
Antispasmodic	Baclofen	• Drowsiness possible, but usually minimal at 5–10 mg every 6 hours dosing • Many drug-drug interactions • After long-term use must be weaned to avoid withdrawal, including possible seizures
NMDA antagonists	Ketamine	• Improves pain scores and has a 50% opioid-sparing effect, though equivocal reduction of opioid-induced side effect • Sedation, dreams, and hallucinations possible but infrequent at analgesic (low) dose
	Amantadine, Dextromethorphan	• Effective dosing usually limited by sedation
	Memantine	• Low incidence of side effects and drug-interactions
Alpha-2 agonists	Clonidine	• Hypotension and sedation possible, but usually minor • If used for >1 week, monitor for rebound hypertension on stopping
	Dexmedetomidine	• Opioid sparing effects • Analgesic effects only occur at sedating doses
Antiarrhythmic	Lidocaine	• IV infusions for up to 24 hours improve pain after open or laparoscopic abdominal surgery • Utility outside of abdominal surgery poorly defined

NSAID, nonsteroidal anti-inflammatory agent; GI, gastrointestinal; CV, cardiovascular; CAD, coronary artery disease; CHF, congestive heart failure.

analgesia; they should be the primary treatments and opioids should be the adjunct.[2]

Unless absolutely contraindicated, all patients with acute pain should receive acetaminophen and/or an NSAID around the clock. Combining an NSAID and acetaminophen is more effective than either drug alone. No NSAID is more effective than another, but there is interpatient variability in response, thus changing agents may be of benefit if one is not effective.

Gabapentinoids, such as gabapentin and pregabalin, have been used preoperatively to reduce postoperative opioid consumption and pain levels. The peak plasma concentration of gabapentin is 2–4 hours with peak CSF levels occurring much later; thus, if it is going to be used, preoperative dosing likely needs to occur significantly earlier than the day of surgery to exert its full beneficial effects. That being said, it appears that preoperative gabapentinoid administration may not confer any significant postoperative analgesic activity yet increases the rate of adverse outcomes.[4]

Benzodiazepines

Benzodiazepines are *NOT* analgesics and must be used with caution, especially when high doses of opioids are required, as significant sedation and respiratory depression can occur in benzodiazepine-naïve patients. In an anxious patient with pain, adequately titrate analgesics before the addition of a benzodiazepine. Diazepam does have muscle relaxation properties, so it may be useful as an IV agent in patients experiencing muscle spasms who cannot take orals. But, as soon as possible, switch them to a "true" muscle relaxant or antispasmodic.

Opioids

Safe Use. Opioids are first-line therapy for moderate-to-severe pain following major surgery and trauma; however, they should never be the only consideration for postoperative pain management. Determine if the patient has risk factors for opioid-induced sedation, respiratory depression (Table 45-4), and/or opioid misuse (Table 45-5). The Opioid Risk Tool, a five-item clinician-completed checklist, can help predict future aberrant drug-related behaviors. If the patient is on opioids preoperatively, or opioids are to be used on discharge, it is imperative to check the prescription drug monitoring program for any signs of misuse. Co-prescribe naloxone for patients discharged on opioids (especially for doses greater than 50 morphine mg equivalents/day).

Choice of Agent. Other than the patient knowing a particular agent has worked previously, it is not possible to determine which opioid may work best. However, some agents require special mention. Meperidine is not recommended because its active metabolite can accumulate in a day or two and cause nervous system excitation. In addition, it causes a strong euphoric

TABLE 45-4. Risk Factors for Opioid-Induced Sedation or Respiratory Depression	
CLASSIFICATION	RISK FACTOR
Dosing-related	Daily opioid dose >100 MME
	Use of long-acting or extended-release opioid formulation
	Combination of opioids with benzodiazepines or other sedatives
	Long-term opioid use (e.g., >3 months)
Patient-related	Age > 65 years old
	Sleep-disordered breathing
	Morbid obesity
	Renal or hepatic impairment

MME, morphine milligram equivalents.

TABLE 45-5. Risk Factors for Longer-Term Opioid Use or Misuse

CLASSIFICATION	RISK FACTOR
Dosing-related	Daily opioid dose >100 MME
	Long-term opioid use (e.g., >3 months)
Patient-related	Concurrent SUD (including alcohol or cigarettes)
	History of SUD in patient or family
	Prior misuse or aberrant behaviors
	Younger age (especially adolescents)
	Attention deficit hyperactivity disorder and/or obsessive-compulsive disorder
	Depression, bipolar disorder, and/or anxiety
	Significant life stressors or poor social support

MME, morphine milligram equivalents; SUD, substance use disorder.

feeling, especially when given as an intravenous bolus. Morphine is relatively contraindicated in the frail elderly and patients with severe renal insufficiency due to the accumulation of an active metabolite, which can lead to sedation and respiratory depression. Tramadol is also a serotonin–norepinephrine reuptake inhibitor and may interact with antidepressants and migraine medications (i.e., triptans, ergots) leading to serotonin syndrome. Additionally, its euphoric potential is the same as heroin or methamphetamine.[5] A recent study showed that tramadol was associated with a slightly higher risk of prolonged use after surgery, compared with other short-acting opioids.

Opioids sensitize the vestibular apparatus to movement; thus, nausea is especially common in patients with motion sickness. Prophylactic scopolamine or treatment with promethazine or ondansetron is usually effective. Pruritus from opioids is rarely due to histamine and is best treated with nalbuphine (5 mg IV every 4–6 hours) rather than diphenhydramine.

Administration. Whenever possible, the enteral route is best as it is the easiest to use and has the most stable pharmacokinetics. If not possible, or if analgesia is needed quickly, then IV administration should be used. If using IV, patient-controlled analgesia (PCA) offers the best overall pain management option. Intramuscular administration is inadvisable because it is painful and has unpredictable pharmacokinetics.

Patient-Controlled Intravenous Analgesia (PCA). PCA is excellent for the maintenance of established analgesia. If the patient is in moderate-to-severe pain at initiation, loading doses must be used to achieve comfort first. There is no clearly superior opioid for use in PCA devices. Continuous infusions should not commonly be used as they increase opioid consumption, add to the risk of respiratory depression, do not improve satisfaction or pain ratings, and do not improve sleep.[1] However, they may be needed in opioid-tolerant patients, especially those chronically taking continuous/sustained-release agents. If a patient has a continuous infusion and they do not activate the PCA, or if side effects increase, the basal rate should be decreased or discontinued.

Dosing. The pronounced variability in opioid response and disease factors, combined with changes in responsiveness over time, mandates individualization of opioid doses. However, some concepts consistently hold. If a patient is not receiving enough pain relief at a given dose, increase the dose by 25–50%. If they are having pain before the next dose is due, reduce the interval and/or increase the dose.

TABLE 45-6. Equianalgesic Dosing Chart (Doses in mg)		
AGONIST	**PARENTERAL**	**ORAL**
Morphine	10	30
Fentanyl	0.1	n/a
Hydromorphone	1.5	7.5
Oxycodone	n/a	20
Hydrocodone	n/a	20
Oxymorphone	1	10

TABLE 45-7. Opioid Weaning Suggestion
Begin only when the cause of pain is effectively eliminated.
Provide an opioid dose equianalgesic to at least half the prior daily dose, for each of the first 2 days of the wean.
Reduce the daily dose by 25% every 2 days until the total dose is 30 MME/day.
The drug may be discontinued after 2 days on the 30 MME/day dose.

MME, morphine milligram equivalents.

Rotation from one opioid to another may provide better analgesia and/or fewer side effects in certain circumstances: (1) if a few attempts at increasing the opioid dose have been made and the patient is not receiving *any* pain relief, (2) if a patient is somnolent but still complaining of pain, (3) if they are having intolerable side effects not treated with appropriate agents, or (4) if a patient has been on an opioid for an extended period of time and is demonstrating signs of analgesic tolerance. Use an equianalgesic dosing table to help calculate the dose of the new agent (Table 45-6). There is not a single, accepted table, so calculations are estimates and clinical judgment is required. Also, the approximations do not take into account the incomplete cross-tolerance between the various opioids that occurs with chronic dosing, meaning that patients will not be "as tolerant" to a new opioid as they were to the one they were on previously and the new agent will work better than expected based on the equianalgesic amount. Therefore, when converting from one opioid to another (but not when switching routes of the same agent), the calculated equianalgesic dose of the new agent must be reduced to prevent oversedation and/or respiratory depression. The exact percent to reduce by is not known but is suggested to be between 25% and 50%.

Sustained-Release and Long-Acting Agents. Transdermal fentanyl is not appropriate for acute pain, especially in the opioid-naïve. There is a black box warning against its use in the acute setting due to the risk of severe respiratory depression from the delayed peak effect of the drug as the pain decreases. However, if a patient is on it preoperatively, it should be continued throughout the postoperative period.[6]

Methadone is not an appropriate first-line agent in the acute setting. Its use requires a comprehensive understanding of its unique pharmacology, including its extended duration of action and dose-dependent potency.

Weaning. Eventually, patients will be in a position to stop using opioids or reduce back to (or below) their baseline. In order to prevent withdrawal, opioids must be weaned. For very high doses in opioid-tolerant patients, the wean has to be quite individualized, but for most other patients the suggestion in Table 45-7 typically works well. While some patients remain on postoperative opioids long term, the implication that they all have opioid use disorder is unfounded.[7] Longer-term use could be normal variance in pain trajectory, physical dependence (without knowledge of how to wean), or persistent postsurgical pain.

Naloxone Use. Naloxone must be titrated (40–80 mcg IV every 2–3 minutes) because it also reverses analgesia and large boluses can cause tachycardia, hypertension, dysrhythmia, pulmonary edema, and/or death.

PATIENTS WITH CHRONIC PAIN AND/OR OPIOID USE

Patients with chronic pain and/or using opioids (prescribed or illicit) preoperatively have an above-average risk of poorly controlled postoperative pain. More pain complaints and higher pain scores should be expected[7]; therefore, objective assessments (e.g., ability to cough, get OOB) along with subjective measures are needed to determine the endpoint of analgesic therapy. They have slower pain resolution, longer hospital stays, and increased readmission rates.[8,9]

Postoperative analgesia is challenging because of opioid-induced hyperalgesia, opioid tolerance, and the possibility of withdrawal.[9,10] Postoperative opioid requirements up to four times the amount typically used in opioid-naïve patients may be needed.[5,7] Equivalent doses of baseline opioids *plus* additional short-acting opioids to cover postoperative pain will be necessary. Using the opioid the patient takes for chronic pain is preferred. However, with pain that is particularly difficult to control, switching to a different opioid may improve analgesia.[6] Nonopioid analgesics should always be utilized, but they will not prevent withdrawal, thus some opioids will be required (at least 50% of what is normally used).

PATIENTS WITH SUBSTANCE USE DISORDERS/ADDICTION

The stigma, misinformation, and prejudices associated with substance use disorders (SUD) are often a barrier to optimal postoperative pain management.[6,10] Providers fear overtreatment of pain (leading to respiratory depression), that the patient is reporting pain just to acquire opioids for euphoria, and that the patient will divert medications. Patients, on the other hand, fear withdrawal, drug cravings, discrimination, and that their pain will not being taken seriously.[10] Patients with an SUD should have reasoned attempts at pain relief just like any patient. Because they often have trouble distinguishing between pain relief and drug craving, it may be helpful to administer analgesics on a fixed schedule as opposed to only "as needed." The initial postoperative period is not the time to initiate detoxification or treatment for addiction. However, if the pain abates while they are still hospitalized, it may be a perfect time to offer services and/or medication for addiction, if they are amenable.

There is no cross-tolerance between opioids and alcohol, cannabis, cocaine, amphetamines, or benzodiazepines; thus, there is no need to use higher than "standard" initial doses of opioids. If a patient is only benzodiazepine tolerant, giving opioids along with higher benzodiazepine doses can result in significant sedation or respiratory depression.

PATIENTS ON MEDICATION-ASSISTED TREATMENT

Methadone

It is unlikely that an individual will receive any analgesic benefit from a chronic methadone regimen in the setting of acute, postoperative pain. Patients on methadone have cross-tolerance to the analgesic effects of other opioids—they do not work well unless given at much higher doses than what is typically given for someone who is opioid-naïve. Regardless of the indication for methadone use, make sure the patient has taken their usual dose preoperatively.[6]

Naltrexone

A varying degree of resistance to opioids should be expected for 4–5 days after an oral naltrexone dose. However, because of chronic upregulation of opioid receptors, heightened opioid sensitivity could occur as naltrexone clears, which can result in an exaggerated response to opioids, including respiratory depression.[6] Figure 45-1 provides an algorithm to help guide management perioperatively.

Buprenorphine

Up until recently, there has been no consensus as to how to manage buprenorphine perioperatively. The concern has been that it can block full agonist activity with resultant inadequate analgesia. The belief was pain control will be "easier" if it is stopped preoperatively, but potential issues include the possibility of withdrawal, increased opioid cravings, and worsened pain, all of which can lead to illicit opioid use. In addition, if stopped, re-induction needs to occur,

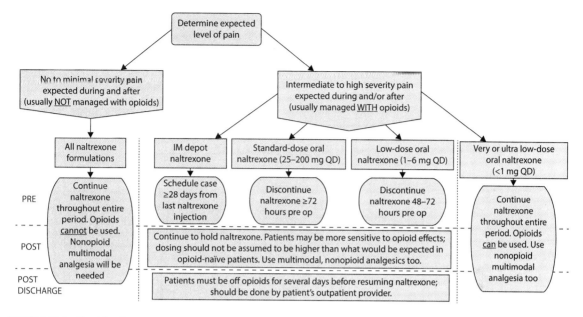

FIGURE 45-1. Algorithm for perioperative management of patients taking naltrexone.

oftentimes requiring patients to first go into withdrawal, which is undesirable. On the other hand, if it is continued and postoperative pain is moderate to severe, "extreme" doses of agonists may be necessary and yet pain may be poorly controlled. This can precipitate drug ideation and be as powerful a trigger of relapse as exposure to the drug of choice.[10]

In recent years, several medical societies have released consensus statements regarding the perioperative management of buprenorphine, although there are some nuances in these guidelines, such as described below, in general, they all recommend continuing a patient's buprenorphine throughout the perioperative period, without adjusting the dose beforehand. They also emphasize the need for a multimodal analgesic plan to improve patient comfort without resorting to exceptionally high doses of opioids.[11]

One idea has emerged to continue "some amount" of sublingual buprenorphine perioperatively to balance the competing issues of pain control and relapse risk.[10] Figure 45-2 offers one possible approach should this be considered. It is important to discuss the risks and benefits of all options with the patient and come to a shared decision preoperatively.

The extended-release subcutaneous buprenorphine injection (i.e., a 100- or 300-mg depot given monthly) results in steady-state plasma concentrations within 4–6 months of initiation, at which time 60–80% of mu-opioid receptors are occupied. Analgesia with full mu-opioid agonists can be achieved with less than 20% of receptors available; therefore, continuing ER buprenorphine perioperatively should be reasonable.[12] The subdermal implant (i.e., four 80-mg rods lasting 6 months) results in plasma concentrations slightly less than that produced by a daily 8 mg SL dose; thus, it may not cause significant issues for perioperative analgesia.

Complete binding of the mu-opioid receptor does not occur with the low doses in transdermal buprenorphine patches and certain buccal formulations. Full agonist opioids for breakthrough pain are effective in patients treated with these formulations, so they should be continued perioperatively.

SUMMARY

Figure 45-3 provides an algorithm to summarize how to approach pain management.

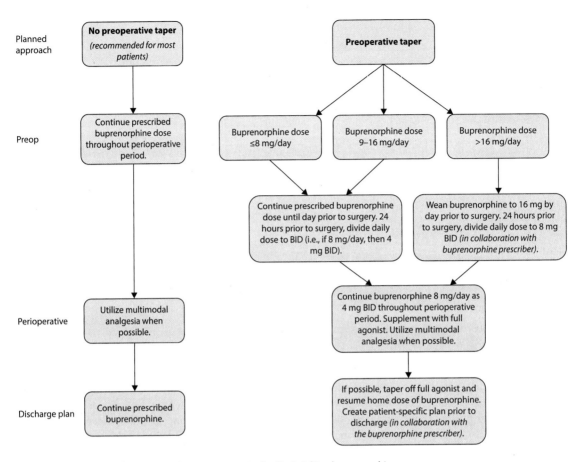

FIGURE 45-2. Algorithm for perioperative management of patients taking buprenorphine.

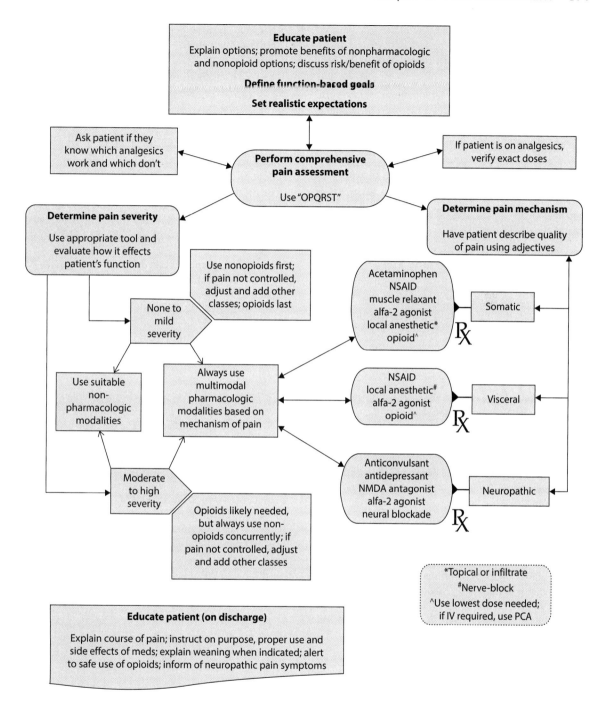

FIGURE 45-3. Algorithm for postoperative pain management.

Clinical pearls

- Have the patient describe the quality of the pain using adjectives.

- Set goals for pain management based on patient-defined outcomes with an improvement in FUNCTION being paramount.

- Risk assessments, or scores from tools, are not 100% diagnostic and not reasons to deny opioids. They suggest when even more caution is needed in terms of dosing and/or provide an estimate of the appropriate level of monitoring.

- If a patient relates that a specific opioid has *never* worked for them, there is little reason to try it again.

- Patients with chronic pain are often viewed as being very challenging and difficult to care for; however, if they are fully engaged in decisions they generally do well.

REFERENCES

1. Chou R, Gordon DB, de Leon-Casasola OA, et al. Management of postoperative pain: a clinical practice guideline from the American Pain Society, the American Society of Regional Anesthesia and Pain Medicine, and the American Society of Anesthesiologists' Committee on Regional Anesthesia, Executive Committee, and Administrative Council. *J Pain*. 2016;17:131. PMID: 26827847

2. U.S. Department of Health and Human Services: Pain Management Best Practices Inter-Agency Task Force report: Updates, Gaps, Inconsistencies, and Recommendations. Washington, DC, 2019. Available at https://www.hhs.gov/ash/advisory-committees/pain/reports/index.html. Accessed on November 29, 2024.

3. Powell RA, Downing J, Ddungu H, Mwangi-Powell FN. Pain history and pain assessment. In: Kopf A, Patel NB, eds. *Guide to Pain Management in Low-Resource Settings*. International Association for the Study of Pain. 2010:67.

4. Verret M, Lauzier F, Zarychanski R, et al. Perioperative use of gabapentinoids for the management of postoperative acute pain: a systematic review and meta-analysis. *Anesthesiology*. 2020; 133(2):265-279. PMID: 32667154

5. Zhang H, Liu Z. The investigation of tramadol dependence with no history of substance abuse: a cross-sectional survey of spontaneously reported cases in Guangzhou City, China. *Biomed Res Int*. 2013; Epub Sep 12. PMID: 24151592

6. Coluzzi F, Bifulco F, Cuomo A, et al. The challenge of perioperative pain management in opioid-tolerant patients. *Ther Clin Risk Manag*. 2017;13:1163. PMID: 28919771

7. Malik KM, Imani F, Beckerly R, Chovatiya R. Risk of opioid use disorder from exposure to opioids in the perioperative period: a systematic review. *Anesth Pain Med*. 2020;10:e101339. PMID: 32337175

8. Rapp SE, Ready LB, Nessly ML. Acute pain management in patients with prior opioid consumption: a case-controlled retrospective review. *Pain*. 1995;61:195. PMID: 7659429

9. Chapman CR, Davis J, Donaldson GW, Naylor J, Winchester D. Postoperative pain trajectories in chronic pain patients undergoing surgery: the effects of chronic opioid pharmacotherapy on acute pain. *J Pain*. 2011;12:1240. PMID: 22036517

10. Quinlan J, Cox F. Acute pain management in patients with drug dependence syndrome. *Pain Rep*. 2017;2:e611. PMID: 29392226

11. Kohan L, Potru S, Barreveld AM, et al. Buprenorphine management in the perioperative period: educational review and recommendations from a multisociety expert panel. *Reg Anesth & Pain Med*. 2021;46:840-859. PMID: 34385292

12. Hickey TR, Hery JT, Edens EL, et al. Perioperative management of extended-release buprenorphine. *J Addict Med*. 2023;17(1):e67-e71. PMID: 35862898

Index